"Should be required reading for all those committed to winning the battle against one of the world's biggest problems."
> —Lamar Alexander, former U.S. Secretary of Education and former Governor of Tennessee.

"Ira Lipman is a unique person who has led his company, in a difficult field, to a position of high prominence. This book should be useful to everyone, not just those in the security business."
> —Howard H. Baker, Jr., former U.S. Senate Majority Leader and White House Chief of Staff

"If you are concerned about becoming a victim of crime, then this book is mandatory reading. Ira Lipman has made a major contribution to assist all of us make our communities safer places to live. Ira is the 'Dr. Spock' of crime control in America."
> —Dr. Lee P. Brown, Professor, Rice University; formerly: Director, White House Office of National Drug Control Policy; New York City Police Commissioner; Police Chief of Houston; Public Safety Commissioner of Atlanta

"With good reason we are more worried than ever about the safety and protection of our families, homes, cars, and property. Armed with the right strategies and proven common sense prevention measures, we can actually prevent crime, enjoy personal safety, and help keep our homes and property crime-free. Ira Lipman's book is a prescription for self-help for all citizens."
> —Dr. Lee Colwell, Professor of Criminal Justice, University of Arkansas at Little Rock, former Associate Director of the Federal Bureau of Investigation

"Congratulations to Ira Lipman for authoring a book on crime prevention that is logical, intelligent, and nonexploitative."
> —Michael Douglas, actor and film producer

"This extraordinarily well-researched book, by the nation's leading authority in the security field, can be a real lifesaver... literally. Each and every chapter offers sound and practical advice on enhancing the security and safety of your family, home, and property. This detailed guidebook on lower-risk living is a must read for all. Study it and keep it handy! Indeed, my only disappointment is that this gem of a book is not available in a pocket-sized edition."
> —Dr. James Alan Fox, Dean, College of Criminal Justice, Northeastern University

"Every woman who has walked fearfully toward her door at night should read this book. So should her family, friends, and children. Its advice is clear and compelling, practical and personally relevant."
> —Dr. Kathleen H. Jamieson, Dean, Annenberg School of Communication, University of Pennsylvania

"A great book. Should be in the home of everyone. If you apply the wisdom contained herein, you will be safer and more comfortable. Read it, use it, and be better off."
— H. Stuart Knight, Director, U.S. Secret Service (retired)

"The very readable book is a gold mine of practical information on how to make our communities safer. Based on solid research and experience, *How to Protect Yourself from Crime* is a valuable resource."
— Barry Krisberg, President, National Council on Crime and
    Delinquency

"Taking back our nation's streets from criminals must involve all of us. Ira Lipman's authoritative guide identifies the various threats we face and uses straightforward language to show what we can do to protect ourselves. *How to Protect Yourself from Crime* is required reading for anyone who cares about the safety and well-being of our communities."
— Carl Levin, U.S. Senator of Michigan

"Crime in the United States is an everyday, serious concern for the American people. Ira Lipman has done a splendid job responding to that concern in *How To Protect Yourself from Crime*. Whether it's setting up the best security system for your home, offering special tips for apartment dwellers or protecting yourself and your family from violent crime, this practical book has what all of us need—sound advice from a pro. Having *How To Protect Yourself from Crime* is like having an extra insurance policy on your house and family. Those who follow Ira Lipman's excellent counsel will not only sleep better at night, they'll sleep—and live—safer."
— Joseph Lieberman, U.S. Senator of Connecticut

"A careful analysis of research on crime and the wisdom of someone who has significantly advanced personal and corporate security in our country are combined to produce the most comprehensive, balanced, and useful guide to crime prevention I have ever read. In a time when many citizens, especially in our largest cities, seem to accept crime as an unavoidable aspect of their environment, this book presents an alternative—reasoned self-protection."
— Charles F. Wellford, Ph.D., Professor, Institute of Criminal Justice
    and Criminology, the University of Maryland at College Park

"The best antidote to criminal victimization I can recommend to my family, my friends, and all citizens of America."
— Dr. Marvin E. Wolfgang, Professor of Criminology and of Law,
    University of Pennsylvania

How to Protect Yourself from Crime

Fourth Edition

Ira A. Lipman

President, Guardsmark, Inc.

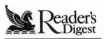

THE READER'S DIGEST ASSOCIATION, INC.
Pleasantville, New York/Montreal

A Reader's Digest Book

Original Copyright © 1989 Ira A. Lipman

Updated Edition Copyright © 1997 Ira A. Lipman

Library of Congress Cataloging in Publication Data

Lipman, Ira A.

   How to protect yourself from crime / Ira A.Lipman.—Updated ed.
      p.   cm.
   "Fourth edition"—Fwd.
   ISBN 0-89577-931-5
   1. Crime prevention. 2. Crime prevention—United States.
3. Dwellings—Security measures. I. Title.
HV7431.L56 1997
362.88—dc21   96-52242

This is a revised and updated edition of *How to Protect Yourself from Crime*. This title was first published in hardcover by Atheneum Publishers in 1975, was published simultaneously in Canada by McClelland & Stewart Ltd. and was reprinted in paperback by the Law Enforcement Assistance Administration in December 1980. Portions appeared in Reader's Digest in August 1981. The second edition was published by Avon Books in 1981. The third edition was published by Contemporary Books in 1989.

Reader's Digest and the Pegasus logo are trademarks of
The Reader's Digest Association, Inc.
Printed in the U.S.A.

ACKNOWLEDGMENTS

Indicative of my position as chairman and president of Guardsmark, Inc., my name on the title page of this book simply reflects the names of the many Guardsmark people responsible for this collective effort. The fine work of those who assisted with the previous editions has been greatly enhanced in this fourth edition by the efforts of Dr. Bernard Cohen, a noted criminologist and sociologist. Also contributing their expertise were world renowned criminologist Dr. James Alan Fox and security experts Barry Boaz and D.J. Ryan. Our appreciation goes to Carol Lynn Yellin, another editor. I am grateful to all those who made this book project possible.

—*Ira A. Lipman*

ABOUT THE AUTHOR

Protection of people and their property has been a lifelong career for Ira A. Lipman. As chairman and president of Guardsmark, Inc., one of the world's largest security services companies, he directs an international network of protection professionals. Guardsmark personnel are responsible for the security of thousands of people and billions of dollars in assets. Following many of the procedures personally developed by Mr. Lipman, the firm serves many leading multinational corporations and institutions, protecting such diverse operations as manufacturing plants, oil refineries, banks, hospitals, and corporate offices.

Known throughout the industry for his innovative approach to security problem solving, Mr. Lipman is frequently sought as a source of information on crime prevention techniques. He has been editorially praised by the *New York Times* for his leadership in disarming the security industry, and his and Guardsmark's achievements have received acclaim in such publications as *The Wall Street Journal, Reader's Digest, Business Week, People,* and *U.S. News & World Report.* Guardsmark's reputation for excellence has led author Tom Peters to describe Guardsmark as the "Tiffany's of the security business" in his book *Liberation Management.* In addition, *Time* magazine has referred to Guardsmark as the company "which many security experts consider to be the best national firm in the business." Mr. Lipman is also publisher of *The Lipman Report,* a monthly newsletter that focuses on security problems ranging from terrorism and sabotage to computer crime, drug abuse, and employee theft.

Mr. Lipman was a principal force in the formation of the Committee of National Security Companies and currently is Chairman Emeritus of the National Council on Crime and Delinquency and Honorary Chairman and past National Chairman of the National Conference of Christians and Jews. He and his wife, Barbara, divide their time between residences in New York and Memphis. They have three sons: Gustave, Joshua, and Benjamin.

For Barbara, Gus, Josh, Benjamin,
and my parents, with love

CONTENTS

〜

PART TWO: SECURITY AWAY FROM HOME

PART THREE: FAMILY SECURITY

PART FOUR: COMMUNITY SECURITY

PART FIVE: PROTECTION FROM VIOLENT CRIMES

PART SIX: **CORPORATE SECURITY**

PART SEVEN: **THE CRIMINAL JUSTICE SYSTEM**

FOREWORD

Crime, like death and taxes, exists in every society. The amount and character of crime and the distribution of victims vary over time and place. Every citizen is aware of these generalizations. But most citizens are uninformed about the specific theories of the causes of crime, the details of the operation of the criminal justice system, and the scientific studies of the modes of crime prevention and treatment of the offenders.

Criminology is the scientific study of crime, criminals, and society's reaction to both. As a criminologist, I have studied delinquency, criminality, law enforcement, and punishment of criminal behavior. My colleagues and I have analyzed abstract theories of crime and punishment, and produced detailed historical reviews and elaborate, quantitative, highly sophisticated statistical studies of patterns of crime, personalities of criminals, and the effectiveness of prevention and therapeutic programs.

For nearly 30 years, criminologists have also been carefully studying the victims of crime, ever since the focus on victims was creatively introduced by Bernard Mendlesohn, an Israeli scholar, and by Hans Von Hentig, a German scholar who escaped from the Nazi period. A new subfield of criminology known as victimology has been developed, devoted to the scientific study of victimization, especially of victims of crime. Studies in victimology cover legal, philosophical, sociological, cross-cultural, macroeconomic, and psychological aspects of the subject. All of this scientific research has shown the importance of the relationship between the criminal and his or her victim.

However, the pragmatic analysis of how we, as individuals, might best protect ourselves against crime, against becoming victims of crime, has been neglected by both criminologists and victimologists. That vacuum has now been greatly filled by this fourth edition of Ira Lipman's *How to Protect Yourself from Crime*.

I first came to know Ira Lipman about 20 years ago when he sought my advice on some matters associated with his private security organization, Guardsmark. I immediately perceived him as an intelligent, humane person who knew his business well, who knew the problems of crime and the practical way of managing those problems on a day-by-day basis in business, in private institutions, and in the private lives of individuals. I came to know the efficiency and the effectiveness of Guardsmark, one of the largest private security organizations in the country. I admired Ira Lipman's managerial capacities and his understanding of the criminological literature he had begun to absorb.

Because of my respect for his pragmatic acumen and intellectual integrity, I, as president of the American Academy of Political and Social Science, encouraged him to be a special editor of *The Annals,* the bimonthly publication of the academy. The issue he edited, "The Private Security Industry: Issues and Trends," Volume 498, July 1988, has been one of our most highly regarded and widely distributed volumes in the recent history of the academy.

This fourth edition of *How to Protect Yourself from Crime* is the most comprehensive treatment of the topic I have ever read. I can think of no significant concern of individuals or groups that is not covered in this volume with thoroughness, precision, and accuracy. I mention accuracy especially, because the descriptions of various kinds of crimes and the recommendations for protection against them are solidly, firmly based on the best available evidence in the scientific literature.

On controversial issues, such as owning and using guns, discussions are carefully balanced and must be applauded. The checklists at the end of each chapter are especially useful as reminders of the details. These lists should be consulted on specific occasions, such as taking a vacation or a business trip, moving a residence, or traveling overseas. All of these summaries should be reread as time and circumstances permit and require. The reader should feel confident that the data, analyses, and information are as current and up-to-date as careful research can provide.

This is not an alarmist book, but there are alarming changes occurring in the amount, character, and violence of crime in our nation. For example, the chapters on robbery and rape are outstandingly grounded in scientific research and provide the best guides to prevention and protection to be found anywhere.

To be alert to these changes, to be aware of protective strategies helps us reduce our chances of being victimized, and ensures our greater safety.

How to Protect Yourself from Crime is the best antidote to criminal victimization I can recommend to my family and my friends, indeed to people everywhere.

Dr. Marvin E. Wolfgang
Professor of Criminology and of Law
University of Pennsylvania

PREFACE
TO THE
FOURTH EDITION

In the 20 or so years since *How to Protect Yourself from Crime* was first published, thousands and thousands of ordinary people have benefited from
the crime prevention know-how contained in this book. We began this
project with one central message in mind: Crime is so pervasive that it de-
fies traditional controls. Police ranks then, as now, were stretched too thin
to control the vast numbers who had selected crime as a career. We said
then, as we do now, that if there is a recurring theme running through this
book, it is that we are making crime too easy for the criminal. In fact, not
only are we victims of crime, we are also, in effect, accomplices.

During the intervening years, our crime rate soared dramatically; then,
in the early 1980s, it began to fall. In 1983, a 7-percent decline, following
declines of 3 percent in 1982 and less than 1 percent in 1981, signaled to
some the end of the "Great Crime Wave" of the twentieth century. Crime
rates continued to fall—if not precipitously, at least steadily. Then, in 1985,
the trend reversed itself, and for the next 6 years the crime rate grew once
again. By 1991, the crime rate had risen 17 percent over the 7-year period
since 1984. But it was the 40-percent increase in the rate of violent
crime—murder, rape, robbery, and aggravated assault—that placed crime
at the top of the national political agenda. In America's battle with crime,
1991 became a turning point. The next 3 years saw reductions in crime
rates—a 9-percent decline from 1991 to 1994. The most recent reprieve
may have been relatively small, but it has given many Americans hope for
a better future.

Many observers were not surprised. The turnarounds, downward
in 1980 and upward in 1986, were predictable. It was a simple matter of
demographics.

One of the major contributors to the Great Crime Wave was the large
population of young people (the group most likely to commit crime). But
in the early 1980s, the baby boomers were getting older, marrying, and
settling down.

The consequent drop in crime rates led some to anticipate a long
period of relative freedom from crime. Unfortunately, that was not to be.

The perpetrators of the crime waves of 1985 and 1986 were the children of the baby boomers, a group that, according to the nation's leading criminologists, is much more crime-prone than their fathers and mothers.

Perhaps we need to accustom ourselves to fluctuations in the crime rate, with continuing periods of viciousness and brutality followed by periods of relative reprieve. In 1993, there were an estimated 43.5 million victimizations in the United States, including almost 11 million violent incidents. Of all households, 23 percent were victimized in that same year, at a loss of $17.6 billion in direct costs. In nearly two decades (1973–1992), serious crime increased 66 percent. We have seen violent crime increase more than 121 percent.

According to recent *New York Times*/CBS polls, crime remains one of the most significant problems facing Americans, along with other concerns over health, the economy, unemployment, and the deficit. A recent CNN/Gallup poll reported that 9 of 10 Americans believe the crime problem is growing worse. More than ever before, people feel personally threatened by the country's mushrooming crime problem. A 1994 *New York Times*/CBS poll revealed that 4 of 10 people fear they or a family member will be raped or sexually assaulted; 1 in 3 fear burglary, and 1 in 4 expect to be mugged. As a result, more and more people were taking protective measures. In a single year, some 7 percent of the nation's population purchased a house alarm, 5 percent bought or carried a gun, many purchased dogs or tear gas, but most just became more aware about crime and possible safeguards against it. Currently, 51 percent of the nation's citizens keep guns in their house, and there are over 210 million guns in the hands of private citizens.

The recent series of high-profile murders and assaults hasn't helped dissuade the average citizen's increasing concerns involving crime. The father of basketball superstar Michael Jordan was murdered when he stopped by a roadside to rest. In San Diego, three people died as a result of a Navy murder. A jogger in Coney Island, Brooklyn, was attacked by a roving gang. Florida tourists were senselessly gunned down. A 4-year-old in Washington, D.C., was shot and killed in a deadly spray of bullets meant for others. New York City and Houston, Texas, like so many other American cities, announce body counts involving victims of homicides reminiscent of the body counts incurred during the Vietnam War. The increase in crime is likely to continue until we as a nation can do something about guns and illegal drugs.

A book like *How to Protect Yourself from Crime* is therefore all the more needed today. Its primary function is to encourage you to take a positive, preventive approach to your own safety. Where possible, the stress is on psychological and physical readiness—that is, *proaction* rather than reaction.

Each year the Federal Bureau of Investigation (FBI) publishes statistics on eight classifications of personal crime. Four are considered crimes against property: burglary,* larceny, auto theft, and arson. Four are considered crimes against the person: murder, forcible rape, aggravated assault, and robbery. It's somewhat consoling to learn that nearly 8 of every 10 crimes as defined by the FBI are crimes against property—that is, incidents during which the victim and the perpetrator do not come face to face. In reading this book, bear in mind that you are unlikely ever to be subjected to a violent crime against your person. Though the possibility does exist, there is no reason for undue alarm. (Clearly, robbery is a crime directed at property as well as the person, but there is the threat, at least, of bodily harm.)

How prevalent is crime in the United States today? We can now expect murder at the rate of 1 every 22 minutes, a rape every 4 minutes, a robbery every 26 seconds, and an assault every 6 seconds. Property crimes occur at even faster rates: a household burglary occurs every 7 seconds, a theft every 4 seconds, and a car theft every 16 seconds. Overall, one serious crime happens every second, and a crime of violence every 5 seconds.

As mentioned earlier, the Baby Boom Aftershock is posing a serious challenge to the forces of law and order; but this demographic bomb is by no means the only cause of our troubling crime rate. Other important contributors are our national involvement with drugs, especially cocaine (notably crack); a lack of trust in many of our national leaders; disintegrating values; racism; the glorification of violence in TV, videos, radio, and magazines; serious difficulty making ends meet; and the mounting numbers of broken families. Solving the problems ahead requires a fresh approach. We can no longer depend on the old approaches, which seem largely to be failing us.

On a national scale, crime bills that propose expansion of the death penalty for numerous federal crimes, banning various assault weapons, increasing the number of police officers, building more prisons, and erecting boot camps for "shock incarceration" are unlikely to have an impact on crime. The "three strikes you're out" measure, which calls for a mandatory life sentence without parole for a third serious felony, is another strategy likely to have minimal impact. Obliteration of root causes and conditions is the best way to minimize violence.

---

*To understand how to protect yourself, you'll need to be clear about some of the terms used repeatedly in this book:

Robbery is the taking of money and/or other valuables under the threat of physical harm or force, with or without a weapon. An example is a holdup with gun or knife. *Burglary* is breaking and entering with no personal threat involved and usually no confrontation between burglar and victim. The traditional "second-story man" is an example of a burglar.

Theft or *larceny* is the act of stealing, in which neither illegal entry nor the threat or use of force is present. Shoplifting is an example of theft.

A complete solution to our crime problem is not just around the corner, and until and unless we reach that point, most of the responsibility for your protection is yours. You needn't arm yourself or organize a vigilante group. Nor should you undertake unrealistic acts of "heroism" that may in fact increase your peril and loss. Instead, simply take a series of common-sense preventive measures.

How to slow down a potential criminal or influence him or her to seek another "mark" (or, better yet, deter that person altogether) is probably the major lesson that this book has to offer. For example, it is estimated that half of all auto thefts result from keys left in the ignition, and a comparable proportion of all illegal entries into homes are made through unlocked doors.

We can't expect somebody else to take care of our security needs. We must handle them ourselves. Read this book carefully and often, and periodically review the security checklists at the end of each chapter. Teach your family good security practices, and reinforce the messages so that you and yours can respond automatically in an emergency. Add notes of your own to fit security precautions and practices to your lifestyle. Before we can completely protect ourselves from crime, we must, in many respects, change our attitude toward it. We must be vigilant, we must be prepared, and we must endure the inconvenience that simple and sensible day-to-day precautions entail. Self-protection is a way of life. Good security practices not only make life safer but also make compensation easier if a crime does occur.

The fourth edition of *How to Protect Yourself from Crime* has been thoroughly revised and updated. For example, new developments in crime in the workplace, computer crime, defenses against rape, and school and campus crime required a complete rewriting of the chapters dealing with these subjects. Other new or expanded topics include family violence, violence in the workplace, carjacking, abducted and missing children, child abuse, battered women, acquaintance rape, campus sexual assault, sexual harassment, and stalking.

This book offers two types of suggestions: routine, day-to-day preventive measures to decrease your exposure to crime, and practical, step-by-step recommendations to guide you through the unhappy and sometimes bewildering experience of being a crime victim. May you never need to put the latter suggestions to use, but genuinely learn to protect yourself from crime.

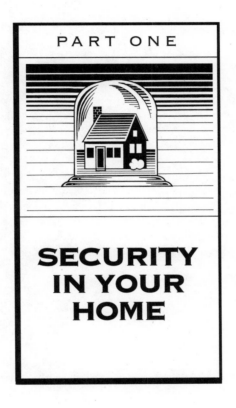

PART ONE

SECURITY
IN YOUR
HOME

1

DOORS AND WINDOWS

Walter, a machinist and bachelor, came home from work Thursday night and discovered that he had been "visited" by a burglar. "A window was all busted out," he commented, "so I knew right away that somebody had been inside." He went into his small, rented house and found a wreck—the whole place was in shambles. His TV was gone, as were his VCR and stereo, some cash, and a few other possessions. No arrest was made, nor did Walter recover any of his possessions.

DOORS

The easiest and most common way for someone to enter your home is simply to open an unlocked door. In fact, 55 percent of all burglars enter homes through an unlocked door or window. Of all break-ins, 37 percent occur during the day. In 1993, over 500,000 homes were burglarized while at least one family member was inside. Very few families take the number-one precaution of locking exterior doors at all times, whether someone is home or not. Children who are in and out of the house all day leave doors unlocked, as do people who go next door for a neighborly visit.

While doors should always be locked, this in itself is actually small defense against the determined criminal. Here's why:

❖ Doors often have small glass or light plywood panels, which can easily be broken or cut with a rasp or a keyhole saw. Someone could then open the lock very easily by simply reaching through the hole.

❖ A door that doesn't fit its frame properly can easily be forced open by wedging a tire tool or prying bar between it and the frame and then "spreading" the door away until the bolt moves free from the strike (the hole in the door frame into which the bolt slides when the door is locked).

❖ Some older homes and apartments have doors that open outward. These can often be opened simply by removing the hinge pins and lifting the entire door from the frame. The Multi-Lock, mentioned later in this chapter, is useful in protecting doors of this type.

❖ Certain locks can be easily picked, removed, or destroyed.

It is virtually impossible to prevent someone from entering your home through an outside door if that person is really determined to do so and has enough time and skill to accomplish the deed.

If you can't entirely eliminate the possibility of criminals breaking into your home, then what's the next best thing to do? Make breaking in as difficult and as time consuming as possible. And if the burglars still succeed, at least you will have forced them to destroy the lock or a part of the door, or in some other way to leave clear evidence of illegal entry. This will be very important when you file an insurance claim to recover your loss. If nothing else, it will at least minimize the likelihood of your claim's being denied on the grounds of negligence.

Strengthening Doors

Strengthening doors—and these comments apply to all outside doors—is not difficult. First, the door itself should be as sturdy as possible. A hollow-core metal or solid wooden door is best.

For aesthetic purposes, however, many prefer doors with heavy glass or wooden panels. These types of doors offer considerably less protection than those just mentioned, but there is one thing in particular that you can do to make them more secure: You should install double-cylinder locks. This kind of lock requires a key to open it from the inside as well as from the outside, which prevents an intruder from unlatching the lock by reaching through broken glass or a hole in a wooden panel. That much delay—unless the burglar is especially determined—will very often send an intruder off to easier pickings. A word of caution, however: In the event of fire or other emergency, double-cylinder locks can delay occupants from getting out of the house. Consequently, a key to the inside lock should always be kept conveniently at hand. In some jurisdictions, double-cylinder locks are illegal in multiple dwellings. Check the local laws in your community before installing these locks. (Nonbreakable glass should be installed at least 40 inches from the lock, especially where double-cylinder locks are prohibited.)

Unfortunately, most doors come with a light-duty strike plate. An insecure strike plate results in a vulnerable residence. These should be replaced with heavy-duty strike plates and 3-inch screws.

There may be a reason why one of these measures won't be practical. For example, your landlord might not want you to replace an existing door or permit you to do so; or you, as a tenant, might not want to go to the expense of installing a really good door on someone else's property. In this case, consider reinforcing your door with a sheet of steel or heavy plywood. It may not be a thing of beauty, but it might save your TV and VCR.

In securing all outside doors, be particularly meticulous with those that offer an intruder cover—such as doors inside vestibules or enclosed porches. Here a criminal could work at leisure, safe from observation by neighbors or passersby. Be aware that these protected areas often are of less sturdy construction than other parts of your home. Ideally they should be finished off with exterior walls as sound as the rest of the house.

Door hinges should always be placed on the inside. If the hinge pins are on the outside, a burglar can easily remove the pins, and with them the door. This can be prevented by removing one pair of parallel screws on each of the leaves that connect the door to the door frame. Then insert a single screw or concrete nail that protrudes about ½ inch from the leaf on the door. When the door is closed, the protruding screw or nail will connect into the screw opening on the hinge leaf connected to the door frame. Even if the hinge pin is removed, the door will be held in place by the protruding screw or nail.

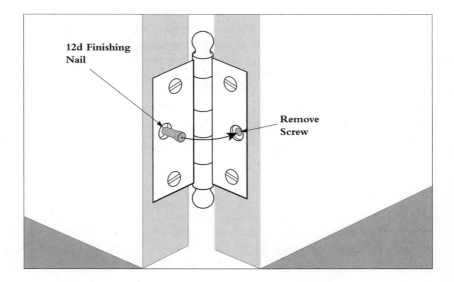

12d Finishing Nail

Remove Screw

Figure 1. Door hinges properly installed on the inside.

Every exterior door should fit its frame snugly. Most don't. House-builders sometimes take shortcuts by making the openings oversized, and even a well-fitted door can develop problems as a house settles on its foundation. The best way to remedy a poor fit is to reinforce the door frame or to replace the door with one that fits. If you don't want to go to that much expense, at least use locks with bolts that slide a minimum of 1 inch onto the frame, or attach a common thumb lock with a long bolt to the inside face of the door. Or better yet, ask a locksmith about an L-shaped metal strip that can be attached to a door frame to protect an inward-swinging door from being jimmied with a crowbar.

A flat plate attached to an outward-swinging door can be used to cover such an opening, but it should be attached with flat bolts or nonretractable screws so that it cannot be removed from the outside.

Storm doors are good energy savers, and when equipped with adequate locking devices, they add an element of security by introducing a delay factor. The glass and/or wrought-iron features serve as another deterrent.

Chain Locks

In general, chain locks are not effective in preventing someone from entering your home. A good kick might easily pull the lock away from the wall. Furthermore, the chain itself can be cut with a hacksaw or a bolt cutter. To maximize the effectiveness of such locks, anchor them with long screws or, better yet, bolts. A wedge-shaped rubber doorstop inserted beneath a door can add substantial additional protection against unwanted entry.

One advantage of a chain lock is that, when it is engaged, it indicates to a burglar that someone is at home, generally causing the burglar to move on. One distinct disadvantage of a chain lock is that burglars, once inside your house, can become relatively free from being surprised on the job simply by engaging the lock themselves. The value of a chain lock is thus debatable, but on balance a good one is worthwhile, if for no other reason than its effect of delaying entry into your house. Also, if you have solid doors without peepholes, a chain lock allows you to speak to visitors without fully opening the door.

Peepholes

A solid exterior door should be equipped with a peephole (or interviewer or optical-viewing device), simply to allow you to ascertain who is outside before you open your door. Ideally, the peephole should have a wide-angle lens. If at all practical, a convex mirror should be installed opposite the door. With this device, you should be able to see anyone attempting to hide beyond the vision range of the peephole.

Night Latches and Doorknob Locks

The night latch or rim spring latch commonly found in most older houses, and the cylindrical lock or doorknob lock found in many apartments and newer houses, do not offer a great deal of security. The doorknob device is easily defeated by prying the entire assemblage loose with a crowbar. Night latches are very common because they are inexpensive and convenient and because they can be engaged simply by slamming the door shut. But often they can be opened by sliding a credit card or similar piece of plastic into the gap between the door and the frame.

Newer night latches have protection to prevent the "credit card entry" into a structure. This represents little, if any, protection, however, as doors of this type can often be compromised by forcing them open with a screwdriver. This can be prevented by equipping the lock with an effective deadlatch plunger, which prevents pushing back the latch's beveled edge. Unfortunately, the faceplate can be pried loose and the cylinder removed quite easily. Thus, this type of lock isn't a satisfactory locking device.

Deadbolt Locks

The remedy for these problems is a deadbolt lock. Such a lock usually features a square-faced (rather than beveled) bolt, which is engaged from the inside by the second turn of a key, or else is operated by turning a thumb knob. Unquestionably, the deadbolt is superior to the common night latch, inasmuch as it cannot be forced open with a knife blade, spatula, or similar implement. The shape of the bolt and the pressure required to move it in any way other than through the normal use of a key or knob make these burglar tools useless. If the bolt is long enough (a 1-inch throw is recommended), the door becomes very difficult to jimmy open.

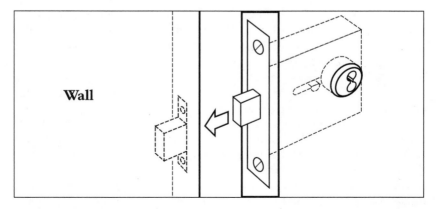

Wall

Figure 2. Deadbolt lock.

Variations on this theme, the rim- or surface-mounted vertical deadbolt lock or the ring-and-bar lock, are even more effective protection measures. For high-risk situations, the Multi-Lock is a deadbolt lock that, when engaged, bolts into all four edges of the door frame.

A deadbolt is, dollar for dollar, the best means of defense that you can enlist in securing your home. You should install one on each outside door, either in place of, or supplementary to, whatever locking devices you are now using.

Other Locking Devices

There are a number of virtually pickproof locks available, but they are expensive and, except in the most extraordinary of circumstances, unnecessary for the average homeowner. Few burglars are skilled at picking locks, so unless there are items of unusual value in your home, installing pickproof locks generally would constitute overprotection.

Push-button combination types of locks are also generally available and are secure from lock pickers, but a drawback is that the combination can be read even from great distances. Such locks are therefore much more effective for interior security than for exterior use. A five-pin tumbler lock is considered adequate for home use.

No lock can prevent a door from being opened by brute force, especially if there is a weak door frame. The wooden door frame itself can present a problem. In many cases when a forced entry is made through a door, the deadbolt itself has held, but the door frame around the strike plate has splintered. This can be overcome by ensuring that there is proper bracing in the wall behind the door frame. If you push against the door frame on the strike-jamb side and it bends outward, it is not well supported.

The proper combination for preventing the wooden door frame from splintering without determined attack is by using a high-security strike box or plate and screws long enough to anchor the strike device into 2-by-4s bracing in the wall immediately behind the strike device. A police brace, a long steel bar that reaches from the floor to the door at an angle, serves as an effective anti-intrusion device in much the same way as does wedging a piece of furniture under a doorknob. The top edge of the bar fits into a lock mechanism installed on the door, and the bottom fits into a metal socket in the floor. Another version of the police brace is a horizontal steel bar that is mounted across the center of the door. This fits jamb braces attached to both sides of the door frame. It can be removed or put back in place in a few seconds. Of course, these devices can be used only when you are on the inside. They do, however, have the very real advantage of being completely pickproof.

Another type of device favored for a high level of home security is the tubular keyway lock. You have almost certainly seen the round locks found on many vending machines. Perhaps you have even seen the service person open the vending machine, using a small cylindrical key. This locking device has the advantage of being extremely difficult to pick and, for all intents and purposes, impossible to force open with a screwdriver or wrench. Other locks have similar advantages, and the configurations of the various available locking devices are many.

Choosing a Locksmith

Choose a locksmith with great care. Some are unlicensed or dishonest and can do more harm than good. Always select a well-established locksmith business that is bonded and insured. Then check with your local Better Business Bureau. Ask the locksmith for recommendations, and make certain you follow them up. One final check: Compare prices before you make your final decision.

Sliding Doors

Of all the doors giving access to your house, probably the most hazardous are the patio doors—typically of the sliding-glass type. In general, such doors have locks that are not very effective. Even if they hold up against an intruder, a piece of glass can easily be cut or broken from the doors and the lock disengaged.

One safeguard is to attach locks with vertical bolts that fit into holes in the floor and upper frame and hold the door in place when it is engaged. Another safeguard is to substitute the panes of plate or tempered glass with polycarbonate or other shatterproof glass, or other types of impact-resistant glazing material. An inexpensive auxiliary means of securing such doors is to cut a broom handle to fit the track in which the doors slide. Thus, even if the lock were forced, the door would not slide open.

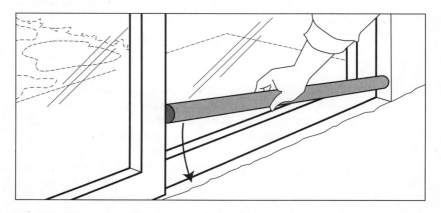

Figure 3. Sliding door and use of broom handle.

These highly susceptible openings into your home may be further protected by inserting screws into the upper track of the door assemblies. Properly placed, these screws can prevent the lifting and removal of an entire door, glass, frame, and all.

Garages and Outbuildings

Garage doors that lead directly into the house are, in fact, entry doors, in the same way as the front door. However, they represent a more serious threat to your security, because an intruder, hidden from sight in the garage, could leisurely breach your security and rob you of your assets. At the very least, such an opening should be protected by a solid-core door, a deadbolt lock, secure hinges, and, if warranted, an intrusion alarm.

Obviously, you should keep your garage locked shut whenever practical. A trip to the grocery store could result in an intruder's use of your unprotected ladder to gain access to a substantially more unprotected upstairs silver chest.

All garages should be protected with *good* padlocks. A good padlock has a hardened (or, better yet, a stainless) steel shackle (the loop). This should be no less than $9/32$ inch in diameter. It should have a double-locking mechanism (heel and toe), a five-pin tumbler, and a key-retaining feature. This last feature, sometimes difficult to find, prevents you from removing the key unless the lock is engaged. Cane bolts and sliding hasps, installed on the inside, are inexpensive but highly effective means to increase the security of your garage.

Roll-up garage doors should have two good padlocks for acceptable security, one on either side of the door. Sometimes upward pressure on one side of the door will cause the other side to rise enough for someone to crawl under. Many garage door assemblies, electric or mechanical, have predrilled holes on the tracks for a padlock, which, of course, will substantially increase your safety and your peace of mind. Also, if you have an electric garage door opener, change the factory designated code to a personal code immediately.

WINDOWS

The primary aim of window precautions is to secure permanently every window that is not needed for ventilation. Windows that are used for ventilation or as an emergency exit, particularly those on the ground floor, should be secured by the installation of key-operated locks, which are easily available from hardware stores and locksmiths.

As a general rule, an intruder will not break a window—first, because the noise would be likely to attract attention and, second, because the sharp edges present the risk of injury. This does not mean, however, that he or she will not remove a small piece of glass with a glass cutter and reach through to unlock the window. Thus, the use of laminated glass or the special impact-resistant plastics developed for schools and store

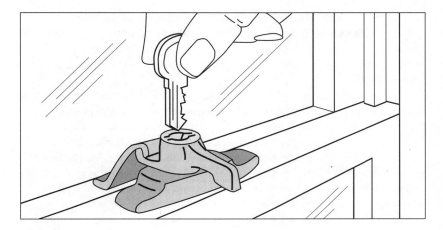

Figure 4. Key-operated window locks.

windows is an excellent extra precaution—if you can afford it.

In many homes, glass is held in windows by putty. This material deteriorates with age, making panes relatively easy to remove with no more than a pocketknife. Usually a contractor will replace all putty when painting your house, but double-check to make sure that this is done.

Double-Hung Windows

The windows of many older homes are of the so-called double-hung construction, made of two panels, one or both of which slide up and down. A two-piece device, resembling a butterfly, locks it shut. This lock can be rather easily opened by sliding a thin piece of metal, such as a knife blade, vertically through the crack separating the two sashes.

Windows become considerably more secure when a hole is drilled completely through the lower window sash and halfway through the upper while the window is in the closed position. A bolt or nail inserted into the drilled hole will effectively lock the windows in the closed position only. Similarly, nails or bolts may be driven into the window tracks to prevent the window from being raised high enough to admit an intruder. For maximum security, such stops should be employed on both sides of the tracks to make removal more difficult and time consuming for a potential intruder.

When a window has been "frozen" shut by paint and is not needed for ventilation, a simple antiburglar precaution is to leave it that way.

Window Guards

Screens made of chain-link fencing are widely used for protecting windows, particularly in industrial applications. Aluminum curtains are available from suppliers of security hardware in sizes suitable for window protection. Bars (horizontal, vertical, or a combination of both) are similarly available. These may be enclosed in a frame attached to the window frame, or they may extend through the frame and into the walls. These more secure applications should be considered for windows on the ground floor of an urban residence.

For windows opening onto fire escapes, fire department regulations usually prohibit the installation of permanently placed bars or guards, but folding or hinged guards may be used on these openings if they are not locked in place. For residential application, however, these items will be considered by many to be aesthetically unappealing. Metal window guards, also called burglar bars, may be more pleasing to the eye, but, like nails in window tracks or paint-frozen windows, they could hinder you when you need to evacuate a building threatened by fire or other danger.

Lockable folding metal screens provide excellent security, yet still provide for emergency evacuation of the home, as long as the key to unlock the screens is readily at hand. It should not be placed within reach of the would-be intruder on the outside. Lockable folding metal screens also work well for windows on the ground floor. Ground-floor windows should be covered with blinds, shades, or curtains to obstruct a potential thief's view of your home's contents. A burglar may look in your windows and see valuables that may be an incentive for a break in. Miniblinds should be closed tightly, with slats up, so, at most, the only view available from outside is your ceiling.

Storm windows, in addition to being valuable savers of energy—and thus money—provide an impediment to the would-be intruder. Although they can usually be removed with little more than a screwdriver, this takes time and can create noise, which will generally send the typical intruder on to easier targets.

Casement Windows

Casement windows are more secure than most double-hung windows in that they are opened with a geared-crank arrangement and often are too small to allow human entry even when they are successfully opened. Intrusion is usually possible only after smashing or cutting the glass. For those who want to be doubly sure, a number of key-operated locks are available for casement windows.

Windows Above Ground Level

Second-story windows pose less of a problem than do ground-level windows, but they still require attention because they may be accessible from the outside staircases, from the fire escapes, from the roofs of porches, or even from trees. Don't store ladders where they are available to a potential intruder, unless secured by a padlock and chain.

In some city areas, windows may be near enough to neighboring buildings to allow a plank to bridge the gap between the structures. In some high-rise apartment buildings, intruders might gain access by lowering themselves from a rooftop or higher floor to an unprotected or open window. Protection in these cases can best be accomplished through the same measures as for ground-level windows; it is a matter of personal judgment to decide how much security is necessary relative to installation costs.

In evaluating your window security, also pay special attention to basement and storeroom windows, attached garages, ventilation exhausts, access to crawl spaces opening into partial basements, coal chutes, storm cellars, attics, and all other spaces that give you access to little-used areas inside the house. In all your security precautions about doors and windows, there must be definite evidence of forced entry if you are to recover theft losses on your homeowner's insurance policy. Similarly, it is difficult to substantiate a claim for loss when you file income tax returns without evidence that the loss was sudden and unexpected, unless you have filed a report with the local police.

Window-Unit Air Conditioners

A particularly vulnerable illegal-access location that is often overlooked by the homeowner is the window-unit air conditioner. One way to thwart the potential intruder here is to ensure that a unit is secured by long screws to both the window and the window frame. When this is not possible, consider placing a bar across the face of the unit, again ensuring that it is very firmly secured to the window frame and/or to interior walls.

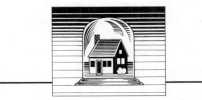

DOORS AND WINDOWS:
A CHECKLIST

1 Exterior doors should be locked at all times.

2 All outside doors, including enclosed porch or vestibule doors, should be protected.

3 Every outside door, without exception, should be equipped with a deadbolt lock.

4 Doors should be sturdy. If they are not, they should be replaced or reinforced.

5 Glass doors and glass- or wood-paneled doors should be equipped with double-cylinder locks.

6 If the walls of enclosed porches are inadequate to prevent through-the-wall entry, they should be made secure. At least, brightly light such areas.

7 Doors should fit frames snugly, even if this means reinforcing the frame or replacing the door.

8 Locks with extra-long bolts can offer additional protection.

9 Chain locks, especially cheap dime store versions, provide little security. Such devices should be limited to permitting the partial opening of a door to establish the identity of a visitor.

10 Peepholes, ideally with wide-angle lenses, should be installed in all solid exterior doors.

11 Night latches and doorknob locks are easily compromised and offer little protection.

12 Patio and sliding-glass doors should be secured with vertical-bolt locks and equipped with shatterproof or impact-resistant panes. A length of broom handle cut to fit the door track can provide an effective, inexpensive auxiliary "lock" for such doors.

13 Roll-up garages require two locks, one on each side of the door, because upward pressure on one side will raise the other side enough for a person to slide under through the opening.

14 Some garage door assemblies have holes predrilled in the tracks. Padlocks inserted through them will provide excellent and relatively inexpensive protection.

15 Cane bolts and sliding hasps, also used for the garage, are inexpensive and highly effective auxiliary interior locking devices.

16 Doors of attached garages should be equipped with locking devices as secure as those protecting the front door. Automatic garage door openers should be turned off when you are away from the house for long periods of time.

17 Attached garages are especially hazardous: If the security of the garage is breached, an intruder could gain entry to the house with little chance of being seen.

18 Garages often contain tools, ladders, and other equipment that would make breaking into the house relatively easy. Make sure yours is locked.

19 All garages should be protected with good padlocks that have the following features: hardened shackle, $9/32$- inch or greater shackle diameter, double locking (toe and heel), and a five-tumbler key-retaining feature.

20 All windows should be equipped with adequate locking devices, preferably key operated, and should be kept locked at all times.

21 Iron window guards can offer protection, but provision must be made to allow the use of windows for emergency evacuation of the building. Interior removable or folding guards are recommended for this purpose.

22 Casement windows, though less hazardous than double-hung windows, nevertheless require adequate locking devices, preferably key operated.

23 Windows above ground level require less protection than ground-level windows only if they are generally inaccessible. If in doubt, protect them as if they were at ground level.

24 Windows used for ventilation should be lockable both in closed and in partially open positions.

---

25 All wall openings large enough to admit a person should be protected.

26 Putty securing windowpanes should be periodically checked and replaced as necessary.

27 Impact-resistant glazing material, though expensive, can be an effective burglar deterrent.

28 Window-unit air conditioners should be adequately anchored to prevent their removal; otherwise these unprotected openings through the walls would easily admit intruders.

2

INTERIOR SECURITY

There are a number of commonsense rules you can follow for protection inside your home.

DON'T ADMIT STRANGERS

First of all, don't admit anyone into your home until you know who it is. If you have a peephole or glass panels in the door or a window nearby, you can see visitors. If you have a solid door, fit a good chain lock to the door, and always use it. As an added precaution, keep at hand a wedge-shaped rubber doorstop, available at variety or discount stores, to slip beneath the door. This will add support to your chain lock if a caller tries to crash through the door. Also, since he or she will probably recoil from the initial thrust, it will give you a chance to slam the door and seek help. If you live alone, consider installing an intercom so that you can communicate with front-door callers without opening the door.

New high-tech security devices are available. You can install in your home an all-in-one security set including a camera, monitor, and phone, so that you can view and communicate with the person who is at your front entrance ringing the doorbell. Or you can install weather-resistant cameras that will allow you a view of your driveway, home entrances, backyard, patio, guest house, garage, or pool area. This system can be connected to your television monitor, so that simply turning to the designated channel will offer you the view transmitted by your security camera. This interior security system can even be hooked up to a VCR and programmed so that selected areas and activities are captured on tape when you are not at home. When you return, you can find out if anyone accessed your property while you were away.

A few simple steps will keep a would-be intruder away from your door. A radio is an excellent crime fighter. A turned-on radio, preferably to a talk show (versus music), and positioned so that it may be heard from outside the front door may persuade an aspiring thief to believe that someone is at home. Another radio, this one near the rear, will add to the thief's plight. Tuning the radios to different stations could easily lead the thief to believe that two people, at least, are at home. The burglar would probably seek an easier target.

On the other hand, leaving your drapes drawn during the day tells a thief one of two things: Either you are not at home, or else you're simply not concerned about the security of your home. This laxity may send a thief looking avidly for an open door or window or some other easy way into your home and belongings.

Return now to your front door, where you are confronting an unknown caller. Once you think you have determined your visitor's identity from what you are told, don't believe it! Assume that the caller is lying, and ask for proof of identity. Insist on two or three items of clear identification. This applies even to a person in police uniform. Even though a police officer with a warrant, if denied admittance, can forcibly break into your home to carry out the task described in the warrant, you are always entitled to see proper identification.

If an unfamiliar person in another kind of uniform appears—to read your gas or water meter, for example—ask him or her to wait while you call the utility company to determine if readings are being taken in your neighborhood that day. Beware the door-to-door salesperson. Call your neighbors on either side to see if they have been visited. If they haven't, the caller will probably be gone by the time you put down the phone.

Don't trust any casual or unexpected caller. Ask for a business card, driver's license, or other identification. If you are still suspicious, suggest that he or she call for an appointment. An unexpected caller might actually be a potential thief or a con-artist (see Chapter 30).

Many legitimate salespeople will call you in attempt to set up an appointment to see you at home. If you do agree to an appointment, be sure to check with the caller's office, using the phone directory number rather than the number given to you by your visitor.

DON'T BE LURED AWAY FROM YOUR HOME

The ways in which burglars or confidence tricksters attempt to gain admission to homes are legion. Many of them are equally skilled at getting people out of their homes.

For example, a friend's purse was stolen at a restaurant. The next day she received a call from a woman who apologized profusely and said that she had taken the purse by mistake. The caller indicated that she was at work, but if the victim would care to meet her at a convenient location, she would be happy to return the purse. Naturally, the friend was overjoyed at the prospect of recovering her property—to the point of even buying lunch for her benefactor. When she returned home, she found her home burglarized. It had been entered by an accomplice, who had duplicated a key from the one in the victim's purse.

CHANGE LOCKS

Whenever you mislay or otherwise lose keys, get your locks changed. Entirely new hardware is rarely necessary, and usually a residential-lock's pins can be realigned on the site by a locksmith and a new key made at minimal expense.

The friend in the preceding story had a hard time recovering her loss on her homeowner's insurance because there was no evidence of forced entry. She could have avoided the burglary simply by keeping her house keys separate from any form of personal identification. Failing that, she should have taken the trouble to have had her locks changed immediately. She still might have lost her TV, stereo, silverware, and Oriental rug, but at least she would have had an easier time recovering on her insurance, because there would have been proof of a genuine forced entry.

HOUSEHOLD INVENTORY

Another form of burglary insurance is a household inventory. Set aside a Saturday or Sunday to go through your home, room by room, and list every item therein, noting also the approximate value of each and, where possible, serial numbers and receipts. Use a form like the inventory sheet provided at the end of this chapter. Items of extraordinary value such as jewelry, silverware, and art objects ideally should be photographed. Then take the inventory to your insurance agent, and discuss your existing coverage, not forgetting items that need separate scheduling for adequate insurance protection. It is also a good idea to videotape each room in your home in order to have a visual record of contents.

Keep this inventory list up-to-date, and retain a copy in your safe-deposit box or nonbank depository or with a trusted friend or relative. Do not keep a copy at your office or anywhere else where it might serve as a shopping list for a burglar.

Another way to protect your belongings is to etch in your name, Social Security number, or driver's license number with an electric pen that has a hard tip capable of scratching most metals. These pens are readily available. Call or visit your local police precinct; many precincts let you borrow these instruments.

Identifying all items of value that are likely to be stolen—such as TV sets, stereo equipment, radios, computers, cameras, and binoculars—makes life a lot tougher for burglars. One reason to do this is that etching makes your household goods harder to fence. Also, etched goods must be defaced to remove any evidence of etching. People are less likely to buy such defaced property, and fences will either not handle damaged goods at all or only at ridiculously low prices. Finally, when thieves are caught with etched merchandise in their possession, they are practically convicted then and there. Some thieves are smart and will avoid etched property entirely—that's really the best reason for etching household items.

Some of your assets defy etching, though, and other protective measures may be necessary to protect you from a thief. Paste copies of expensive gems may fool your adversary; marking the skin side of furs (after loosening the lining, of course) may lead to a recovery if your mink or sable is retrieved by police. Some auto manufacturers may attach unique identifiers to automobile components. You may protect your vehicle's highly desirable, easily removed accessories by etching CB radios, T-tops, and similar items.

Operation Identification is a nationwide project encouraging citizens to mark their property to combat burglary and theft. In one large city, burglary rates for Operation Identification households were 18 times lower than those of nonparticipants. A major reason for the success of projects like these is the character of the participants. People who join a communitywide crime prevention activity like Neighborhood Watch and Operation Identification are the same ones who install adequate lighting and good deadbolt locks and who use and practice overall self-protection.

Many people attach decals to their front doors advising welcomed and unwelcomed visitors alike that the premises are protected by a patrol service, alarm service, or other type of security device (see Chapter 3). In many cases, the homeowner purchased only the decals. No other services or devices were added to the security of the structure. A really accomplished thief is not fooled: It's his or her profession. A young thief, just starting to make his or her mark, might be fooled. So the decal won't hurt, and it may help.

Many police departments throughout the country have specialists who advise on ways to improve the security of homes and belongings. By all means, make use of these services if they are available to you.

SAFEGUARDING VALUABLES

It is sometimes difficult to determine which items should be protected by off-premises secure storage, whether a nonbank depository, a bank safe-deposit box, or your attorney's custody. Your attorney should be consulted in this regard. However, there are a few basic rules.

Never carry a lot of cash with you or keep cash around the house. Pay by check, or use charge accounts. If you have to carry "mad money" or emergency funds, use traveler's checks—you don't have to be traveling to cash them. Also, never leave checks or credit cards lying around. Lock up or hide them at home.

Home Safes and Security Closets

Some people take the sensible precaution of using a small safe to protect valuable items. It can be especially effective against fire. However, most home safes can be physically removed by a skilled and determined burglar and thus do not offer a great deal of protection against theft. Also, most such safes cannot protect larger items like furs.

Some of these objections can be overcome, of course. A small safe may be hidden, bolted to the walls or floor, or otherwise made a permanent addition to a structure. Setting the safe in concrete in the basement is one approach. Installing an alarm on a safe is also a fine additional security measure.

One excellent alternative to a safe is the home security closet. This requires lining the floor, walls, ceilings, and door of a suitable space with fire-retardant or fire-resistant material and then providing adequate locks for the entry door. Fire-resistant building material and adequate locking devices are generally available, so an accomplished handyman could fabricate a personal elementary security closet. Usually, an ordinary closet door must be rehung because the hinges of most are on the outside. Bracing or otherwise strengthening the door frame also will usually be necessary so that it cannot be removed along with the door.

It would be difficult, if not impossible, to construct a safety closet with walls as impenetrable as those of a safe. Thus, an alarm system is highly recommended. Or, for a more sophisticated installation, consult a general contractor or bank vault/safe installer.

Bank Services and Nonbank Depositories

One particularly valuable service offered by banks is a safe-deposit box. There are also specially secured 24-hour-a-day nonbank depositories. Such locations are often better secured than bank boxes—many have around-the-clock armed guards—and they have the convenience of being accessible at any time, day or night. Some nonbank depositories have the added advantage of being owned outright, rather than leased. Virtually all these services are insured for the protection of clients, and when you arrange for this type of service, you would be wise to investigate the extent of any insurance coverage. Both kinds of deposit boxes are recommended for storing valuable jewelry, stock or bond certificates, and all other valuable or important documents.

One document that should *not* be placed in a safe-deposit bank box is your letter of last instruction, commonly known as your will. The law in many states requires that a safe-deposit box, to safeguard its contents, be sealed after the owner dies. It may take several days to obtain the necessary court authorization to open the box, so your family would not have immediate access to your will.

The best strategy may be to leave it with your lawyer. Attorneys have special safes that can easily accommodate and secure these documents, and they can make your will available when necessary. It is a good idea to keep a copy of your will at home in a strongbox or in a nonbank depository.

Securities and Valuable Documents

Do not assume that stock certificates are not negotiable simply because they are issued in your name. Stolen stock certificates are frequently used as collateral for loans, which are then, of course, defaulted. Obtaining reissuance of a stock certificate to replace one that has been lost or stolen is a laborious and time-consuming process, for the issuee is generally required to post a bond to indemnify the transfer agent for any possible loss resulting from the sale of the stolen certificate. There is also the distinct possibility that you might suffer a loss from being unable to sell a security while it is tied up for months in a reissuing process.

The best means of protecting certificates is to leave them in your safe-deposit box, in a nonbank depository, or in the custody of your broker. A federally sponsored insurance program protects investors from loss, within specified limits, of securities held by brokers for their clients. This arrangement certainly is preferable to keeping certificates around the house, even though recovering on the federal insurance can embroil you in an administrative nightmare during which your assets may not be liquid.

Bearer bonds and other freely negotiable securities should be avoided in favor of registered equivalents. If, however, there is no alternative to owning bearer instruments, they should be kept in a bank safe-deposit box or specially secured 24-hour nonbank depository.

HANDGUNS

However comforting a gun might be to you, it is important you realize that it also increases the chances of an accident or homicide. Unless you and every member of your household know exactly how to keep and use a firearm safely, it is probably more hazardous to you than to any intruder.

At least 210 million firearms are to be found in the homes of Americans, many of them handguns. And these figures will increase by the year 2000. Approximately a third of the states have passed legislation that requires a permit to carry a concealed firearm for protection. Citizens who have passed a background check and completed a course in the safe use of firearms can get a permit. There is one matter agreed on by all parties to the controversy over the ownership and use of handguns: Guns are deadly. About 30,000 Americans die each year from gunshots due to suicide, homicide, or accidents. Over 80 percent of these deaths are due to handguns. Guns kill more people between the ages of 15 to 24 than all natural causes. Of all murder victims, 82 percent aged 15 to 19 were killed with guns. One side of the controversy feels that it is important to preserve the constitutional right of citizens to keep and bear arms, and that the ultimate protection of the people of this country may rest in the protection available within the family unit. The other side insists that the loss of lives in the United States from handgun use and abuse is too dear a price to pay. They also point out that other constitutional rights have been modified to accommodate changing conditions. In 1993, Congress passed the Brady Bill, mandating a 5-day waiting period for handgun sales.

Regardless of our handgun biases, we all realize the awesome potential that these weapons have for taking human life. One study charted the use of handguns in the commission of three serious crimes—rapes, robberies, and assaults—over a 10-year period. Of more than 65 million of these attacks, handguns were involved in more than 8 million. In 1992, some 931,000 violent crimes were committed with handguns, the highest number ever. More than two-thirds of the nation's homicides were committed with firearms, and in over 50 percent of the incidents, a handgun was employed. About a quarter of all aggravated assaults involved a gun, and in 4 out of 10 robberies, a gun was present. A robbery victim is three times more likely to be murdered when a gun is employed than in robberies where a knife—the next most lethal weapon—is used. About 21,000 gun victims are wounded each year. This figure is in addition to an annual average of about 11,100 people murdered by handguns. A gunshot victim will spend more than twice as long recuperating in a hospital as the average patient: 16 days as opposed to 7 or 8.

The overwhelming reason for having a handgun in the home is for protection. Unfortunately, far more people in the home are injured by firearms than are intruders. Half of all firearms fatalities occur at, or very near, the victim's home. Tragically, 40 percent of the lives lost are those of children, many of whom found where "Daddy kept his pistol."

According to the United States Department of Justice, more than 341,000 firearms were stolen between 1987 and 1992. About two-thirds of all firearms theft occurred during burglaries and larcenies. The more guns in possession of private individuals, the more likely they will fall into the hands of hardened criminals.

The number of innocent bystanders of stray gunfire is substantial. In New York City, for example, a total of 1,212 passersby—318 under 18 years of age—were victims of random shootings between 1991 and 1993. The risk of random shootings increases in warm weather when large numbers of people congregate outdoors. Also, as semiautomatic handguns, Uzis, and assault rifles fall into the hands of criminals, the number of victims of random shootings is likely to increase. These weapons, when pointed at an intended target, widely spray gunfire, often striking people nearby. The majority of random shootings occur in high-crime neighborhoods and in public-housing projects where guns are abundant.

The National Rifle Association (NRA), the organization most celebrated for its defense of our rights to keep and bear firearms in a legal manner, offers a number of commonsense suggestions for safeguarding a weapon kept in the home. The NRA suggests that firearms be kept out of the reach of children, the immature, and the irresponsible. Unloaded firearms should be kept locked up in the home. Under most circumstances, it is preferable that the weapons be out of sight, so that a thief who may be in your home or see into it is not tempted. Similarly, the ammunition for your weapons should be locked and out of sight.

There is but one reason for keeping a loaded gun in your home: protection of lives and protection of assets. If it is assets you feel the need to protect, consider securing them in a bank or, more conveniently, in a nonbank depository. Some authorities suggest that the safest way to keep a weapon in the home is to store the weapon and the ammunition apart from one another. Without question, this will provide a safer home environment most of the time, but without ammunition, you may be defenseless when you really need the weapon for the protection for which it is intended. How to store your weapon is a difficult decision. For both handgun and shoulder-fired weapons, several companies manufacture steel-sided combination-locking or key-locking containers that can be bolted to the wall or to a closet shelf. That way, a weapon will not be readily available to an intruder or a child. Ask yourself this question: What do I fear more than the possibility of my child's having access to a loaded firearm? Your answer to this question, based on your knowledge of your family, will dictate your course of action.

If you have a weapon in your home, you have the responsibility of ensuring that it is available to you when you need it but, at the same time, denying it to anyone for whom you wish otherwise. Toward this end, you should take these precautions:

- ❖ Keep it unloaded until you're ready to use it.
- ❖ Keep all ammunition in boxes that are clearly and accurately marked.
- ❖ Keep your finger out of the trigger guard unless you are ready to fire.
- ❖ Provide childproof storage.
- ❖ Check your weapon before you use it or store it.
- ❖ Open the action immediately on removing the gun from its case or rack.
- ❖ Ensure that your weapon is free of rust.
- ❖ Treat all weapons you touch as if they were loaded.
- ❖ Carry your weapon with the muzzle under control at all times.

- Ensure that the bore is unobstructed.
- Make certain that all metal parts are free from accumulations of heavy grease.
- Be certain that the action works freely.
- Be certain that the trigger works freely.
- Be certain that the safety works properly.
- Be certain that you store *only* the ammunition prescribed for your weapon.
- Ensure that your weapon is cased, or its action opened, whenever you enter or leave an automobile.
- Follow local laws when transporting firearms, and be certain they are unloaded.
- Enroll in a weapons safety course if you have a gun or plan to acquire one.
- Study your instruction manual thoroughly before using your firearm.
- Never handle firearms while under the influence of alcohol or drugs.
- Never give your child a toy that looks like a real gun.

At the very least, all firearms in the home, including hunting rifles and shotguns, should be equipped with lockable trigger guards. *You should remove the firing pins* of guns that are part of a collection or are used for decorative purposes. A firearm capable of, and intended for, firing should be maintained in good condition—it may be needed on short notice.

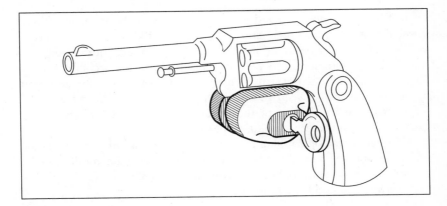

Figure 5. Trigger lock.

Firing a defective weapon could cause injury or death to the user. Firearms should be stored in a safe place, away from children and where an intruder would be unlikely to find it.

ENTERING AN EMPTY HOUSE

A woman of our acquaintance who lives alone has a rather active social life. When she leaves the house, she invariably leaves a $50 bill on a lamp table near the front door. She reasons that an intruder would be satisfied with this take, which is sufficient to purchase a round or two of most popular drugs. She believes that the thief will be deterred from carrying off the other valuables in the house. More importantly, she earnestly desires to avoid confrontation with an unwelcome visitor.

Another tactic she uses is based on most burglars' wish to avoid confrontation as earnestly as their unwilling hosts. When she arrives home, she presses her own doorbell. This should cause any intruder to vacate promptly. She once was asked what she would do if an intruder answered her ring. She had learned the name of an individual who lived on the next street, with a house number the same as her own. Her intention is to tell the intruder—if he or she answered the door—that she was seeking that person. She reasoned that the intruder might check the address in a telephone book and, satisfied that her story was plausible, remain to continue the theft. Perhaps the intruder would remain long enough for the arrival of the police, which she would have called.

There are two lessons to be learned from this extraordinary woman. First, through proper planning, it is possible to react appropriately to virtually any problem one might face. The second lesson is that you may encounter an intruder in your own home, and if you do, you are in substantial danger.

If You Encounter an Intruder

Even if you have done a good job of securing your home, it is entirely possible that you may return and see someone inside. Your first reaction will almost certainly be fright, plus an impulse to protect your possessions, leading to the temptation to yell or otherwise bring on a confrontation. Such confrontation is not a particularly good idea, if only because you might be directly between the intruder and his or her only avenue of escape. You are an obstacle to the intruder's survival—a very dangerous situation if the intruder is armed, desperate, or violent.

A far better way of handling the situation is to go as quickly and as quietly as possible to a neighbor's house and call the police. Then call a neighbor on the other side, and enlist his or her assistance in watching your house while you await the police.

LIVING ALONE

The person living alone, especially a woman, must take special precautions because she or he is often thought by criminals to be vulnerable. If you live alone, your home will most likely often be empty, and you'll need to take extra measures to make it look occupied. Timers can turn on lights, radios, or televisions at preset times, which is more economical than just leaving them on when you go out. An answering machine is a good idea, as callers can't be sure whether you're home or not. If you would like one, and your apartment house allows pets, you can get a dog; it serves as an excellent deterrent. You can fake it, if need be, by buying a barking tape sold by an alarm company, placing a "Beware of Dog" sign on your door or window, and leaving a water and food bowl outside.

The person living alone should always have a telephone in the bedroom and a strong deadbolt lock on the bedroom door. A cellular telephone is your best bet, because it allows emergency calls even if the telephone lines are cut. The bedroom door lock should be key operated, and a duplicate key should be left with a friend or a trusted neighbor in case of sudden illness or other event necessitating quick assistance.

Keep doors locked at all times even if you're home and be especially cautious about strangers at your door. If there isn't already a peephole on your door, install one and use it to verify the identity of visitors before opening the door. If your building has a locked entrance, don't let strangers in behind you, and avoid getting into the elevator with a strange person. If you are embarrassed and need an excuse, say something like "I forgot my mail" or "I forgot to buy something at the store." If your building is lacking in security measures, complain to the building manager, and persuade your neighbors to do so as well. Try to live in a building or complex that provides adequate security. Be sure that the locks on the doors are changed with every new tenant.

In both the telephone listing and on your mailbox or intercom, list your last name and only a first initial so as not to disclose your gender. If possible, make your schedule unpredictable, and don't reveal it to anybody. Avoid telling people you don't know very well that you live alone. Tell them you have a roommate, or that you live with a relative. *Never* let anyone into your home whom you don't know very well. Doing so is very dangerous, because once entry is gained, the "polite" guest may turn into an attacker. One woman invited a man she had been seeing for a while into her home. After he left, she realized that two gold chains and a pair of pearl earrings had been taken. This woman was relatively lucky; another woman did the same and was raped at gunpoint. Obviously, not everyone is untrustworthy; the point is that there are many risks involved in living alone, and you should do your best to be prepared and aware.

WOULD YOU BE ABLE TO RECOGNIZE A BURGLAR?

It is doubtful that you would be able to recognize a burglar if you saw one. First of all, you would probably be expecting a hardened criminal, not the fuzzy-cheeked teenager who came around last week to see if you wanted your lawn mowed. You would not believe that the Swiss Army knife your neighbor carried could be used to remove a small pane of glass from a front door, providing access to the night latch (as opposed to the deadbolt lock, which would provide more reliable protection). You might even think that the nice kid who dates your daughter really did buy the stereo he gave her for her birthday.

REPORTS TO THE POLICE

There may be a time when you will find it necessary to report a criminal or crime to the police. These are the statements they will be interested in hearing from you:

- ❖ "I wish to report a crime."
- ❖ Where—the address or the street intersection.
- ❖ What—the type of crime, injury, shots, fight, etc.
- ❖ Who—the persons involved, including how many, their descriptions.
- ❖ How escaping—if in an auto, give license number, make, and model.
- ❖ Where to—the direction headed, whether the car turned around, toward what nearby intersections, etc.

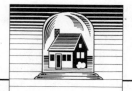

INTERIOR SECURITY:
A CHECKLIST

1. Don't admit anyone into your home unless you know that the caller has verifiable identification and valid reasons for calling on you.

2. Use a chain lock and a rubber doorstop while identifying a stranger at your door.

3. Do not assume that a stranger in uniform is legitimate. Verify the stranger's status with his or her employer.

4. Before you admit a stranger who has phoned ahead and made an appointment to see you at home, verify that the stranger is employed by the organization that he or she claims to represent.

5 Be particularly wary of people claiming to be building or fire inspectors or door-to-door salespersons. Check with their place of employment before admitting them.

6 Beware of people attempting to get you away from your home.

7 Turn on at least one radio when you leave, so that an aspiring thief will think someone is at home.

8 If you lose your keys, get your locks changed.

9 Make an inventory of all your belongings, and keep your list up-to-date. Protect the list carefully.

10 Use the nonbank depository type of safe-deposit boxes for the convenience of around-the-clock access to your valuables.

11 Identify appropriate items of property with an etcher or similar device.

12 Consider installing a security closet in your home.

13 Never keep a lot of cash in your home or on your person.

14 Never leave checks lying around, and lock up or hide your checkbook in the home.

15 Use a safe-deposit box or specially secured nonbank depository for storage of valuables and valuable documents.

16 Observe all precautions for safe handling and storage of firearms in the home.

17 Equip any firearms you own with lockable trigger guards.

18 If you surprise a burglar or robber in your home, try to escape and avoid a confrontation. If that is not possible, cooperate, don't try to be a hero.

19 Install locks on your bedroom door, and have a telephone in the room.

Inventory Sheet

Include cars and items such as lawn mowers that are not normally kept inside the home. Cover attics, basements, garages, and so on. Prepare lists for contents of lockboxes. Photocopy this page for additional record keeping.

Room:_____   Date:_____

Item	Serial Number	Date Purchased	Cost	Approx. Value	Amount of Insurance Coverage	Comments

3

ALARM SYSTEMS

"I was sound asleep, and all of sudden this wailing sound woke me up," Don said to the fire marshal. "I didn't know what it was at first, but then it occurred to me that it must be the alarm. The alarm had just been installed that day! We lost a lot, but, thank God, no one was hurt."

More than ever, citizens are investing in home security, and a residential alarm system is one of the top priorities.

SECURITY FUNCTIONS

An alarm system does two things: It detects and it communicates. The alarm system that might be installed in your home would probably function both as a fire alarm and as an intrusion alarm. So-called panic or silent duress buttons would add a third function, that of manually communicating the need for some sort of assistance. The system could also have other functions; it could monitor a vital piece of equipment, such as a home furnace or wine cellar temperature control.

A chronic problem with alarm systems, especially home alarm systems, has been a very high false-alarm rate. In most cases, however, the false alarms have been due to misapplication of sensors or to user error.

Fire Detection

You're more likely to have a fire than an intruder, so this chapter covers that function of the alarm system first.

Fires develop in four stages: the incipient stage, the smoldering stage, the flame stage, and the heat stage. Different sensors on the market are designed to detect the fire in these different stages. Naturally, the earlier in its development that a fire can be detected, the better are chances to limit the damage it will cause. No sensor, however, is the proper one for all applications.

In its incipient stage, a fire doesn't produce any smoke or flame. It does, however, generate products of combustion, microscopic particles that rise on air currents. Ceiling-mounted ionization detectors have an inner chamber that contains a small amount of radioactive material. An outer chamber is open to air. Air passing through the outer chamber becomes ionized or electrically charged. When particles of combustion enter the chamber, the electrical charge between the two chambers is altered, setting off an alarm. This is the most expensive of the sensors available. Due to its method of detection, it may sound a false alarm in a dusty atmosphere.

The photoelectric detector will sound an alarm during the fire's smoldering stage. Smoke or visible products of combustion enter the detector's sensing chamber and interrupt a light beam, causing an alarm. This type of detector, however, is not good for areas that may normally have smoke, such as a kitchen or areas near a fireplace, since the detector will cause a false alarm if excessive but nonthreatening smoke is produced. These units are relatively inexpensive.

A rate-of-rise or temperature-change detector senses the rapid temperature increase that occurs as the fire progresses from the smoldering stage to the flame stage and then to the heat stage. A heat or fixed-temperature detector, which activates when the air around it reaches a designated temperature, may be incorporated into a single unit with the rate-of-rise detector.

Generally, no single type of detector is used exclusively in a home. For example, the heat detector is usually used in conjunction with an automatic sprinkler system and is inappropriate for most home uses. But one or another of these systems provides a relatively inexpensive means of fire protection. Many insurance companies discount premiums for customers who install them.

Intruder Detection

There are two broad categories of devices to detect intruders: point protection and space or volumetric protection. Point-protection devices detect an intrusion through a specific location, such as a door or window, even through a wall. Space protection devices detect movement within a particular area.

The magnetic contact switch uses a magnet to hold one of the contacts of a switch away from the other. Contact-switch sets can be either surface mounted or concealed. When the magnet is attached to a door or window, and the switch is attached to the door jamb or window frame, the magnet keeps the two switch points apart. When the door or window is opened, the magnet can no longer hold the spring-loaded contact to prevent the switch from engaging, and the alarm sounds.

However, one problem with the surface-mounted version of the switch is that it can be defeated by using another magnet to hold the switch contact, even though the door is opened. Using either a balanced switch set or a concealed contact set can negate this possibility.

Virtually everyone has seen glass-break sensors attached to store windows. These sensors, activated by the shock of breaking glass, are also replacing the silver-colored foil tape used in the past on residential windows.

There are shock or seismic detectors that provide protection for the specific object upon which they are mounted, such as walls, safes, file cabinets, and closets. They also guard window frames, glass panes, and patio or French doors. Any vibrations resulting from pushing, knocking, banging, touching, or kicking will upset the equilibrium of the device and sound the alarm.

A fourth type of device, the pressure detector, uses something like a doormat that is installed under the carpet inside the doorway, in a hallway, or on stairs. An individual's weight on the mat brings electrical contacts together and activates the alarm. Some self-opening doors at supermarkets and discount stores employ the same principle.

A fifth type of detector uses a beam of light shining across the inside of a door or window to a photoelectric sensor, like those that prevent some elevator doors from closing on passengers. The alarm is activated by the interruption of the beam. In the past, however, an intruder could circumvent a photoelectric sensor merely by stepping over or sliding under the beam or by shining a light beam at the sensor. To overcome this vulnerability, many photoelectric sensors use infrared light, which is invisible to the human eye, moving at a given number of bursts of light per second between the transmitter and receiver, marking an advance over "visible spectrum" light sources. In either case, a transmitter sends a ray of light (visible or invisible) to a receiver and sounds the alarm when the light's passage is interrupted or changes rhythm. This technology can also be used for space protection by placing the transmitter at one end of a room and the receiver at the other. In especially sensitive areas, such as a silver closet or safe room, a fiber optic wire mesh built directly into the walls can be useful. The breaking of the wire triggers the alarm.

Space Protection

The ultrasonic sensor generates high-frequency sound waves. Such a device can protect a three-dimensional teardrop-shaped area approximately 25 feet out from the sensor. These waves are too high in pitch to be heard by the human ear, so any intruder is unaware of their existence. When the waves bounce off an intruder, the pattern of the waves is altered, activating the alarm.

Unfortunately, some individuals—and many pets—are irritated by these ultrasonic "noises," and these sensors are also subject to false alarms caused by the flapping of a curtain, a ringing telephone, or even a rush of air from a heater starting up. Loud noises in adjacent spaces might also activate such a system. Two sensors, tuned to different frequencies, may cause false alarms if installed too near one another.

A similar system uses electromagnetic microwaves rather than sound waves. While this eliminates the irritation to sensitive ears, if not installed correctly these waves will penetrate walls, rather than bounce off them like the ultrasonic waves. This means that movement in the next room or outside the building can activate such a detector.

A passive infrared sensor detects an intruder's presence by sensing his or her body heat. There are numerous detection patterns available with passive infrared sensors. These detection patterns range from a ceiling-mounted unit with 360-degree field to a long narrow zone, to a "curtain" to protect a wall.

When an intruder enters a protected space, the passive systems can detect alien presence immediately. A person's body temperature will be roughly 25 degrees hotter than the ambient room temperature. As with all intrusion detection devices, there are drawbacks with a system such as this. Obviously, such a system would be impractical for protecting an area often frequented by people. Animals, heating ducts, electric motors, and even a television receiver would be capable of emitting sufficient heat to affect the operation of a passive infrared detection device. Similarly, these devices become less reliable at room or ambient temperatures approaching normal body temperature, because at such levels the body's temperature would be masked by that of the surrounding air.

Audio detectors are used to protect entire rooms. These detectors consist of wall- or ceiling-mounted microphones. The detectors are set at a certain noise level, and if that level is exceeded, a signal is sent to a central station. One problem with this system is that the central station operator can open a circuit and listen in to activity in the monitored space.

In an effort to overcome the problem of false alarms, which affect the reliability of space detection sensors, manufacturers now combine them into single units known as dual-technology sensors. In these, a passive infrared sensor is paired with an ultrasonic or a microwave sensor. Both sensor types must trip before an alarm is sent. In effect, each half of the unit questions the other half, compensating for the weaknesses in each technology that result in a false alarm.

In most cases, the sensors are connected by wires to the alarm control unit, which houses the alarm's off-on switch and the part of the system that sends the alarm signal to an on-site sounder or out to a response center. In more and more cases, systems are now using wireless technology, in which each sensor has a small battery-powered transmitter that sends the signal to the control unit. An internal alarm in the system will tell the control unit if the sensor's battery is running down or if the sensor is being tampered with.

No single sensor technology can be considered effective on its own, thus the concept of concentric rings of security. A free-standing residence may have magnetic contact switches on all exterior doors and windows, space protection in hallways or areas where there is a large amount of peripheral glass, and a magnetic contact on the door to a silver cupboard. A good system uses a mix of techniques, so that an intruder who defeats one layer of protection will be caught by the next one.

Again, a qualified professional can help determine which mixture of sensing or silent-duress alarm system devices is best for you.

COMMUNICATING THE ALARM

Once a detector has sensed a fire or intruder, the system must be able to communicate that fact. The detectors can be set to activate a bell or siren on the premises or to activate a radio that transmits an emergency message. Many installations use a telephone line to transmit a signal to a contract central station where personnel on duty telephone the police or fire department to respond.

As stated at the beginning of this chapter, false alarms—as high as 90 to 95 percent of all alarm signals transmitted—have traditionally been a major problem. The alarm industry has made a determined effort to reduce this rate by improving the products and by educating dealers, installers, and users.

In many communities, due to high rates of false alarms and limited response resources, police and fire departments no longer will accept alarm signals directly from residential or most commercial alarm control units. Instead, the signal must travel from the protected premises to a contract central station, where personnel then telephone the appropriate public agency. Even with such a system, in many communities the police allow a given number of false alarms per year and then assess a fine for each alarm call exceeding the limit.

Also, some radio-operated devices violate Federal Communications Commission (FCC) regulations. Bells or sirens that go off repeatedly can cause neighbors to ignore the alarm—perhaps at the time of a true emergency. This is unfortunate, because most alarm systems signal in the immediate area, rather than transmit to a remote location.

Cellular telephones can be used as independent signal transmitters, especially if the residential or business telephone lines have been cut. A few years ago, during a jewel heist, the "bad guys" cut an entire trunk link so that the central alarm station was overwhelmed with alarm signals. The alarm company was not able to sort out the source of the legitimate alarm until it was too late. A cellular telephone would have averted this problem. An earlier edition of *How To Protect Yourself From Crime* said that the opening up of many communities to cable TV creates an exciting possibility for alarm systems. Cable lines can connect homes to the system on a two-way basis, bringing TV into the home and transmitting emergency information from the home to a central station on the same cable. Transmitting signals through cable lines is less expensive than sending them over telephone lines. Not only fire and intrusion detectors, but respirators, boiler-level monitors, or virtually any type of sensor could be a part of such a system. This promise remains; reality however, is still some time away.

ARMING AN ALARM

Unfortunately, regardless of how well planned and sophisticated your alarm system may be, there is always one problem—you. You are in and out of the home all day. Whatever the alarm system, it must be told when it's you turning it on and, especially, off, and when it's someone or something else. This is called arming the system.

Obviously, you don't want your alarm to "cry wolf" every time you enter the house, so you must be able to turn it on and off and enter your home without triggering the alarm or compromising its effectiveness at detecting an intruder. Following are the three arming (or disarming) mechanisms generally used with an alarm system.

The key-armed system uses a key to arm and disarm the system. This can be inconvenient if your arms are full; and, moreover, if your keys fall into the hands of a burglar, your entire alarm system becomes valueless.

Push-button keypad arm/disarm systems are more convenient and secure than key-operated systems, but if the code numbers are discovered then the security of your system is compromised. A time-delay feature is part of this intrusion alarm systems. Time-delay allows the user to activate the system from inside the residence and then have a set amount of time to exit before the system is armed. On reentering, the time delay allows a certain amount of time to shut off the system before an alarm is activated. The system will sound a pre-alarm tone to remind the user to disarm the system and to let an intruder know that an alarm has been activated.

Some systems use a portable, hand-held keypad that resembles a calculator or a television remote-control to arm/disarm, bypass selected parts of the system, transmitt a silent duress (panic) alarm, and query the system from distances up to 100 feet from the system control unit that is within the protected perimeter. The user's personal code must be entered before the system will acknowledge commands.

Other alarm systems enable users to telephone in from anywhere in the world to arm/disarm, bypass, and query the system. Again, the user's personal code must be entered for the system to acknowledge commands.

The greatest false-alarm hazard lies in your failure, on reentering your protected premises, to identify yourself properly to the alarm control unit, either with a key or your code number, within the allotted time.

HOW TO BUY AN ALARM SYSTEM

When you set out to purchase an alarm system, begin by seeking objective advice. Many police crime prevention units and fire departments have alarm system specialists. Your casualty insurance carrier probably has a specialist who will not only be able to recommend special equipment but also be able to tell you how to lower your insurance premiums by installing it. If you aren't satisfied, contact a master locksmith, who may be able to steer you away from some of the fly-by-night firms. At the same time, you might get the locksmith to replace all your night latches with dual-keyway deadbolt locks equipped with 1-inch-long throw bolts. Of course, alarm manufacturers and installers will be more than happy to offer advice. It may not be totally objective, but if it is the only advice available, it is better than nothing.

Some alarm systems are worse than none at all. You obviously cannot afford a system that delivers only false security. In selecting a source for your alarm system, remember that the equipment is complex and that you must have good service available for it. Generally, this would rule out buying a system by mail from a distant supplier or from any firm other than one that specializes in the sale, installation, and service of such systems. As a rule, the longer the warranty, the better the system. But if the system is issued by a "here today and gone tomorrow" firm, the warranty, regardless of terms, is suspect.

Check parts inventories. If a critical part is available only from a single manufacturer located in Yokohama (or Yonkers, if you live on the West Coast), you may be asking for trouble. If your dealer doesn't have the parts on hand, your system may well be useless to you.

Certain features should be a part of your alarm installation. Among these is the system's self-check capability. This enables you to check the "health" of your alarm system and be certain it is in proper operating condition. Of course, you must remember to make these capability checks. Even if you should forget, an alarm with a system-in-trouble warning signal will probably jog your memory.

One feature that is most important is a provision for emergency power for your system when normal power supplies are interrupted. In the event of a fire, which may have interrupted your power, your auxiliary power could save your life. If an intruder deliberately interrupts your power, auxiliary power could prevent loss of property, injury, or death at the hands of the thief.

Some auxiliary power systems employ nonrechargeable batteries. If yours is such a system, it is absolutely essential that you follow the manufacturer's recommendations for battery replacement to ensure the viability of the auxiliary power system. Rechargeable batteries can malfunction, too; if your system has this type of backup, you should determine proper testing procedures. It may be necessary to write to the manufacturer of the batteries to obtain the information, since the equipment installer may not have it or may represent that the batteries never need replacement.

Make certain that your alarm's signal horn sounds loud enough to be effective. Ideally, the horn should be mounted in the attic and sound through a vent to the outside. Before you sign any contract, try to arrange to see an actual installation that has been performed by your chosen contractor. Check for its appearance, workmanship, and customer satisfaction.

Finally, check with your tax accountant. Certain types of installations may affect the tax treatment you receive when you sell your home. A hard-wired, through-the-wall installation, for example, although more expensive initially, might be the least-expensive choice in the long run.

CAVEAT EMPTOR

Let the buyer beware! The proliferation of crime is perhaps matched only by the proliferation of opportunists preying on the near-paranoid reactions of some sectors of the public. The use of scare tactics to sell alarm systems is deplorable. Be especially cautious about such an approach, particularly from unsolicited, direct-mail advertising or door-to-door salespeople. Don't allow yourself to be stampeded into immediate action. The best response to a now-or-never sales approach is "Never!"

Find out whether your state requires an alarm company or dealer to be licensed. If so, make certain that the company or dealer has such a license. Determine whether the establishment has its own central station. If not, ask who manages the central station and its location. Find out who it is, exactly, that is expected to respond to an alarm signal. Does the alarm company have its own security force, or are the local police expected to respond? And, of course, you should be aware of the average response time to an alarm signal.

Beware of installation charges. If at all possible, contract a firm price, installed. Many unscrupulous operators will quote absurdly low prices (for, as a general rule, absurdly inferior equipment) plus a "nominal installation fee." Your definition of *nominal* may be a lot different from theirs.

Many buyers will have to finance an alarm system. The dealer may offer to arrange financing for you and hint that he or she will carry your note. In most instances, the dealer will carry it no further than the discount window of the nearest bank or finance company, where it will be sold to the bank or finance company, which becomes its holder in due course. The dealer is then responsible for carrying out the contract, but the holder in due course is entitled to payment. If the dealer defaults on the contract or even skips town, you will probably still be liable to pay the holder in due course. You could very well get fleeced under such an agreement, especially if there is collusion between an unethical contractor and equally unethical holder. Thus, it is absolutely necessary to deal with a completely reliable, ethical contractor.

Take care, too, in selecting the communication phase of an alarm's operation. Find out how the alarm signal will be carried from the protected premises to a response point. If you buy a system that the installer programs to dial the police or fire department with an emergency message, make sure your town's departments will respond to such calls. Be certain that radio-transmitted messages don't violate FCC regulations. Check out every angle before you sign anything.

One last word of warning: Beware of service contracts. While good service from a reliable contractor is the main consideration when you purchase an alarm system, contractual prepayment for this service may be unnecessarily expensive. Be certain to investigate total costs before making your commitment.

KEEP YOUR SECURITY SECRET

The less that people know about the steps you take to secure your property, the more secure you will be. Do not advertise everything you do to make your home secure because virtually every defensive action you might reasonably take can be countered, subverted, or bypassed when a would-be intruder knows exactly what to expect. (In one case, a burglar alarm installer serviced homes for 2 years, until he was arrested for burglarizing several clients.) This may seem a little contradictory in light of the earlier suggestion that decals be used. But the fact is that many houses display alarm decals when, in reality, they are not protected by an intrusion alarm. Unfortunately, the professional burglar generally knows this—and, furthermore, knows how to determine for sure whether such a system has been installed. Should there actually be an operating system, the professional possibly can circumvent it, given enough time and the absence of disturbance. The amateur burglar, on the other hand, is generally not as well schooled in the mechanics of theft and thus is more easily deterred by exterior warnings.

Your interest is obviously to avoid being burglarized. You thus need to strike a balance between deterrence and total disclosure—revealing enough to discourage the random burglar but not so much that you make it easy for the skilled and determined pro who singles you out.

It is important that you be guarded in what you tell people. Suppose a neighbor has a valuable collection of cut glass that is stolen while she is out of town. Later, when police crack the burglary ring, it is discovered that one of its members is a young man who lives in the neighborhood. It is hardly coincidental that the neighbor remarked that the thieves "seemed to know exactly what they were looking for."

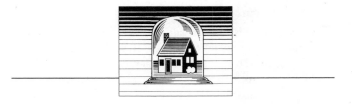

ALARM SYSTEMS: A CHECKLIST

 Give serious consideration to installing an alarm system with panic buttons that is backed up by auxiliary power sources.

2 In considering alarm systems, investigate multipurpose systems that detect both fire and intrusion incidents.

3 The ionization type of fire detector is probably the one best suited for most home uses; however, it is also the most expensive.

4 An intrusion system might employ several types of detectors, depending on your requirement. Explore these possibilities with a qualified professional before settling on an alarm system.

5 Some equipment may be adaptable to other detection and communication functions, for example, monitoring items of equipment such as home furnaces, wine cellar coolers, and heaters.

6 Alarms are communicated locally (for example, a bell rings), or remotely (for example, they are transmitted via phone lines to the fire department, police, or commercial alarm central station). Be diligent in determining which is most cost effective for you.

7 Seek objective advice in determining your alarm needs. Fire departments, police, or insurance carriers often have specialists who can advise you. You may also find that installation of certain equipment can reduce insurance premiums.

8 Use exterior deterrent signs, but do not reveal anything about your security system.

9 Avoid disclosures that indicate you own items of special value.

10 A warranty is only as valuable as the person or entity guaranteeing its performance. Beware of the "here today, gone tomorrow" installer. Beware, also, of high-pressure sales tactics. Beware of unspecified installation charges. Beware of service contracts: Some are good, while others add considerably to the total cost of a system.

4

YOUR TELEPHONE

Every day for the past 6 years in a Miami suburb, Barney, 85 years old, has dialed the same telephone number just before 9:00 a.m.

"Good morning, Dorothy," he says to police complaint clerk Dorothy.

"Good morning, Barney. Have a nice day," says Dorothy.

This daily conversation is part of a police service originally named Reassurance Program and later called Operation Good Morning. Police say the program, started in 1968, has saved the lives of elderly people living alone. The more than 50 people on the other end of the line say it helps save them from loneliness.

ESSENTIAL RULES

The telephone is a marvelous invention that has been adapted to many uses, most of them benign, like the one in the opening example. But the telephone is also an instrument of crime—in fact, possibly the most widely used criminal instrument. The cardinal rule is that you should always use your telephone on your terms, not those of the caller. Moreover, never talk on the phone unless you do so willingly.

Guard What You Say

Here's a very important lesson of telephone security: Never say anything over the telephone that you do not want a stranger to know. For example, a caller who asks for the man of the house should never be told that there is not one or that he is out of town. Far better to tell the caller that your father or husband "is asleep right now and will return the call when he awakes." It is vitally important that this lesson be taught to children, as well as ingrained as a habit in adults.

Every caller who hangs up when the phone is answered is not a burglar attempting to find out if anyone is at home. Telephone equipment can malfunction; calls can be disconnected; callers can become flustered when an unfamiliar voice answers the phone and hang up as a reflex action. However, there is always the possibility that the caller is a would-be burglar, and it is a good idea to assume just that and to check immediately to see that all doors and windows are properly secured.

Know Your Caller

Occasionally you may get a call from a person claiming to be a peace officer or government agent making an inquiry. Unless you are subpoenaed by a court of law, you are not required to give information. Generally, as law-abiding citizens, we do have an obligation to cooperate with law officers, but that obligation does not extend to cooperating unquestioningly with people who merely represent themselves as such on the telephone.

When you get a suspicious call of this nature, insist that your caller visit you in person so that you can properly examine his or her identification. Say something like, "May I call you back? It isn't convenient for me to talk right now." Then return the call at his or her office, having first checked the number against the telephone directory to ensure that the caller is actually who he or she claims to be. If you are unable to verify the telephone number in the directory, call the directory number of the agency that the caller claimed to represent. If the agency cannot identify your caller, report the incident to the police, and give them the number that your caller gave you.

A final warning: Beware of the caller who claims that your name has been given as a reference. You have an obligation to your friends and neighbors not to reveal information about them indiscriminately. You should always arrange to return a call requesting such information so that you can first verify that the call is legitimate. Alternatively, you might check with the acquaintance who submitted your name as a reference, or you might agree to respond only to a written request for such information.

It is, incidentally, a good idea to advise anyone whose name you give as a reference that you have done so, so that time will not be taken up unnecessarily in double-checking a call received on your behalf.

SUMMONING EMERGENCY ASSISTANCE

Emergency numbers for police and fire departments should be available at every phone in the home; however, under the stress of an emergency, people sometimes lose their composure to a point where they forget how to take otherwise routine actions. Thus, as a further precaution, place a small note (using a label maker is ideal) on the phone saying: "Dial 0" or "Dial 911," if your local police department has adopted this special emergency number. And if you or yours are highly excitable, it isn't a bad idea to include your own address as well!

TELEPHONE-ANSWERING MACHINES AND SERVICES

A telephone-answering service is a valuable security measure, especially if there is no one at home for considerable periods of time. Under no circumstances should the service tell callers that the user is out of town or away from home or give a time when he or she is expected to return. Likewise, the service should be instructed not to reveal that the operator is, in fact, an answering service, but rather to give the impression that the operator is a domestic employee.

Telephone-answering equipment that delivers a prerecorded message and records a caller's message can be used advantageously as a security device if you always indicate in your messages to callers that you cannot take their call at the present time. Do not indicate that you are away from home. For a strictly residential phone, it is usually a good idea to use first names only to avoid revealing your surname to a caller who doesn't already know it. Similarly, it isn't necessary to repeat the phone number the caller has reached. Never leave seductive messages and always use "we" instead of "I." An excellent deterrent to harassment if you are a woman is to have a male relative or friend record your message.

If you travel extensively, consider buying an answering device that enables you to receive your messages from another telephone. In this way, you can return your calls, even from far away, and still avoid revealing that you are out of town. Of course, never disclose that you are out of town, or leave your arrival date on an answering machine. This is an invitation to burglars.

Incidentally, don't be alarmed if you get a lot of calls in which no messages are left. Many people simply object to talking to a machine, and hang up as a result.

CELLULAR TELEPHONES

Cellular telephones generally have a great deal of security built in, much of it resulting from the nature of the system's operating parameters. Cities are divided into hexagonal areas called *cells*, which provide a number of frequencies and various levels of power output which change as vehicles and pedestrians traveling through them. As phone users leave one cell, powerful computers switch their cells to the neighboring one without interruption.

Stealing a cellular phone from a car would be relatively easy, b ut using it would not. Built into the system are theft-prevention protocols, including a user-entered code without which the systems will not operate. If, however, a careless owner leaves the code on a scrap of paper behind the sun visor, a thief can make all the free calls he or she wishes. Even in this instance there would be some protection for the owner. When the cellular service provider was notified of the theft, the service could be deactivated.

Portable cellular phones are a convenience offering mobile security but are harder to protect. The added security cellular phones offer is well worth the expense of batteries and AC chargers.

Although cellular phones are designed with security in mind, be aware that today's state of the art is tomorrow's garage sale. In protecting this convenience, you must be aware that someone will devise a method or piece of equipment to defeat your safeguards. You must continually upgrade the safety, sanctity, and security of your possessions and those of your loved ones.

TELEPHONE SECURITY WHILE YOU'RE AWAY

The telephone is one service that you should *never* have disconnected while you are away from home. A temporary disconnection message delivered by a special operator is a clear indication of one of two things: You haven't paid your bills, or you are out of town. You don't wish to leave either impression on callers.

HANDLING SPECIAL PROBLEMS

Nuisance and Obscene Calls

Under federal and most state laws, it is a crime to make harassing or obscene telephone calls. For these offenses, penalties of up to a year in prison and/or fines of up to $1,000 are prescribed. A typical state law would read: "It shall be unlawful for any person or persons . . . to telephone another person repeatedly, if such calls are not for a lawful business purpose, but are made with intent to abuse, torment, threaten, harass, or embarrass one or more persons." Similarly, the statute generally prohibits obscene phone calls, described as any "lewd, obscene, or lascivious remarks, suggestions, or proposals, manifestly intended to embarrass, disturb, and annoy the person to whom the said remarks, suggestions, or proposals are made." On the local level, 9,000 obscene telephone call complaints are received by NYNEX every month. An additional 6,000 are reported as threatening and abusive.

If you do receive an obscene call, hang up immediately and forget it! Most obscene calls are isolated, one-time occurrences, possibly placed by someone dialing numbers at random. Often the callers are adolescents, putting forth a display of bravado for their friends, although annoyance callers can also include neighbors, acquaintances, or fellow employees. Should the calls continue, do not broadcast your displeasure. If you are not expecting important calls, remove the receiver from the hook, if only for a short time. The caller will likely be frustrated and turn his attention elsewhere. Maintain a log of the calls, and notify your telephone company immediately. Usually a pattern of calls must be documented before action can be taken. Report calls to your local telephone company's Annoyance Call Bureau. The methods the telephone company will use to bring an end to this nuisance can vary widely depending on the particular equipment serving your home. Thus, you shouldn't feel shortchanged if your nuisance-call problem is handled differently from your neighbor's.

Not all callers are adolescents or people with "nothing better to do." Experts claim that 75 to 90 percent of repeated harassing calls are from someone you know. Some are apparently upstanding members of the community. A university president in Washington, D.C., was forced to resign after numerous obscene calls were traced to him. He victimized women who placed ads in their local newspaper for home day-care services. He, like other obscene callers, was driven by a sexual desire to shock his victims verbally.

Under no circumstances should you attempt to debate or get into a shouting or cursing match with your caller—unless, of course, you are requested to do so by law enforcement or telephone security personnel to assist in their investigation. Be certain who is requesting your assistance, since some obscene callers get someone to call first and pretend to be from the phone company. To excite or inflame anyone, especially one demonstrating such antisocial behavior, is a certain invitation for a repeat performance. Also, do not talk to or reason with the caller or ask why the caller is doing this. Anything other than your hanging up or leaving the receiver off the hook encourages the caller to continue. The most effective means of avoiding a series of obscene or nuisance calls is to get an unlisted number. However, doing this is inconvenient. Changing your telephone number won't be effective if the caller is an acquaintance who will learn your new number. One expert suggests having two numbers: an additional number and an answering machine to pick up your former number, so that your harasser will not be able to contact you. After a while, he or she may give up.

If you are a woman living alone, have your telephone number listed with only your first initial. Never disclose personal information about yourself. If you answer the phone and nobody responds, hang up. Repeated hang-ups or wrong numbers may come from someone checking if you are home, including a criminal. A common tactic to discourage such calls is blowing a loud whistle into the receiver. However, some experts caution that this will agitate the caller and make the problem worse. If someone calls and asks for your name or what number they have reached, do not tell them. Tell them they have a wrong number. Some women have brought their obscene calls to an end by having a male friend answer their telephone.

A number of devices and services may be offered by your telephone company that can be used to thwart nuisance or obscene callers. One such device is *Caller ID*. A screen displays the telephone number of your caller, so that you can repeat it to the unwanted caller or choose not to answer the telephone. *Call Block* or *Call Rejection* enables you to block undesirable numbers from getting through. The telephone company is able to note the phone number, date, and time of specific calls if you have *Call Trace*. You can enter an access code to trace a call. *Call Return* allows you to enter certain digits to "call back" your caller. Unfortunately, most of these services are effective only for certain calls and may not work for cellular or public telephones. Another less costly option is for you to pretend you have one of these services by pressing the disconnect button, requesting that an operator trace the call, and then hanging up. A nuisance or obscene caller may believe you and be discouraged from calling back.

As with making obscene phone calls, taping or otherwise deliberately gaining access to a telephone call without being a party to the conversation or gaining permission from one of the parties is a crime. Federal and some state law officers, of course, may do so, but only when they have a court order covering a specific telephone for a specified time. If you feel your life is being threatened by a caller notify police.

Telephone Surveys

The use of the telephone for sales purposes, often through the gimmick of a so-called survey, can be very annoying to some people, but unless there are serious misrepresentations, it is not illegal. There are, however, other types of "surveyors" who are gathering intelligence information for illegal purposes, and thus it pays never to give confidential information over the phone unless you are certain about the person to whom you are speaking. Do not, for example, spontaneously answer questions concerning where you work, what you look like, your income, any items of value you may have in the home, your sexual habits, or anything else of a personal nature. A good tactic is to say that the caller has reached an answering service, and that she or he may leave a name and number. If the caller is illegitimate, he or she will most likely hang up. If an unwanted call continues, simply hang up yourself. You may wish to respond to legitimate surveys, but do so only after you have determined that their objectives are worthwhile and beneficial. (Read Chapter 27 for protective measures against telephone fraud.)

Unwanted Telemarketing Calls

Many of us are bothered by unsolicited telephone calls from telemarketing firms and promotional mailing material. While some people find this a satisfactory way of shopping, others find it highly intrusive. People who wish to have their names removed from telemarketing and promotional mailing lists should send their names to:

Telephone Preference Service
c/o Direct Marketing Association
P.O. Box 9014
Farmingdale, NY 11735-9014
(for telephone solicitations)

or

Mail Preference Service
c/o Direct Mail Association
P.O. Box 9008
Farmingdale, NY 11735-9008
(for mail solicitations)

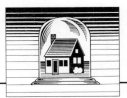

YOUR TELEPHONE: A CHECKLIST

1 Beware of people who contact you by telephone, seeking information about you, your associates, your friends, or your neighbors. Call back to verify that you are talking to a person with a legitimate reason for such information.

2 A caller who hangs up without speaking may be attempting to determine whether or not your home is occupied. Consider such a call a reminder to check your security measures.

---

3 Be wary of callers identifying themselves as law enforcement officers or government agency representatives. Check with the agency first, then return the call rather than cooperate unquestioningly.

4 Keep emergency numbers available at all telephones. If you are easily excited, have your address available as well.

5 Consider getting a telephone-answering service or a telephone-answering device.

6 Never record precise information on an answering device about when you will be away from home or when you anticipate returning, and never give such information to an answering service.

7 Cellular phones have a number of built-in protections; don't fail to utilize them.

8 Never cancel your telephone service when on vacation or on an extended trip.

9 Report repeated nuisance or obscene telephone calls to the telephone company. Do not talk to an obscene or nuisance caller.

5

YOUR DOG

Police Dog Patrol Officer Block today reported the fourth burglary suspect caught in a week by her dog, Max. Officer Block said she was cruising in the area of a burglary at the Southside Liquor Store, about 2:30 this morning, when she saw two suspects running, arms loaded with bottles. She said that when she shouted for them to halt, one stopped, but the other continued running. She sent Max after the man. Max quickly overtook the suspect and brought him down.

Along with the boulder rolled across the mouth of the cave, the dog was high on the list of people's first security measures. The dog became an ideal pet, subservient to its owner but inherently with an urge to protect its owner's property.

If you don't already have a dog, you should give serious consideration to owning one. Convicted rapists and burglars suggest that a dog is an effective deterrent to crime. Dogs have considerably better-developed senses of hearing and smell than do people, and dogs can detect the presence of would-be intruders well ahead of human beings. Dogs are especially helpful to senior citizens who may have hearing or vision impairments. By warning you of the presence of intruders, a dog allows you time to take protective or defensive measures—while at the same time letting the intruders know that their presence has been detected, which will usually be enough to persuade them to move rapidly elsewhere. Criminals know that most dogs rarely hesitate to attack, whatever the odds, in defense of their owner's and their own territory.

Never get a dog only as a security measure. You must be prepared to give your animal the care it requires, including regular walks, adequate food and water, veterinary needs, and, perhaps most importantly, lots of love. A "security" dog, like any other pet, deserves your affection and respect. Your special relationship will reenforce your dog's natural desire to protect you from harm. Even dogs who are usually absolute "sweeties" may turn into protective attack dogs when they sense danger.

YARD DOG OR HOUSE DOG?

The question of whether a yard dog or a house dog is better from a security standpoint is moot. A yard dog is likely to be a better deterrent, but a house dog is likely to be a better defense if an intruder actually gains entry to your home. Consider also that yard dogs are more susceptible to being poisoned or to being set loose by would-be intruders.

What breed of dog you select is largely a matter of personal preference. In general, for security purposes, a big dog is better than a small one. Rottweilers, doberman pinschers, and German shepherds are most frequently preferred. Pit bulls have also become popular due to their immense strength, despite some widely reported incidents involving them in unprovoked attacks. Perhaps even more important than size and strength, however, is the dog's "voice"—the louder and more persistent its bark, the better. A small dog that barks a lot, especially when people approach your residence, can be a great deterrent. Female dogs are reputed to be more territorially protective.

Like the wolves and foxes from which they descend, dogs are nocturnal animals by nature, but they often adapt to the rest patterns of their masters. Nevertheless, their innate sense of nighttime hunting makes them particularly valuable protectors while the rest of the household is asleep.

For this and other reasons, dogs have been used in police work for more than 40 years. In the 1960s, as the nation's "drug culture" developed, dogs were used to detect drugs. So effective are they for this purpose that the U.S. Customs Service considers them to be the very best means of locating drugs. "Dope dogs" are a select group, with senses of smell half again as acute as that of the typical pet dog. These dogs are recruited not from fancy kennels but from urban animal shelters because customs officials prefer the streetwise city dogs.

SPECIALLY TRAINED SECURITY DOGS

This discussion has purposely avoided referring to specially trained security or attack dogs, because, except in extraordinary circumstances, these animals are not suitable for the average household. They are expensive, they require periodic retraining, and they must have constant practice and handling in order to retain their specialized skills. And the owner/handler's training is as important as the dog's training. Also, these dogs must be kept away from welcomed visitors to your home.

A security-trained dog who gets loose and roams the neighborhood can become a menace, especially if it becomes confused in unfamiliar territory. Lack of regular training and handling can cause such a dog to lose, totally or partially, some of its "fail-safe" restraints. Thus, only people who are subject to extortion, kidnapping, or other very serious crimes, or those who keep extremely valuable items around the house, should consider keeping these animals. Even then, owners should be aware of the risks involved, including the very heavy liability they face if the dog attacks an innocent person. Trained guard dogs must never be treated as the family pet. Unfortunately, many dogs raised as attack dogs can "snap" at any time, even against their owners.

If you consider getting this type of animal, for whatever reason, be sure to investigate thoroughly before buying. The recent increase in crime—especially aggravated assaults, rapes, and robberies—has given rise to charlatans who pass off ill-trained or untrained animals as trained security dogs. Unscrupulous kennels may sell you an overtrained dog, aware that you lack the ability to handle the animal. When you try to return the dog, you may be offered an inferior animal as a substitute at the same price.

These specially trained dogs can be hazards, both to their owners and to other people, especially to young children. One 7-year-old girl was petting a big dog tied to a parking meter. The dog jumped up on her, licked her, and bit her cheek, breaking through the skin. Tell children not to touch dogs they don't know. Sadly, many hostile dogs have been abused by disreputable trainers or even their owners. Dogs can be trained in a humane manner, thereby developing a more calm and stable disposition. The personality of most dogs reflects their upbringing, so enlist the aid of a veterinarian, the head of the police dog squad, and other qualified individuals before deciding where to buy an attack dog.

Undoubtedly, a big dog is a formidable foe and can, under certain circumstances, be excellent security. It can, however, be a neighborhood menace if not properly cared for. Even if you must risk alienating a neighbor who owns a hostile dog, do not allow any dog to threaten you and your family. Humane shelters will pick up not only neglected pets but also nuisance animals, and may also subject the owners of offending animals to sanctions. Cayenne pepper spray should be used against attacking dogs. Mace may not be effective.

In recent years, there has been a significant increase in the number of gunshots police have fired at dogs. For example, in New York, 96 bullets were fired in 1992; this number rose to 155 in 1993. According to the annual Firearms Discharge Assault Report of the Police Department, 113 of these targets were pit bulls attacking people, including police officers. As a result, some officers are being taught how to deal with attacking dogs more effectively.

At the risk of offending the millions of cat owners in the world, we must point out that cats do not offer much security protection, both because of their small size and because they don't bark. The dog's primary weapon is its bark—and it's probably just as well if that bark is worse than the dog's bite.

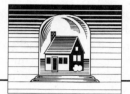

YOUR DOG: A CHECKLIST

1 A dog can be a very effective security weapon, and you should seriously consider owning one. Large dogs provide excellent security when carefully trained and monitored.

2 The dog's principal security use is to serve as a warning device and as a deterrent.

3 Don't buy an animal solely for protection. Be prepared to love and take good care of your dog.

4 Do not get a specially trained security dog, especially an attack dog, except in the most extraordinary circumstances. Always investigate very thoroughly before buying such a dog.

5 The quality of training of the owner/handler of a security dog is as important as training of the dog.

6 Specially trained security dogs must be regularly schooled to maintain their skills.

7 The best-trained dog will not be effective if its handler cannot interpret its actions.

8 Dogs that have been improperly trained may often be more vicious and uncontrollable than totally untrained dogs.

9 Call the humane shelter to pick up any neglected or hostile dog that has become a neighborhood menace.

10 If your neighbor owns a vicious dog, do not allow it to imperil you, your family, or your own dog. Cayenne pepper spray should be used against an attacking dog.

6

SERVICE EMPLOYEES AND INVITED STRANGERS

Detective Sergeant Ernest LaFay today announced the arrest of four persons, including a former newspaper carrier, in connection with a series of daylight burglaries in Newport.

Milk or grocery delivery persons, dry cleaners, baby-sitters, repair workers, pest control personnel, decorators, carpenters, remodelers, meter readers, mail carriers, and even part-time housekeepers or housecleaning services are typical types of service people who are permitted access into the home or apartment.

All these people who call on you have one thing in common: They have the opportunity to pick up a key ring or leave one of your doors or windows unlatched. Many of them may know where items of value are kept in your home. And at least one category, the domestic employee—whether full-time or part-time—may know practically as much about your household habits, idiosyncrasies, income, savings, and many other personal aspects of your family and your family's lives as you do yourself. And there is one more important thing that all these people have in common: the possibility of developing a real or imagined grievance against you, which gives them a rationale greater than greed for jeopardizing your person or property.

RISK PROTECTION

How do you protect yourself against such risks? Let's break the problem down into categories, dealing first with people who will be in your home regularly, sometimes when you are not there. This group includes domestic employees such as cleaning staff, housekeepers, children's nurses or governesses, chauffeurs, gardeners, and baby-sitters.

Check References

Remember this primary rule of thumb: Do not let anyone into your home unless you know who he or she is, and always check references completely. If a prospective employee can't provide references, then do not hire that person under any circumstances. If it is warranted, have a background investigation conducted by a reputable investigative agency, plus a retail credit check if this was not a part of the employment agency's investigation.

If you are still left with even the slightest doubts, it is worth going to the trouble of requesting a records check from the police departments of areas where the applicant has previously lived. You may encounter some difficulty here, because right-of-privacy legislation can prohibit police from releasing information. Do your best, however, because the truth of the matter is that an alarming number of applicants for domestic positions are actually subjects of outstanding arrest warrants!

Wherever possible, your investigations should extend also to immediate members of the applicant's family. A maid whose spouse has had a number of convictions for breaking and entering is hardly an ideal employment prospect.

Bonding

The bonding of domestic employees is not cheap, but the benefits will outweigh all other considerations if you are really concerned about security. In simple terms, a fidelity bond is a contract in which a bonding company will protect you against dishonest acts by an employee. A bond differs from insurance in that it covers acts that the principal (the person bonded) has control over, while insurance covers uncontrolled events such as accidents and natural disasters. Your insurance carrier can provide you with information on bonding employees. Bonding also gives you a valuable by-product, in that it requires yet another investigation into the background of the employee, one independent of your own.

Employment Agencies

One word of caution about domestic employment agencies: Some are very good, and some are not. If you deal with an agency, investigate it as thoroughly as you do the individual it recommends. A relative or friend who has had a satisfactory experience with an employment agency is certainly the first person you should contact when checking out an agency. Consult the Better Business Bureau for complaints. Check past editions of the Yellow Pages (at the phone company or at the library) to determine which firms have stood the test of time.

BABY-SITTERS

Typically, baby-sitters are either neighborhood teenagers or mature women, quite often widows whose own children have already been reared. Nice and trustworthy as they may seem to be, either type of baby-sitter can present genuine security problems.

You may have known the teenager down the street all your life, and you may be a friend of the family. What you may not know, however, is that the teenager's boyfriend or girlfriend happens to have a drug problem and that, despite any objections on your part, as soon as the children are asleep, this person may visit your house and remain until just before you are expected home.

A mature woman, on the other hand, might pose quite different problems. Just suppose, for instance, that she finds her Social Security benefits or the small pension she receives inadequate to meet her living requirements. It is common sense to recognize that she will have the same survival instincts that we all do.

Also, it should be pointed out that not only the young are given to abusive or violent behavior. Recently, a nanny admitted in court that she had fractured the skull of a 10-month-old boy in her care by hurling him forcefully to the floor because he had pulled her hair. The baby died as a result of the injury.

This discussion will not try to assess which type of baby-sitter offers the lesser risk because in the long run that always depends on the individuals involved. But there is no doubt at all that the best baby-sitter is the indulgent grandparent or the favorite aunt. Beyond that, in the selection of a baby-sitter, your best defenses are thorough investigations of whomever you choose and confidence in your own instincts. At least, always obtain and check references. Conduct an extensive interview, and be sure to ask your potential baby-sitter how she disciplines children and what she would do if the child gets angry.

A clear understanding about responsible behavior with the baby-sitting teenager's parents, and perhaps their occasional check on daughter or son, can be beneficial, as is a request to a neighbor to keep alert on your behalf. These simple steps might prevent someone from backing a truck up to your home and stripping the place.

Regardless of the age or experience of the baby-sitter, you must leave clear, complete, and written instructions, including such matters as where you will be and the phone number; the name and phone number of a neighbor to contact in an emergency; the name of your physician and directions to the nearest hospital emergency room; phone numbers of fire, police, and poison information hotlines and other emergency phone numbers; medications to be administered and instructions on administering them; locations of aspirin, bandages, or similar supplies; and names of callers who may stop by. Ask the sitter for help in compiling your list of information.

If you are a teenager who is asked to baby-sit, accept jobs only from people you know. If you do not know the caller or feel uneasy about a job offer, ask your parents to speak for you. They should ask the caller who recommended you, and then they should contact the reference. Ask a friend to accompany you to the interview. Once you report to the job, lock all doors and windows. Never open the door to anyone except in an emergency when you need assistance. If you go outdoors, neither you nor your charges should talk to strangers. Be alert for suspicious persons or happenings. If in doubt, call the police.

When the baby's parents return, report to them all suspicious or unusual occurrences or telephone calls. If you have made plans to have one of the children's parents take you home but that person appears intoxicated, insist on calling your own parents, or make other arrangements.

REPAIR WORKERS AND COMPARABLE VISITORS

Don't disclose information about your comings and goings to route people or service personnel who regularly visit your home. Irregular or semiregular visitors—such as in-home salespeople, movers, carpenters, painters, decorators, and repair workers—are an even greater security hazard. Almost without exception, they are in the employ of others who are providing services to you under some form of contractual arrangement, which means that you have virtually no control over the selection or investigation of the people who will actually be entering your home. The work they will be doing usually creates some confusion and probably a lot of inward and outward traffic of people and commodities. Unless you can be everywhere at once, with eyes in the back of your head, you are vulnerable.

Consequently, well before the first worker shows up, you need to do some careful planning. Move jewelry, furs, art objects, valuable documents, and any other portable valuable items to your safe-deposit box, security closet, or some other secure place, such as a neighbor's home. Do the same also with liquor, wine, medication, firearms, and small appliances.

Deal only with reputable companies or individuals that can furnish ample references, and check those references. Make certain that someone you trust is present to check up on things and generally to look after your interests. If you plan to look after activities yourself, do not try to do the job alone; it is more than a one-person task at best, and there is much truth in the old saying about safety in numbers. Consider engaging a security officer or patrol service in the evening hours, especially if there are ladders lying around the yard or windows that must remain open to allow paint to dry. If you move out until the work is completed, hire a house-sitter or security officer to protect your residence.

Once things get back to normal, make an inventory check. Someone may have had the opportunity to duplicate a key found in your home. Consider changing your lock cylinders—including window locks, if you neglected to remove the emergency keys from their places near those locks. Indeed, these are ideal occasions for making a thorough check of all your safety and security procedures.

WHEN AN EMPLOYEE LEAVES

When an unhappy domestic worker leaves your employ, you should take even more precautions. First, check your home inventory; second, change your locks. Even if you do not have a spare door key somewhere around the house—even if you've never left a key lying around the house that might have been duplicated—change the locks.

Although you may keep most of your valuables in a safe-deposit box or nonbank depository, over the years you will have developed special hiding places at home for valuable items you use on a day-to-day basis. Your 1-day-a-week housekeeper will have found these caches. An employee who hasn't stolen from you during his or her time of employment may not be so honorable on departure. Periodically changing your hiding places will minimize this risk. Don't simply trade places—change them. Move the good silver from the dining room to a spot in the kitchen or to an upstairs bedroom; transfer the diamond ring from the powder box in the bathroom to the toe of an evening shoe in the closet. And make absolutely certain that you change the entry on your home inventory list; otherwise, there's a chance that you yourself will forget the new location. Also, find a new and secure spot for the inventory list itself, unless you want to present a burglar with a nice, neat shopping list.

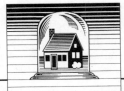

SERVICE EMPLOYEES AND INVITED STRANGERS: A CHECKLIST

1 Remember that domestic employees have a great opportunity to case your home and thus offer valuable information to burglars.

2 All domestic employees, including baby-sitters, should be thoroughly investigated before being hired.

3 If you use domestic employment agencies, investigate them thoroughly.

4 Consider fidelity bonding for domestic help and all employees, including baby-sitters.

5 Do not permit baby-sitters to entertain visitors in your home.

6 Ask a neighbor to keep an eye on your house when it is entrusted to a baby-sitter.

7 Leave clear and concise instructions for baby-sitters; be sure you include appropriate phone numbers.

8 Do not provide route people and service personnel with information about your comings and goings.

9 Workers in your home pose a particular hazard. Deal with only reputable contractors and service organizations. Arrange for someone to check on the progress and activities of the workers in your absence.

10 If workers will be in your home for more than a day, or if more than two or three will be present, remove or lock away all easily movable items of value.

11 If work done in your home seriously impairs your security measures, consider hiring a guard or a security patrol during the hours of darkness.

12 When an unhappy domestic worker leaves your employ, make an inventory check, change locks, and reevaluate all of your security and emergency measures.

13 When work in your home is completed make an inventory check, change locks, and reevaluate all of your security and emergency measures.

7

LIGHTING YOUR HOME

"My front porch light had burned out about a week ago," said John D. Sloan, of 1828 Iroquois, "and I never got around to changing the bulb. When I came in, that sucker was waiting for me, and he really rang my bell. I must have been out for 45 minutes. I guess I was lucky, though; I only had about 10 bucks on me, and a lot of that was in change. He took every nickel of that, though, he sure did."

The first chapter of this book conceded that, given enough time and determination, an intruder could break into your home regardless of any security measures you might take. By not lighting your house and ground adequately, you give would-be burglars one of their two basic requirements: time. Theoretically, at least, a burglar has all night to break into a dark house in a darkened setting.

The first principle of lighting for security is that it should be sufficient at all wall openings (doors, windows, exhaust ducts, crawl space and accesses, and so on) to deny an intruder the cover of darkness. The second principle is that all other hazardous areas should be adequately lighted.

BUILDING EXTERIORS

In a few instances, two lighting elements on opposite corners of a house can be sufficient to illuminate all openings in the walls of a structure. Generally, however, some degree of lighting on all four sides of a house is necessary to light it adequately. In all cases, lighting should be intense enough so that your neighbors can see someone trying to break in, but not so strong that it disturbs their peace and privacy.

If your street is adequately lighted, so much the better. If it is not, consider lighting your entranceway in such a manner that you can be certain not to encounter any unpleasant surprises when you arrive late at night. Lighting as much of the front part of your property as possible at night is an excellent idea, and you should encourage your neighbors to do the same. Report any burned-out streetlights, and ask your neighbors to do so, too.

Shadowed Areas

Trees, heavy shrubbery, bay windows, cul-de-sacs, enclosed porches, and many other natural or constructed features of a house create shadowed areas; these should be illuminated. In many cases, adequate light can be provided by burning a lamp inside the house close to a window. In most instances, however, one or more windows or doors will be so situated that they are effectively screened from the street and from neighbors as well, irrespective of interior lighting. These are principal areas of vulnerability that definitely should be specially illuminated.

Alleys

Alleys servicing the rears of homes are invariably hazardous areas. They are usually dark, not particularly well kept, and seldom traveled at night, and they often harbor large numbers of trash containers, which provide convenient cover for the would-be intruder. Typically, such alleys are separated from houses by solid fences to hide their unsightliness, but fences also prevent residents from seeing what's going on. Adequate illumination of the entire area between the fence and your house is thus essential for maximum security.

Consider the placement of trash receptacles, especially if you're a homeowner who has an adjacent alley. Trash receptacles offer excellent hiding places from which a would-be intruder—or even a passerby acting on impulse—could surprise and overpower you, especially at night. Few people bother to lock the house door behind them on short trips to the garbage can, so if you are at home alone, you might put off taking out the trash until morning or, alternatively, call a neighbor and ask that he or she watch you on your errand.

Adequate lighting is essential not only in alleys but also adjacent to the gates of all fences around your property.

How Much Lighting Is "Adequate"?

If you can see well enough to read a wristwatch by the light around any high-hazard exterior area, the lighting is satisfactory from a security view-

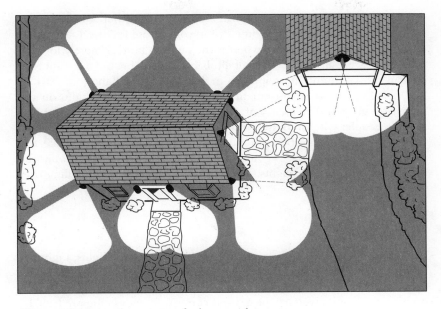

Figure 6. Lighting the exterior of a house and garage.

point. If you can't easily read your watch, or if you have any doubts, add more lighting.

INTERIOR LIGHTING

Many people are in the habit of leaving a light burning in the front part of the house or on a front porch at all times during hours of darkness. There are both advantages and disadvantages to such practices. Certainly the front door should always be adequately lighted. On the other hand, a porch light left burning periodically, rather than all the time, indicates to anyone who may have been casing your house that you are out but that you expect to return soon, an indication that might cause a potential intruder to pass you by. Probably the best technique is to alternate lighting sources so as to confuse the would-be intruder.

Front-room lights raise a similar problem. Without qualification, we recommend that lights be left on in apartments where only the light from under the door shows in the hallway. In a freestanding house, however, one look through the window into a well-lighted interior can show the potential intruder that the coast is clear. Drawing heavy drapes helps somewhat, and it is always a good idea to draw the drapes when you are home at night. The experienced burglar, however, knows that when the room is occupied, he can expect to see an occasional shadow when a person passes between the light source and the drape.

Here again, it is six of one and half a dozen of the other. A burglar who has singled you out and spent time casing your house isn't likely to be deterred by a living-room light, whereas the random burglar merely looking for someplace—any place—to hit probably would be. So once more, a general rule of thumb must apply: If in doubt, light the light.

During your normal movements about the house, turning lights on and off as you go, you give plenty of evidence that you are at home. Burglars are shy people, with absolutely no desire to meet their victims face-to-face. You can generally be assured that if you're at home and awake and moving around, a burglar is going to skip you. When you move about the house at night, use your lights for more reasons than to avoid falling over your furniture.

Night-Lights

When you retire for the evening, do not turn off all the lights: Lighting, remember, is a major enemy of the burglar. But do not leave the same lights on every night, because if your house is being cased, you do not want to give your adversary the aid and comfort of your being predictable.

When you have to get up during the night, make some noise and turn on some lights. It is unlikely that a burglar who isn't reasonably sure that you are asleep will attempt to enter your home while you are in it. Even then, you in turn can be assured that the intruder has a very quick escape route from any point in your home and will use it the moment it is apparent that you are awake and moving around. So give the burglar all the encouragement to leave that you can by lighting lights and banging doors.

An outdoor light switch in your bedroom, and perhaps in some other room in which you spend considerable time after dark, is a good idea, as is a second switch to turn on all (or many) inside lights simultaneously. A sneak thief cannot sneak very well when bathed in light.

When your house is unoccupied during the hours of darkness, always leave some lights on—not the same lights every time but enough to ensure your safety in returning. If you're going to be gone for several hours, consider using timers that will periodically turn lamps on and off. (Chapter 9, on home security while on vacation or an extended trip, discusses some of the dangers of timers. This discussion refers to your being absent for only a few hours.)

LIGHTING FOR PARKING AREAS

When you come home at night, be sure that you park in a well-lighted area. This is especially important if your routine is such that you return at the same time or at a predictable time each night. If the lights illuminating your garage or parking place aren't burning—and you know you left them on—keep right on going, and find a police officer or neighbor to accompany you back to your home.

Readily available are outdoor lights with sensors that turn on when motion is detected, for example, in the backyard, pool, or driveway. These lights can also be adjusted to function as ordinary lighting. Moreover, you can purchase outdoor lights that automatically turn on when it gets dark.

Good protective lighting is available today, and at such inexpensive prices that it is well within the reach of every homeowner. Timers capable of handling four or more separate instructions cost less than a pullover shirt. Several of these, distributed throughout the home, should be capable of completely confusing a nighttime prowler. Typically, these timers are equipped with a dry-cell battery, which will keep the memory intact in a power outage. The instructions of the timer will continue once line power is restored.

Another, even less-expensive, item—a rechargeable emergency light that can be plugged into home outlets—is readily available and can be a godsend when the lights go out. If there is an interruption in utility power, these lights will provide sufficient light so that you can leave the building safely. Most of these lights can be used as flashlights when the power in the home is normal.

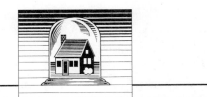

LIGHTING YOUR HOME: A CHECKLIST

1 Provide sufficient lighting at all doors, windows, and other openings in the walls of your house to deny the cover of darkness to an intruder. Lighting is generally sufficient when you can read a wristwatch by it at night.

2 Light the front of your property, and encourage your neighbors to do the same with theirs.

3 Report nonworking streetlights immediately.

4 Illuminate all shadowed areas caused by trees, shrubbery, or construction features of your house, being particularly attentive to any doors or windows that can't normally be seen from the street or from neighboring homes.

5 If an alley serves your home, illuminate the entire area between the alley and your house.

---

6   Provide additional illumination for areas where trash containers are located, especially if they are adjacent to an alley.

7   If you are home alone at night, wait until morning to take out your trash.

8   Light all gates in fences surrounding your property.

9   Turn lights on and off when you move from room to room at night.

10   Leave some lights burning all night.

11   Draw your drapes at night.

12   When you get up during the night, turn on lights and make a bit of noise.

13   Return to a well-lighted house.

14   Use timers to turn lights on and off during brief absences.

15   If you believe someone is in your house when you return, go to a neighbor and call the police. Do not attempt to be a hero.

16   Park only in well-lighted places.

17   Prepare emergency lights in the event of an interruption in utility power.

8
⟊

OUTSIDE SECURITY

High walls, dead-end driveways, and heavy shrubs or foliage provide protective cover for night intruders. Such barriers should be lighted, shrubs trimmed, and areas generally opened to maximum visibility consistent with usefulness and aesthetics.

—Katzenbach et al., The President's Commission on Law Enforcement and Administration of Justice. Task Force Report: The Police (Washington, D.C.: U.S. Government Printing Office, 1967)

BASIC PRECAUTIONS

Security is certainly not the prime consideration when you consider your home's outside appearance. A house surrounded by an 8- or 9-foot fence, brilliantly illuminated with high-intensity lighting, with closed-circuit television scanning a remote-controlled gate, and with large, vicious dogs roaming the yard, looks more like a prison or a top-secret missile base than a home. Nevertheless, there are various ways to maintain good security without sacrificing aesthetics.

From 1985 to 1994, the FBI reported more than 30 million burglaries. Burglars can be extremely dangerous: They are responsible for three-fifths of all rapes and robberies in the home and a third of all household assaults.

Perimeter Fencing

If you'd like a decorative hedge or a neat fence surrounding your property, by all means have it. In fact, a clear delineation of your property line will help you establish trespassing if a would-be intruder were apprehended on your property, even though the intruder was not attempting to break into your house. On the other hand, you don't want a hedge or fence so high that someone on the street couldn't see an intruder attempting to break in.

It is common sense to do whatever you reasonably can to limit access to your property. For one thing, an injury to a child taking a shortcut through your property could involve you in lengthy litigation. So install and use latches with self-closing mechanisms on all gates.

Whether gates should be locked or not is debatable. If the lot is very large, they probably should be, at least after dark. But locking the gates whenever you leave the house is a giveaway to criminals. One compromise might be always to lock all gates except those in front, which could be locked only at night.

Don't Flaunt Valuables

If you have valuable art objects, collections, antiques, or similar treasures, place them on inside walls where you and your guests can enjoy them, but don't put them near windows through which they can be removed. At night, draw your drapes.

Good Housekeeping Is Good Security

If you let the shrubs outside your house grow high enough to conceal an intruder, you are asking for trouble. The same holds for large accumulations of limbs cut from trees or other piles of rubbish. Another safety precaution is to knock down and flatten large shipping cartons or other containers before you put them out with the trash.

Many of us enjoy wood-burning fireplaces, but we should learn not to store firewood at a point adjoining the house where it might serve as a good hiding place for an intruder or as a stepladder up to our windows. It is far better to store the firewood some distance from the house.

An open garage and nobody home, and bicycles or expensive toys lying around the yard, are an open invitation to a thief, as well as an indication of a careless homeowner—the thief's delight. A lawn in need of cutting or a sidewalk of unshoveled snow is also likely to catch the burglar's eye, giving the impression that the house is unoccupied. The family may just be at work, but the daylight burglar won't care. An intruder is as capable of entering your home and removing its valuables while you are out for a few hours as when you are gone for a few days.

No Names, Please

A thief, walking randomly down the street, sees your liquor cabinet through an undraped window. The thief gets your name and address from your mailbox and calls from a nearby telephone. If you aren't home to answer your phone, you're likely to experience a break-in then and there. Your name on the mailbox is all too often an invitation to a confidence man or a would-be intruder to fabricate a plausible-enough story to persuade you to open your door, so don't give him or her ideas. Of course, if you're not home, the thief will just break in and probably start with the liquor cabinet.

Swimming Pools and Other Outside Structures

A swimming pool presents several security problems. A high, sturdy fence is essential to prevent children from falling into the pool. Even when it is fenced off, however, a pool poses some lighting problems. All-night lighting around the pool might discourage nocturnal swims by strangers, but it is also a signal to a thief that your home is one of some affluence, especially if your neighborhood has few pools.

Even if your house is secure, substantial pool lighting is advantageous. But a yard dog or a neighborhood patrol service, or even an organized Neighborhood Watch group, may be able to deter visitors enough to enable you to do without the use of attention-drawing lighting.

Toolsheds, storm cellars, greenhouses, and other appurtenant structures should be equipped with strong padlocks, as well as top-quality hasps and hinges. If the hinges are exposed, weld them in place, or insert set screws through the hinges at an unexposed point (see page 7 and Fig. 1). Garage doors should be locked; key-operated automatic devices are especially recommended.

Watching over the Neighborhood

One aspect of being a good neighbor is getting to know your neighbors—and knowing who isn't your neighbor. A stranger going through the neighborhood, perhaps driving around and around the block, could well be cause for concern. If in doubt, take down the car's license number. Remember, a community where neighbors care and watch out for each other is immeasurably more secure than one where neighbors hardly know or talk to one another (see Chapter 23).

Don't demand a reason for every stranger seen on your street, and don't phone the police every time you encounter an unfamiliar face. But do take notice, and make it clear that you are taking notice. The stranger who doesn't have a legitimate reason for being around will probably keep moving—away.

One group of thieves achieved spectacular success by staging fights in residential neighborhoods. Spectators would get so carried away by the mock hostility that they wouldn't notice one or two members of the crowd stealing away to nearby open-doored houses and coming back out, loot in hand, in less than 15 seconds.

Many thieves also market their hauls. Usually, the goods are not hawked in the same neighborhood that they came from originally. Rather, they are sold in poorer neighborhoods, where people tend to ignore their neighbors, particularly those who may be involved in criminal activities. Such buyers are also less likely to question the origins of bargain-priced goods.

If you notice strangers in your neighborhood taking undue interest in an automobile that you know to be the property of a neighbor, be on your guard. You may have to notify police. The same is true if you should hear breaking glass or an explosive noise that you can't account for.

And if you do have to phone police, take a few seconds to compose yourself and rehearse what you intend telling them. First of all, *where:* "1235 Fifth Street, between Maple and Sycamore." Second, you will want to tell the police *what:* "A burglary, I think. I heard breaking glass, and their alarm went off." *Who involved:* "Two men, Caucasian, both average height, both wearing jeans and T-shirts." *Autos:* "They left with two pillowcases full of lumpy objects, and drove away in a 1977 brown Pinto, Minnesota plates, first three numbers are 2G7." *Where headed:* "They turned south on Sycamore, probably heading for the interstate ramp."

In actual practice, it is unlikely you would be reciting a litany such as this one. The police officer answering your call will, perhaps, switch you to the proper bureau. In any event, the police will be interested in the types of information outlined (where, what, who involved, autos, and where headed), and they will probably ask questions, rather than allowing you to go through your spiel. But you should be prepared, just in case.

TRESPASSERS IN THE NEIGHBORHOOD

If you see a prowler or a trespasser in your yard or a neighbor's after dark, turn on lights—the more, the better. Should the prowler take off running, activate the alarm if you have one, and phone the police. Don't attempt to chase down a fleeing suspect even if you do have all the help you need. It is better—and safer—to try to keep a suspect in sight than to try to apprehend him or her. Leave the chasing to the law enforcement officers, who know what they are doing.

SECURITY PATROL SERVICES

This book periodically refers to neighborhood security patrol services. A good one is a valuable addition to your security arsenal, but it is only a supplement. Capable burglars will see to it that they are working behind the patrol officer. Also, your dog is as likely to sound its canine alarm at the patrol officer's approach as at the burglar's. Patrol officers should vary the starting point of their route and occasionally double back, so that the times of their appearances at your place aren't predictable.

The costs of patrol services vary according to frequency and quality of work. But all things considered, a good security patrol is a worthwhile investment. Be sure to investigate the company thoroughly, check references, and determine if the patrol officers are licensed or commissioned by the police.

It's not neighborly to piggyback or free-ride on a neighbor who has a security patrol service, although a patrol officer showing up next door would no doubt help deter a burglar from your place as well. Why not pool your resources and double the exposure of officers around your property and your neighbor's?

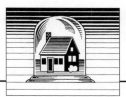

OUTSIDE SECURITY:
A CHECKLIST

1 Delineate your property line with fences or hedges.

2 Keep hedges or fences low enough for a passerby to see an intruder attempting a break-in.

3 Use latches on all gates.

4 Don't display valuable possessions so that they can be seen by passersby.

5 Don't display valuable possessions where they might be accessible to and removed through a window, without a burglar's even being inside.

6 Keep garage doors locked; key-operated automatic devices are especially recommended.

7 Remove your name from the mailbox.

8 Secure toolsheds, greenhouses, and other appurtenant structures adequately.

9 Protect swimming pools from unauthorized use.

10 Don't call unnecessary attention to a pool, especially if it is the only one in the neighborhood.

11 Keep your grounds in good order: lawn mowed, walks shoveled clear of snow, and so on.

12 Don't store firewood against the house.

13 Be aware of—but not foolhardy with—strangers in the neighborhood.

14 While you are out, never leave your door unlocked even for a few seconds. Criminals can loot your home in less than 15 seconds.

15 Do not attempt to apprehend a trespasser or prowler.

16 Augment other security measures with a neighborhood security patrol if it is called for. Vary security patrol check times, and investigate security patrol services thoroughly.

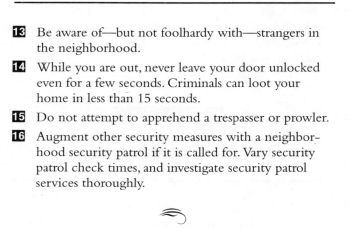

9

HOME SECURITY
DURING VACATIONS

Your home is most vulnerable to an intruder when there is no one home, and a family vacation increases that risk. Don't make it obvious that you are away.

What About Deliveries?

Most advisory services, such as travel agencies, tell us that if we will be away from home for more than a day or two, we should be sure to cancel the newspaper and milk deliveries and even ask the post office to hold mail, because accumulations of all these items are dead giveaways to potential intruders. Is this good advice? Well, if you follow it, you will have told five or six people your plans, including how long you will be away, and they are all likely to be people who know considerably more about you than you know about them. It is thus far better to let the deliveries continue, and arrange with a friend or neighbor to have them brought into the home. If there is no one of whom you can ask this favor, then definitely cancel all deliveries, notifying the delivery people and the offices supervising them.

Don't Kennel Your Dog

When you are away from home on vacation, try, if at all possible, to have a friend, neighbor, or a professional dog walker feed your dog (and walk it, if it is a house dog) rather than lodge it at a boarding kennel. The dog can be extremely valuable as a deterrent around an otherwise unoccupied house.

Avoid the Second-Car Giveaway

If you're a one-car family and you take that car with you on vacation, there's really not much you can do to prevent someone from noticing that there is no car in the driveway. You're in better shape, of course, if you customarily keep your car in a closed garage. If you are a two-car family on a motor vacation, your second car, parked in the same spot day after day, gives further evidence that you are away from home. Ask your neighbor to move it every day or so.

Avoid Pretrip Publicity

If you are prominent in your community and news of your trip might be included in the social or business sections of your newspaper, make certain these items aren't run in the paper until after you return. If for some reason you can't delay this news, arrange for the protection of your home. If you can't find a trustworthy house-sitter, arrange for an on-premises security officer.

Professional thieves and burglars read newspapers, and if they know you will be in New York for the opening of your new play or in San Francisco for your daughter's wedding, they may come calling. Even if you avoid publicity, professional thieves sometimes befriend deliverymen—who may even be paid accomplices—for information, so be prepared to outmaneuver a thorough and professional adversary.

Notify the Police

Notify the police that you will be away, so that they can provide some additional attention to your property while you are gone. If you've arranged for a house-sitter or the assistance of that friendly neighbor, give his or her name to the police to avoid any unpleasant incident. Also provide the police with the names of any other friends or relatives who have keys to your house.

Don't Pack the Car the Night Before

Don't try to get a few minutes' early start on your vacation by packing the car the night before. It's not worth it when you consider the risk of awakening to find everything, car included, gone from your driveway or garage. And even if all is intact, there may be a burglar watching you pull away, waiting to get at all the goodies you didn't take along. Just before departure, check to see that all doors and windows are locked and that you have taken all the necessary keys.

OTHER GOING-AWAY MEASURES

Use your safe-deposit box or nonbank depository for valuables, or entrust them with a friend or relative while you're away. Pay your bills before you leave, or else leave checks with a friend or a neighbor who can pick up your mail and pay the bills soon after they arrive.

If your home is equipped with an intrusion/fire alarm, have it checked before you leave, remembering that there is no need to tell the service representative why you want it checked. Check auxiliary power supplies, too.

Always leave an itinerary with a friend, neighbor, or relative who can reach you in the event of an emergency.

A few toys or garden tools in the yard will make it appear that the house is occupied. However, in order to perpetuate your sham, it will be necessary that your bait be changed and rearranged. Otherwise an experienced thief will see through your ruse.

If you normally leave your drapes open, don't draw them just because you are going to be away. If, on the other hand, you habitually open them during the day and close them at night, ask your neighbor to do the same for you. If you can't arrange this, leave at least the ground-floor drapes open the entire time. You won't fool the experienced burglar, but perhaps you can introduce some element of the unknown.

ON THE ROAD

Finally, while you're en route, your out-of-state or rental-car license plates distinguish you as a "mark." A string of robbery-murders of tourists in Florida a few years ago attests to this. A thief can capitalize on the fact that you're an out-of-towner through a number of methods designed to separate you from your assets. Thieves derive comfort from the belief that, even if caught red-handed, they would probably go free because you will be reluctant to return to testify against them. You should park in a manner that shields your license plate from prying eyes, by parking between two cars. Be especially careful if you are driving a car with special plates or with a decal identifying the vehicle as a rental. This only advertises your vulnerability. Recently, several incidents of rental carjacking have occurred across the country. (Chapter 12 on Vehicle Security and Carjacking provides useful tips on how to avoid this horrendous crime.)

WHILE YOU ARE AWAY

Almost every recommendation made so far in this chapter involves the assistance of a friend or neighbor as the best means for protecting your property while you're away. Unfortunately, in many cases, this becomes just too much of an imposition. Here are some other ways to make your house look lived in.

Lights and Timers

If the lights go on and off at precisely the same time every night, the experienced burglar will notice it. There are inexpensive timers that vary on-off times continuously, including a timer that activates a lamp (or any electric appliance) each time the compression motor of a refrigerator activates.

If a timer isn't practical, at least leave some lights on when you go. They will probably go unnoticed during the daytime, but the total absence of lights would certainly be apparent at night. Turn down the volume control of your telephone so a passerby won't hear the continued ringing of an unanswered telephone. (An answering machine is recommended; see page 43.)

Don't shut down air-conditioning or heating equipment. A still compressor on a muggy night is proof to a skilled thief that the house is unoccupied. Since most vacations take place in the summer, air conditioners also should have thermostats or timers. To conserve energy, you can cut back on the cooling level, but at least arrange to have the fan motor running. An added benefit is that air conditioning removes the humidity from the house, helping to preserve your furniture, floors, books, drapes, and whatever else could be warped or damaged by dampness while you are away. Make certain that timers and related wiring are of sufficient capacity and voltage to handle the power requirements of your air-conditioning equipment.

Lawn Care and Snow Removal

Keeping your lawn cut or the snow shoveled is essential when you're away from home for a long period and you want everything to appear normal. However, unless you usually use a professional cutting service, entrust vacation mowing or snow shoveling to a neighborhood child. Pristine snow is a certain giveaway that you're not at home, so, at the very least, have someone put footprints in the snow on your walk and driveway.

Locking Gates and Trash Removal

While a locked gate will deter a burglar, one locked at noon will assure him or her you're not at home. Ideally, your neighbor—who by this time is surely overworked on your behalf—would lock your gate in the evening and unlock it in the morning while you're away. If this can't be arranged, you probably will just have to play the odds and lock the gate, hoping a burglar will think twice about lifting the loot over the fence, particularly in broad daylight.

It is rare for an occupied home to have no trash for 2 weeks. Ask your neighbor to put out some trash on pickup days. If your pickup is not regularly scheduled, try to arrange for a neighbor to share his or her garbage service with you.

House-Sitters

Consider engaging a house-sitter who will actually live in your house while you're away. A friend, relative, or domestic employee in whom you have complete trust is ideal. A professional or semiprofessional house-sitter can often be engaged through college placement offices. Mature students or even faculty members often make themselves available for house-sitting duties. Other trustworthy house-sitters include people with whom you work, members of your church or synagogue, or people referred by neighbors.

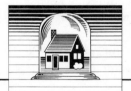

HOME SECURITY DURING VACATION: A CHECKLIST

1 Arrange for a friend or neighbor to bring in the mail, milk, and newspapers. If this isn't possible, cancel deliveries.

2 Arrange to have your dog fed, watered, and walked at home rather than kept at a kennel.

3 If you have a second car, arrange to have it moved occasionally in your absence.

4 Avoid publicity about your impending trip.

5 Leave an itinerary with someone, so that you can be notified in case of emergency.

6 Consider use of a neighborhood patrol service during your absence.

7 Notify police of your absence, providing them with the names of house-sitters or neighbors who will be assisting you and names of others who have keys to your house.

8 Don't pack your car the night before departure; load it quickly in the morning.

9 As a last effort before departure, check to see that all doors and windows are locked and that you have taken all necessary keys.

10 Arrange for secure storage outside your home of furs, jewelry, and other valuables while you are away.

11 Pay bills that come due in your absence, and arrange for the payment of others that may arrive while you're away.

12 Have your alarm system checked before you leave.

13 Leave shades and drapes in the positions they would normally be in if you were home, arranging, if possible, to have them raised and lowered or opened and closed routinely.

14 Use variable on–off timers to turn lamps on at night.

15 Set thermostats, or utilize timers, for air conditioner operation that fits weather conditions.

16 Turn down the volume control on telephones. Install an answering machine, preferably one that allows you to retrieve messages from wherever your happen to be.

17 Arrange to have your lawn cut or snow shoveled as required during your absence.

18 Have fence gates locked, preferably at nighttime only, during your absence.

19 Arrange for garbage and trash to be put out for pickup as usual.

20 If you don't have a generous neighbor, use a qualified and trustworthy house-sitter in your absence.

21 Toys or tools in the yard will suggest that the house is occupied, provided that they are replaced and relocated periodically.

10

SPECIAL TIPS
FOR APARTMENT
DWELLERS

A New York City Housing Authority police officer shot and slightly wounded a 27-year-old man he found lurking on the roof of a housing project. The wounded man, identified as Leonard Brown, was said to have had a knife in his pocket. Brown had advanced toward the patrol officer with his hand in his pocket when he was ordered to halt.

While many of the home security suggestions made so far apply to all dwelling units, some pertain solely to a freestanding house. Other special considerations are more or less the exclusive concern of the occupant of an apartment, co-op, or condominium.

An apartment's limited access may make it more secure, but it also creates some specific problems. For example, the front door has to be better secured, since it is unlikely an intruder will be a passerby. On the other hand, assistance in an apartment can be only a few steps away, rather than many yards.

SECURITY FEATURES TO LOOK FOR

The following is a shopping list of features you will want to consider before renting an apartment, or a list of services you may want to pressure your landlord into providing. An apartment building with maximum security should have these features:

❖ Around-the-clock doorman or security officer who announces all guests and requires proper identification of all visitors and callers.
❖ Fire stairs equipped with one-way doors, which should operate only from inside the fire stairwell on the ground floor and roof and only from outside the fire stairwell on all other floors.
❖ Garages equipped with self-closing outside doors or a guard, or both.

Few apartment complexes have the resources to supply maximum security. But even a small, limited-budget building can follow good security measures, which include the following:

❖ Door-opening systems, equipped with an intercom system or closed-circuit television, with every tenant trained to use the system properly.
❖ Self-service elevators with small mirrors permitting a view of the entire interior of the car before boarding.
❖ Entrance into attached or basement garages controlled by key or magnetic card, and automatic closure of these doors.
❖ Fire stairs equipped with one-way doors.
❖ Adequate lighting throughout the common spaces of the building.
❖ Light fixtures located or protected so that an intruder can't get at them.
❖ Roof doors operable only from the inside.
❖ Well-lighted alcoves or other blind spots in corridors, with mirrors to prevent them from being used as hiding places.

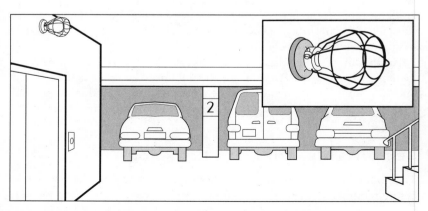

Figure 7. Lighting fixtures placed where they can't be broken.

WHEN YOU MOVE IN

There is one fact that should motivate you to assess the effectiveness of your locking devices. In apartment buildings, most crimes result from the failure to use existing locks, or from their inadequacy or vulnerability. For your own peace of mind, change the locks when you move into an apartment.

Security of Keys

Your building superintendent may insist on having a key to your apartment, in which case point out that a burglar breaking into the super's apartment would then have access to every apartment in the building. If fire codes require the superintendent to have a key, put yours in a sealed envelope with your name signed across the flap. It would be much better, if possible, to leave the key with a friend, than to notify the superintendent where the key can be found. Don't hide your key near the door. Once your keys are protected, your apartment is probably more secure than the typical freestanding house. But there are other things you should do to increase your protection.

You should consider adding a lock of your own to your apartment door. A deadbolt is the lock of choice. You would be protected even if a passkey fell into the wrong hands. It is not unprecedented for building superintendents to misuse keys entrusted to them. Your landlord may object if he or she knows of your protective addition, but after all, your possessions, even your life, might be on the line. The reverse side of this should be considered: In the event of an emergency, police or fire personnel would be unable to protect your belongings without forcibly opening your apartment.

Doors and Windows

Review Chapter 1 for basic precautions concerning doors and windows. Be sure to install outside doors with chain locks and peepholes. Outside doors should be locked at all times, whether you're in or not.

Doorplates and mailboxes should not indicate the gender of the occupant. "M. Jones," for example, is much preferable to "Ms. Mary Jones."

Don't leave notes on doors indicating when you'll return to your apartment or that you'll be returning alone. "We will return soon" is much better than "I will be back at 6:00 p.m."

In an apartment, you almost certainly will have fewer windows to protect than in a house, and it is quite likely that only one or two walls will have windows at all. Some of these windows, though, may open onto fire escapes, which offer access from your apartment to the ground and vice versa. These windows must be protected by lockable metal coverings to keep intruders out. In addition, the keys to these grills must be kept close at hand to enable you to get out if there is a fire. A word of caution: Don't position emergency keys so close that they could be reached from outside the building. The ideal key storage location is someplace where it is out of sight of anyone at the fire escape.

If a fire escape adjoins one of your windows, a folding screen on the inside will prevent entry through the window but will allow exit from it. If this violates building codes, shatterproof glass serves the same purpose.

OTHER BUILDING SECURITY PRACTICES

The most important security measure for any apartment is a sense of neighborliness and cooperation on the part of all the tenants—a keen desire to make the communal home more secure. Know your neighbors, and involve yourself with them in making your building a safe place to be (see page 83). Report anything not operating properly: door closers, burned-out lights, inoperative locks, rotted fire hoses, and so forth. Report any unusual or apparently illegal incidents to the landlord or superintendent and to the police. Don't open the exterior door to anyone unless you either recognize the person or can positively determine the purpose of the visit.

Apartment lobbies can be scenes of serious crime. Picture this scenario: A wrongdoer of some sort rings for admittance. No answer. He or she makes a mental note that the apartment is unoccupied and moves to the next buzzer. Again, no answer, again a mental note. The next buzzer is answered, "What do you want?" A mumbled reply about "special delivery" or "package from the local department store" will usually persuade someone in the building to open the door. Once inside, the wrongdoer can loot relatively safe from detection, especially after having discovered which apartments are unoccupied.

Draperies on lobby windows denote, to many, an air of privacy. But privacy in the lobby is not to be desired. The sight of a doorman, on the other hand, will usually send the criminal elsewhere. Neat and orderly premises speak of residents who care about their surroundings and probably have taken steps to ensure the sanctity of their homes. Draperies also can be a more menacing accessory. An intruder who in some manner gains entry into the building needs only to hide behind the protective drapes to prey on residents who enter.

Intruders often position themselves near the mailboxes. Practically every tenant will visit the mailboxes daily, and will be much more attentive to the mail than to almost anything else. It's likely that the tenant will have left the apartment door open for the short trip downstairs, providing the thief yet another opportunity to do wrong. Traffic around the mailboxes may be especially heavy on days when Social Security or public-assistance checks are delivered. Any person who receives checks in the mail on a regular and predictable basis must—*must*—change to direct bank-deposit services for protection against thieves.

The mailbox area should be well lit. If a stranger is loitering near the mailbox area, wait until he or she leaves, or return later. A surveillance camera provides extra protection. If your building is not equipped with one, suggest this idea to the building manager, and encourage your neighbors to do the same.

In consideration for taking your rent (or your condo maintenance) payments, your landlord (or management) owes you adequate lighting inside and out. One authority lists the three most desirable security features in an apartment to be a 24-hour doorman, closed-circuit TV, and an abundance of lighting, both inside and outside the building. As described earlier, adequate lighting is that sufficient to read a wristwatch by.

A landlord or building manager may ignore, delay, or otherwise attempt to dissuade you from receiving your due. If you aren't able to get satisfaction from those managing your place, perhaps the local building inspector will prove helpful.

Elevators and Other Special Hazards

Elevators can be a potential hazard to the apartment dweller. Don't ride in an elevator with a stranger. Wait for someone you recognize to accompany you. Also, stand near the control panel. If a suspicious-looking character gets on an elevator, get off at the next floor after pushing as many other buttons as you are able so that the door will open on many floors. Do not press your floor number until all strangers have pressed theirs. A criminal will be most interested in your destination and make it appear that he or she resides on the same floor. Always try to position yourself with your back against one of the elevator walls so that you minimize your exposure to muggers and pickpockets.

When you arrive at your destination floor, check the corridor before you leave the elevator. If there is a stranger in the hallway, don't leave the elevator. As a general rule, the basement is the most hazardous location in an apartment building, whether or not there is provision for parking in the basement. Basement parking may increase the possibility of someone's entering the building by driving in along with a car that arrives legitimately to park. Once there, the intruder is free to enter every floor in the building (unless, of course, tenants have keys to the elevator on the basement level or there is a TV camera observing the elevator vestibule and monitored by the doorman in the lobby.

Basement laundry rooms are, perhaps, equally hazardous, in large measure because they are used less frequently than most other areas of the building. For this reason, they are favorite areas for attacks. To the criminal, especially the sexual offender, the lack of activity is beneficial. He can bide his time, awaiting the right moment and the right victim, and once he zeros in, he will likely have the time he needs.

Most of us, at one time or another, have boarded an elevator headed in the direction, up or down, opposite to that desired. Usually, this minor inconvenience costs us nothing but a few minutes. If, however, you find yourself on an elevator descending to the basement, perhaps at the behest of a criminal looking for a victim, you may be facing a serious problem. To avoid this danger, punch the "door open" button on the elevator, then get off before the door closes. You then have only to stand and wait to board an elevator that you know is headed in your direction.

Indoor emergency exits (fire stairs) should generally not be used except for emergencies. Realistically, few people will wait 5 minutes for an elevator just to visit a friend two floors below. But remember, these stairs are built to withstand a fire, and the fireproof doors deaden all sounds on the stairs. Your cries for help may be inaudible outside the staircase.

Basement laundries and apartment vestibules or mailbox areas are also vulnerable locations for assault. Remember, there is some safety in numbers. It is far safer, and much more sociable as well, to go to the mailbox area or the basement laundry room with a neighbor. If you must go alone, keep moving if you are at all uncomfortable with what you see.

Health Clubs and Solariums

To attract the sociable and exercise-conscious yuppies—as well as the down-to-earth, expanding middle class—more and more new apartment houses, especially co-ops and condominiums, include health clubs and solariums. Many of these feature indoor or outdoor swimming pools, saunas, steam rooms, heated whirlpools, restrooms, showers, lockers, rooms for physical fitness, expensive state-of-the-art exercise equipment, areas for aerobics, and even a play area stocked with toys for children. The solarium, often situated on or near the roof, may be equipped with expensive chaises, chairs, and tables. All this paraphernalia may provide easy relaxation for hardworking residents, but it also presents a security nightmare.

For protection in these areas, the first rule is to follow all basic security principles described in this chapter. For example, be sure that all doors to all rooms, storerooms, and utility closets are locked when not in use—with a deadbolt, of course. Rooms with expensive equipment should also be alarmed to signal the doorman or the concierge of unauthorized entry. For the club and swimming pool, the best security consists of an attendant and a lifeguard during scheduled hours. Closed-circuit television should monitor strategic points in each room, plus all hallways and corridors. In all rooms, panic buttons should be available to patrons who are threatened by any intruder who gets by the health club attendant. The solarium should be equally equipped, especially if it is situated far from the rest of the club. Take nothing of value with you to the health club; leave valuables securely locked in your apartment. While you exercise or swim, your purse, pocketbook, or wallet, and all other personal belongings should be secured in a locker.

The children's play area should be kept neat and orderly, with all toys secured in a locked closet when not in use. Do not enter the playroom if you see a suspicious person. Report them to the concierge or doorman, and have him check their identity and why he or she is in the playroom.

Terraces

A terrace, often serving as a surrogate suburban patio in the middle of the city, may offer relaxation and privacy. But it may also attract burglars, who perceive it as a convenient access to your apartment. Even a terrace far from the street on a high floor is accessible to burglars, who may reach it from an unsecured hallway door leading to the outside, or through a neighbor's apartment that was forcibly entered. Not finding anything of value in your neighbor's apartment, the disappointed burglar designates your apartment as the next primary target.

The most important preventive measure is for all windows and doors leading to your terrace to be adequately secured. For sliding glass doors, probably the most vulnerable doors in your apartment, follow the procedures provided in Chapter 1. These include installing a shatterproof glass or other impact-resistant glazing, inserting a broom handle (cut to size) in the track on which the doors slide, and attaching locks with vertical barrel bolts to fit into holes in the top and bottom tracks.

TENANTS' ASSOCIATIONS

The organizations known as tenants' associations assume all levels of formality. A simple arrangement may be nothing more than asking your neighbor to look after your interests if you plan to be away for a few days. Or one tenant may tell another with whom she is going to dinner that evening, just in case. Some neighbors install buzzers between their apartments for quick response in the event of an emergency.

A slightly larger, but equally informal, association would involve your taking the time to meet every person on your floor (or some part of a large floor). In this way, you would be able to identify someone who is not a resident of your floor and thus be warned of a potential danger. If your suspicions persist, call the manager, or else wait a few minutes before leaving the building. This little warning could possibly save you from injury, or worse.

A group of tenants could check with local police to determine the availability of a crime prevention squad. These units have proved highly successful in mobilizing a group of individuals into a cohesive protective element, merely by teaching the group members to better protect themselves. Sometimes tenant groups will band together and form patrols to provide security for the environs. Generally, these units operate only in larger housing complexes, often in problem housing developments.

RENTING OUT YOUR APARTMENT

Mainly for your own protection, all security equipment such as locks, bolts, and alarms should be in working condition, but if you rent your condo or co-op, you must also be concerned for your tenant's safety. In California, a female condo renter was abducted from the condo's parking lot, robbed, and assaulted. Citing fraud and negligence, she sued the condo association for her injuries. She argued that the owner of the apartment had assured her that the private parking lot was protected by a modern key-entry security gate. Yet the criminals who attacked her were able to enter through a defective gate. The court found in her favor because condominium owners are required to take reasonable measures to safeguard tenants, and defective gates abrogated this responsibility. In many states besides California, condo owners are liable for crimes against their tenants if the obligation of protecting them is assumed but not fulfilled.

DIFFERENT LEVELS OF SECURITY

Before you accept varying levels of security at different times of the day, consider possible consequences. If your tenants' association wants to hire a second doorman for only part of the day, when expectations of danger are greatest, check your local laws. A court, questioning why certain shifts are covered by two persons and others by only one, might attribute negligence to the building management during the other hours. For help in determining high-risk hours, call in a crime expert or even your local police department. The police are often willing to provide this expert advice without charge. Taking such reasonable measures could constitute a strong defense in a lawsuit.

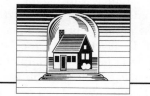

SPECIAL TIPS FOR APARTMENT DWELLERS: A CHECKLIST

1 When moving into an apartment, look for these security-oriented features:

    a. Doormen or security officers who screen visitors
    b. Properly secured interior fire stairwells
    c. Properly secured garages

d. Remotely operated door-opening systems, with intercom systems or closed-circuit television

e. Interior-view mirrors in self-service elevators

f. Adequate lighting

g. Protection against alcoves or other blind spots that may be used as hiding places

h. Roof doors operable only from inside

2 On moving into an apartment, change locks.

3 Protect spare or emergency keys.

4 Equip outside doors with chain locks and peepholes.

5 Do not reveal gender on mailbox or doorplates.

6 Don't leave notes on doors indicating anticipated time of return or using "I" instead of "we."

7 Protect windows, remembering that those adjoining fire escapes should prevent illegal entry but not prohibit emergency exit.

8 Know your neighbors, and work together for your mutual security.

9 Report anything peculiar: faulty equipment or an unusual incident.

10 The three most essential security features for an apartment are a 24-hour doorman, closed-circuit TV, and sufficient lighting inside and outside the structure.

11 If your building has a health club, follow all the basic security measures described for securing your apartment.

12 Do not take anything of value to the health club, and secure all personal belongings in a locker.

13 Make sure to secure all windows and the door leading to your terrace.

14 When renting your condo or co-op, be certain that all security equipment is in working order.

11

≈

SPECIAL OCCASIONS MEAN SPECIAL RISKS

"I'm still in shock," declared Lucia Whittlesby yesterday evening. She had just given a bridal shower for a neighbor, and the guests had recently left. "The silver tea set was missing, and I don't even know what else is gone. I can't imagine who would do such a thing—and to think that I invited them here!"

The special occasions in our lives can also be the source of some rather special security problems. Any occasions that are covered in the local newspapers present special problems, as do any social get-togethers. Holidays are also a time of increased risk of crime.

HOLIDAYS

Holidays are usually a time of celebration, but danger and crime can quickly bring all the fun to an end. Around Christmas time, burglaries and thefts tend to increase. Cash and gifts are more abundant than at any other time throughout the year. Try to shop for gifts early, and don't carry too many packages. An overburdened shopper is an easy mark for a crook. Be sure to keep packages in your car out of sight, placing them in your trunk or under a car seat. Many people have been unpleasantly surprised to find a broken car window or door lock after only leaving "for a minute." (For more tips on security while shopping, see Chapter 14.)

Scams are also rampant during the holiday season. While shopping, don't believe anyone who approaches you with an unbelievable price. Crooks have even posed as sales clerks. Never buy expensive items on the street. The goods are likely to be either stolen or a rip-off. For similar reasons, never buy tickets for holiday shows (or any other show) from scalpers.

Always check if a charity you are interested in is legitimate. Many fraudulent Santas will collect your donations for themselves. If you receive a telephone solicitation, ask the caller to mail you materials about the organization. *Never,* ever, give out your credit card number over the telephone unless you are absolutely positive the person on the other end is legitimate. Sending a check or money order is a lot safer. (Also, see Chapter 27, for additional tips on protection from scams.)

New Year's Eve presents yet another opportunity for thieves and burglars, who don't take holidays off. If you leave home, make sure your residence appears occupied; leave a light and/or a radio or television turned on.

Safety is also an important consideration. Do not fire handguns, and report anyone you see doing so to the police. Never drive while intoxicated (DWI). Have a designated driver, take a cab or car service, or use public transportation. Over one-fifth of drivers are under the influence of drugs and/or alcohol on New Year's Eve, and over half of these are dangerously intoxicated. If you spot an intoxicated driver on the road, call the police immediately and provide a description.

DWI and loud, explosive fireworks are also risks on the Fourth of July. Fireworks sold on the street are illegal and dangerous. They are responsible for countless deaths, injuries, and fires.

Extra caution should also be exercised on Halloween. Be sure to secure your residence and your car. If you have a garage, by all means use it. In addition, always check to see who's calling at your door before you open it. Don't just assume that the caller is another trick-or-treater. (For additional information on how to protect your children on Halloween, see Chapter 20.)

FUNERALS AND WEDDINGS

A death in the family typically is followed by an obituary in the press, listing the time and place of the funeral services. It is expected that every member of the deceased's household will attend these services, and burglars know it. Arrange for a friend or neighbor, or a contract security officer, to house-sit while you are attending funeral services.

A wedding is one of the most important days of one's life and is also a momentous occasion for the parents of the new couple. Make certain that this special day is not spoiled by a burglary during the ceremony. A wedding notice in the newspaper is not the criminal's only tip-off. A burglar may have been alerted by banns of marriage being published at your church, or by an employee of your caterer, florist, jeweler, or someone else providing services or goods who happens to double as a "bird dog" for a burglary ring. Even a passerby seeing a man leaving the house in a morning coat with daughter in a bridal gown can inform a burglar of the valuable wedding gifts on display inside. Protect them with a house-sitter or guard.

Businesses supplying goods and services during these occasions may hike prices to make a profit from your overstimulated emotional state. Always consult a trusted friend or relative before making any commitment.

EVERYDAY SPECIAL OCCASIONS

Occasions don't need to be too special to offer criminals the chance to rifle your house. If you are seen leaving the house with your golf clubs, a burglar knows he will have hours to work undisturbed. The burglar has only to to ring the bell to determine if anyone is at home.

While it isn't practical to get a house-sitter every time you play nine holes of golf, you can arrange with a neighbor to keep an eye out for any unusual occurrences. From the vantage point of security, a nosy neighbor is a jewel. Of course, you should be ready to reciprocate when your neighbor leaves to play golf.

Having a Party

If you're having a big party at home, take some precautions, especially if you don't know all your guests well. There is nothing wrong with the host's and hostess's enjoying their own party as much as the guests do, but your party planning should include some commonsense security planning. Resist the impulse to show off your collection of gold coins. Securely put away any important papers or documents, especially those containing financial information. Check out any help you hire, and take the precautions of safeguarding small, easily portable valuables. You might count the silver, too, after everyone has left.

Hosting a party with a guest list that includes people not known to you, such as an author's reception or a political fund raiser, can be a great deal more expensive than you anticipated at the outset. Thieves attending these gatherings are certain to be on the lookout to steal small, easily concealed items. They may also rifle guests' handbags. As Chapter 14 urges with regard to shopping, you should be in tactile contact with your handbag at all times, unless it is protected in locked storage. Furs, too, are highly sought-after items and can be removed by concealing them under other garments.

Protecting your guests' property requires a bit of planning. You should not use a room easily accessible from outside to store property of your guests. A thief could drop valuable commodities through a window or fire escape to an accomplice waiting on the street below. You probably should not select your own bedroom either to store property. If you're like most people, you tend to keep your own valuables near at hand for protection, usually in your own bedroom. Your best bet for storage is a spare bedroom or that of a youngster.

A Friendly Game of Chance

At what point does your friendly Friday night poker game become a professional gambling operation? More than a few such games will be raided by robbers this year, and some will be raided by the police as well. High-stakes poker games do constitute gambling and, therefore, are an attraction to robbers. The potential for trouble increases if one member of the poker crowd has gotten in over his or her head and might be capable of non-sporting means of getting even.

It is generally best to avoid high-stakes games. But if you'd rather not avoid them, at least take some precautions, such as using chips rather than currency and settling at the end of the game by check instead of cash.

Going to the Movies

When you go to the movies, don't just choose the film of your liking; also pay attention to ensure that the movie theater is in a safe neighborhood. Try to avoid sitting near boisterous or suspicious individuals, and never tell a fellow moviegoer to stop talking or to refrain from smoking cigarettes or anything else. Have an usher do these distasteful tasks. Above all, be sure your children are properly supervised whenever you allow them to go to the movies.

AFTERMATH OF AN EMERGENCY OR CRISIS SITUATION

Personal security in an emergency situation is largely a matter of being prepared. A crisis may befall us at any time; it often comes without warning; and it calls for prompt and proper reaction. So advance planning is essential. In the aftermath of natural disasters, not to mention technological crises such as power brownouts or blackouts, your vulnerability to crime is greatly increased.

Hurricanes, tornadoes, floods, earthquakes, blizzards, and ice storms have at least one thing in common. Any of these catastrophes can result in the destruction of homes and other structures, long periods without electrical power and/or telephone service, and the curtailment or unavailability of customary police protection and medical assistance. To be properly equipped to cope with such situations, you should keep essential emergency supplies on hand in your home at all times. These include a battery-operated radio, spare batteries, one or more flashlights, candles and matches, a clock or watch, a first-aid kit, plus some drinking water and emergency food supplies.

The criminal element is likely to be out in full force during any extended blackout or similar emergency, so be careful to establish your personal security. Remember, the police won't be able to offer you the protection they normally would. They will be tied up keeping traffic moving and other vital services functioning. Battery-operated radios and automobile radios may enable you to keep in touch with the rest of the world, but strive to preserve battery power. You really don't know how long you will be in a crisis, and you must ration wisely. Avoid use of your automobile except in serious situations. To do otherwise could hinder emergency crews.

In certain crises or disruptions, particularly in urban areas, opportunistic thieves may assemble to loot. You might even face the prospect of defending your home or business against a ransacking, avaricious mob at a time when the ranks of law enforcement are stretched tenuously thin. You may or may not wish to add a firearm to your emergency cache. It is not a decision to be taken lightly.

THINK SECURITY

This chapter barely touches the surface of the many special occasions or situations that might require special security measures. The main point is to realize that your security hazard increases anytime you're out of your home or whenever anyone else is in it. Some situations, of course, are more hazardous than others, and only you can properly match resources against risks. If, however, you train yourself to think in terms of potential risk in advance, you will be prepared to take the appropriate protective steps.

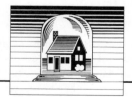

SPECIAL OCCASIONS MEAN
SPECIAL RISKS: A CHECKLIST

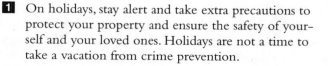

1 On holidays, stay alert and take extra precautions to protect your property and ensure the safety of yourself and your loved ones. Holidays are not a time to take a vacation from crime prevention.

2 Assume that your security needs to be increased whenever you're out of the house or whenever someone else is in it, and take adequate protective steps.

3 Arrange for a house-sitter when you and your family announce a funeral, wedding, or other event that may have been described in a newspaper or given other publicity.

4 Establish agreements with your neighbors to keep alert on your behalf whenever you're away from home. And, of course, be ready to reciprocate.

5 Guard against pilferage of small valuable items if a group of strangers or casual acquaintances are invited into your home. Investigate any part-time help engaged for special occasions.

6 If you are hosting a social gathering, protect your guests' coats and other belongings in a room that is secure from burglars.

7 Don't carry large amounts of money to a high-stakes poker game or similar activity. Use chips while playing, and settle debts by check at the end of the game.

8 Select a movie theater in a safe location, avoid boisterous individuals, and, if required, seek assistance from the theater's staff.

9 Be prepared to cope with increased security risks that may come in the aftermath of natural disasters or other emergencies.

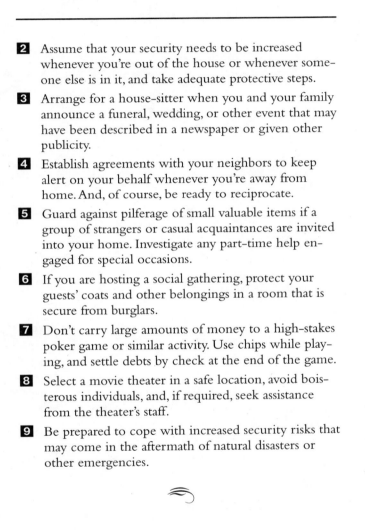

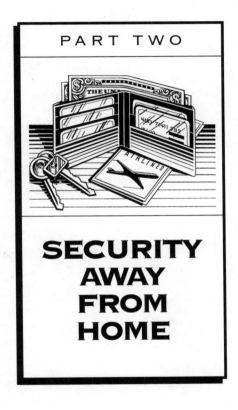

PART TWO

SECURITY AWAY FROM HOME

12

~

VEHICLE SECURITY
AND CARJACKING

A few friends were having dinner in a restaurant. When they returned to the parking lot, the valet attendant was nowhere to be found. They finally found him locked in the trunk of one of the cars in the lot. Two of them discovered that their cars were stolen, a Porsche and a Mercedes-Benz. Four other luxury foreign cars were also taken, for a theft worth about $300,000. The perpetrator was a gunman with the aid of a few accomplices, and the theft took less than 10 minutes.

Motor vehicle theft is a wide-ranging crime that, according to the Bureau of Justice Statistics, has for the last several years touched over 2 percent of the nation's households. Almost 2 million motor vehicles, valued at $7.6 billion, are stolen each year. Two-thirds of attempts at vehicle theft are successful. One of every 130 registered vehicles is taken by a criminal. One of every 98 registered vehicles is stolen in the West, the highest rate in the country. Although there was a 1.5 percent decrease in motor vehicle thefts between 1993 and 1994, this represents a 7-percent increase from 1988 and a 53-percent increase from 1983. Of all vehicles stolen, 80 percent are automobiles. According to the FBI, the owner of one auto has a 9-percent risk of having the car stolen during a 10-year period. This figure increases to 17 percent with two cars. With carjacking still very much a problem on American roads, car owners are finding that they are at risk even while driving.

A motor vehicle is probably the second largest investment most of us make, and there are a number of things we can do to protect this investment. There are obvious strategies: Don't leave keys in the ignition, lock car doors, and park in a safe location. As basic as these precautions are, most car thefts would be eliminated if the tips were faithfully followed. Four out of five cars stolen were left unlocked, and nearly 20 percent had keys in the ignition. Chapter 14, "Security While Shopping," provides additional information about safeguarding your auto against theft—not only the entire vehicle but also the piece-by-piece theft by car strippers. This type of piecemeal theft has an advantage for a thief, as most parts are not identified by serial number. One hubcap is much like another. If you've ever changed a car tire, you know how easy it is for a thief to steal tires and rims with no equipment other than a jack and lug wrench.

Nearly one-half of stolen autos wind up in "chop shops"—garages that dismantle stolen vehicles. A precautionary deterrent is to engrave your Vehicle Identification Number (VIN) on various parts and panels of your vehicle, making it less attractive to car thieves who dismantle for parts, and easier to identify if parts are recovered. A thief can get as much as five times the value of a car by selling parts to "chop shops."

A particularly vulnerable type of car is that which has an outside hood-release mechanism. Thieves can open the hood, cut battery cables with a bolt cutter, and get away in a matter of seconds. Key-operated hood locks are available at auto accessory stores, and heavy chains and padlocks can sometimes be used to prevent a hood from being raised. This method, while effective, is of course inconvenient when you attempt to open the hood for routine maintenance.

ACCESSORIES

If you have an audiosystem, car phone, or a citizens band (CB) radio installed in your car, you are displaying desirable goods to a thief. Get a system with a detachable face, and take it and your phone with you when you leave the car. Most CD players fit right in your pocket. If carrying it is not feasible, lock it in your trunk.

Your driver's license and automobile registration should never be stored in your car. The glove compartment and the area above the sun visor are among the first places searched by a thief. Carry these papers on your person, and handle them as you would any valuable papers. If keeping registration on one's person should prove totally impractical, as would be the case if a number of drivers used the same car frequently, the trunk provides more secure storage for these documents.

If your car is equipped with mushroom-shaped inside door locks, have them replaced with straight or tapered ones. The older kinds may allow a crook to gain entry with a coat hanger. Another accessory in your car that is attractive to thieves is your radar detector. Do not tempt a thief by leaving such a device in plain view.

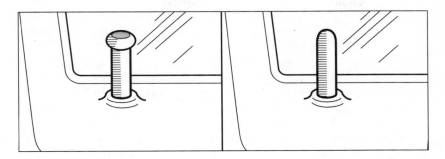

Figure 8. Old mushroom-shaped door lock and new straight or tapered lock.

The prize that more and more thieves want is the computer, or Electronic Control Module (ECM), in the dashboard. These computers are the vehicle's operating center, controlling everything from power door locks to flow of fuel to the engine. It takes an experienced thief only about 30 seconds to steal the ECM, which may be resold for at least a few hundred dollars. Several people have been repeatedly victimized. In Queens, New York, a woman caught a young man in his early 20s breaking into her car. She called police; they found that the thief was carrying a bag filled with computer chips. You may increase your protection by purchasing a metal cage that can be bolted, not welded, to the metal interior of your car.

Air bag thefts are increasing, especially in large cities. When thieves break into cars for parts, air bags are stolen 1.5 percent of the time. When cars were stolen and then recovered, air bags were found to have been taken over 10 percent of the time.

ALARMS AND OTHER SECURITY DEVICES

If you must carry items of value in your car, an alarm device is likely to be a good investment. However, any such system is subject to false alarms, and the system can be circumvented. Only extraordinary circumstances call for car alarms, and even then you may just be letting the thief know that there are valuables in the car. Despite these disadvantages, an auto alarm is useful for security.

Alarms that require a key for deactivation are the least effective, because a thief may disarm the alarm by tampering with surrounding wires. Alarms that require a secret code to be punched in may also be cut off. Remote alarms are the most effective, and the most expensive. Alarm systems that go off immediately after entry are better than those that go off after 30 seconds or more. This may be all the time the thief needs to be off with your car. It is suggested that an expert install your alarm. That alarm is harder for a crook to defeat than a self-installed system. The newest alarms on the market are portable, activated by air pressure; they emit a piercing sound when a door or window is opened.

In Chapter 2, we discussed the use of decals on homes as a deterrent to theft. While most of these decals advertise that the premises are protected by alarm systems, not all of them are. The same thing may be said of stickers announcing vehicle alarms. Not all of them are backed up by hardware. Thus, as with home alarms, auto alarm decals won't hurt anything, and they may even help, particularly if the person attempting to steal the auto isn't very sophisticated. The practiced thief, however, will be able to distinguish between alarmed and unalarmed cars and will act accordingly, probably against your best interests. If you do have an alarm system, experts suggest that decals so advertise, but do not name the particular system, as experienced thieves will know how to bypass it.

One common and highly visible antitheft device is a steering-wheel lock, "the Club," for example, which prevents the steering wheel from turning. There are also locks that go around the steering wheel and hinder accessibility to the ignition. Also available are various types of switches that are not visible. These are known as "passive systems" because they immobilize the vehicle. A "kill switch" prevents your car from being started until this hidden switch is set in the proper position. An ignition cutoff switch will make your car stop dead seconds after it is started. A fuel switch cuts off the gasoline supply; a gas lock is also a good idea—a thief will only be able to go as far as the amount of gas in the tank allows. A new remote device that locks the brakes by stopping the flow of brake fluid operates much like remotes that can lock doors from a distance. It is effective from as far away as 1,000 feet.

The most effective devices are Stolen Vehicle Recovery Systems (SVRS). These send out signals that may be picked up by police so that the location of your car may be traced. However, the distance from which these signals can be detected can be quite short (usually from 2 to 5 miles but also as short as five blocks in areas with radio disturbance). SVRSs are not available in all areas. The device is not visible to potential thieves, so it fails as a deterrent. It also does not prevent vandalism, unless the car is equipped with an alarm. Nevertheless, manufacturers of these devices boast a 95-percent vehicle recovery rate, with a quarter of these incidents bringing about the arrest of the perpetrators. This is even more startling when compared with the national auto theft arrest rate of 5 percent.

Also effective is the installation of a Global Positioning Satellite (GPS) anti-theft/duress system which allows a vehicle to be tracked and also sends out a silent duress signal.

Check if your local police department has a car theft program, such as New York City's Combat Auto Theft (CAT), Philadelphia's Stolen Auto Verification Effort (SAVE), and Stop Cleveland Auto Theft (SCAT). For a small fee, you will receive decals for your window, and the police will stop your vehicle if it is being driven during late-night or early-morning hours to check if the driver has authorized use of the car. These programs and devices may even entitle you to receive a discount on your vehicle insurance.

BEFORE ENTERING YOUR CAR

As you approach your car, make it a habit to check it on all sides for flat tires and obstructions near the wheels and also for persons hiding under the vehicle. Before you get into your car check for illegal entry. If you think your car has been broken into, don't disturb fingerprints or any other evidence that may assist the police.

Next, look in the window and check inside your car. Do this even if the car has been in an attended garage or if it has been delivered to you by a parking attendant. Again, you may discover evidence that you won't wish to disturb. You might also discover someone crouching on the floor. Carrying a small penlight in a pocket or handbag is an excellent security protection. You should use it during hours of darkness to examine the interior of the vehicle thoroughly before entering. If all appears in order, unlock the door. If the door isn't locked and you are reasonably certain that you locked it when you left, be cautious. Before you get into the car, check to see if your radio and tape player are still there and if the glove compartment is in order.

From a security standpoint, a citizens band radio or a cellular telephone is an excellent item for a well-equipped auto. As a matter of fact, there is a good argument for having both devices. There are gaps in the coverage of cellular phones when you leave populated areas. In this circumstance, your CB might help you through an emergency. CB Channel 9 is monitored continuously for emergency radio traffic throughout almost all of the United States.

AFTER ENTERING YOUR CAR

Once you are in the car, lock all the doors, fasten your seat belt or shoulder harness, and start the car. But what if it won't start?

If it is daylight and the car is parked in your driveway or in front of the house, the problem is almost certainly a mechanical malfunction. If it is late at night and you are parked in an unfamiliar or high-crime neighborhood, the car's disability might have been caused deliberately. Look around, and if you see something suspicious, get out of the car, lock the door, and get assistance. The best place to go is probably the place you just left. Even if you are qualified to make repairs yourself, you would be well advised to have someone you know with you.

If, on the other hand, you think that robbery or assault looks likely, and if you are not on a brightly lighted or heavily traveled thoroughfare, you have two choices. You can lock the car and go away, then return for your car in the light of day with assistance of your own choosing. Or you can lock the car and stay inside, being prepared to blow the horn if you are threatened.

Whatever you do, do not accept a stranger's offer of assistance. This may be the person who disabled your car. Ask the stranger who seems interested in helping you to call a friend, a relative, or the police. Don't accept anyone's offer to call a service station for you; an accomplice may be standing by. If you're inside your car and a would-be benefactor attempts to get you to unlock the door, blow the horn and keep blowing it until your "friend" leaves or until someone in the neighborhood gets disturbed enough to call the police.

IF FOLLOWED

Do you think someone in a car is following you? Ask yourself if you have given anyone reason to do so. Did you flash a roll of money in a store? Did you just cash a check? If you think it is likely that someone is following you, take evasive action, and drive in the center lane. If your follower persists, stop at a service station and make a call. While it is true that a service station can be a haven, it is equally true that you might be followed there. Stations, particularly at night, are often staffed by only one person, and it is quite possible that this individual may not wish to be involved. Therefore, you would be better off looking for a service station adjacent to a diner.

If you cannot locate the safe haven you seek, and you still feel threatened by someone following you, drive to the busiest intersection you can find, activate your flashers, double-check that your doors are locked, and honk your horn until assistance arrives. As a general rule, assistance is defined as a uniformed police officer. Infrequently, a person may appear to be a police officer but the car may arouse your suspicion. If in doubt, proceed to a lighted area or a nearby police station where the persons' identity can be determined.

When entering a driveway or a garage, be sure no one is following you. If there are automatic doors, make sure there are no suspicious-looking people or vehicles around. If there are, don't go in. Find out who they are or wait until they leave. If they don't leave, call the police. In addition, make sure the garage door is closed and that nobody has followed you in before you get out of your car.

STALLED-CAR CRISIS

If you are driving with passengers along the expressway and your car stalls, get the car completely off the roadway. Get the passengers out of the car and away from the road. Signal for assistance. Attempt repairs if you are qualified, but do so away from the road traffic.

A more-or-less universal signal that you need assistance on the road is a display of a square piece of cardboard or a flag that can be seen from a passing auto. A white cloth tied to the radio antenna is another widely used emergency signal. Leave lights on at night, using emergency blinkers or turn signals to warn oncoming traffic. A raised hood will also signify that caution is in order and assistance is needed.

Hazards of Towing

Be extremely cautious of towing companies. Consider the following incidents reported by AAA (American Automobile Association). One driver had a flat tire on a busy highway; he parked the car on the shoulder and waited for help. A tow truck arrived unsummoned, and the driver announced that the charge for repairing the flat was $25. The operator of the vehicle decided to repair the tire without assistance. In another incident, a tow truck operator claimed that the car could not be started and insisted on towing the disabled vehicle to the company repair shop. When calling the repair shop for an estimate later on, the customer was informed that the repairs had already been made, at a cost of $741. Similar horror stories concerning illegal towing practices abound throughout the country.

The first thing you should do when the tow truck arrives is to make sure that the towing company is licensed. If the company's name, address, telephone number, tow rates, and license (where required) are not visible on the truck, be suspicious. Inspect your vehicle for damage, and remove all valuables before it is towed. Countless complaints of damage and theft have been made against towing companies. It is best to contact your own repair shop. If this is not practical, do not sign an "Authorization to Repair" unless you are satisfied with the expertise and integrity of the repair shop chosen by the towing company. Request a repair estimate and an itemized bill, which will be useful if you should decide to challenge the charges. An itemized bill will be required if your vehicle is covered by a warranty. Many towers accept payment by credit card.

PROTECTING YOURSELF FROM CARJACKING

Unfortunately, carjacking is a popular (and brazen) crime—your car is stolen while you're still in it, or just as you're getting in or out of it. In October 1992, stronger laws against carjacking, or the use of a weapon to steal a car or other vehicle, were passed by the federal government. A criminal convicted of this crime now has to serve a minimum of 15 years if injury is inflicted on the victim. This legislation distinguishes carjacking from ordinary car theft by subjecting the offender to a harsher penalty.

With new and better alarms and protective devices for cars, it is becoming increasingly difficult for thieves to steal an uninhabited vehicle, a development that has made carjacking more appealing to the criminal element. In addition, the extensive coverage of carjacking in the media has probably encouraged more car thieves to "copycat" this method.

Carjacking Techniques

Probably the most widespread carjacking technique is the "bump and rob," in which you are rear-ended by a driver. While your first instinct after getting bumped is to immediately get out of your car, *don't;* getting out leaves you wide open and extremely vulnerable, especially if you are alone. If you are bumped, stay in your vehicle; through your rear-view mirror, gather information about the car that hit you.

You may also be followed home from a mall, an automated teller machine, or any other place from which you are likely to have taken more then the usual amount of goods or money. Carjackers even have been known to establish fake valet parking setups, where you literally hand your car over to them.

Another widely used technique in an attempt to have you pull over is the thief's impersonation of a police officer. Make sure it's really a police car or, if the car is unmarked, try to determine if the officer is wearing an authentic uniform. An estimated 25,000 citizens are victimized each year by criminals posing as police officers. Assess what the police officer says as he approaches your car. An authorized law officer will tell you why you've been pulled over and immediately request your license and registration. Roll the windows down only an inch or two and ask to see the officer's badge or ID.

Greatest Risk Factors

Carjacking incidents have taken place at all times and in all places, but you may be at a greater risk under these circumstances:

❖ When stopped in traffic, especially at red lights and stop signs
❖ In parking lots and garages
❖ When getting on or off a highway
❖ At a self-service or late-night full-service gas station, carwash, or convenience store
❖ At an automated teller machine (ATM)
❖ When getting into or out of your car

When driving, always keep your windows rolled up—if the weather hot and you don't have air conditioning, keep them at least three-quarters of the way up—and lock your doors as soon as you enter your vehicle. Carjackers most frequently get into cars when doors are not locked. Some automobiles are equipped with a "panic button" that automatically locks all doors and windows in the event of an emergency.

Do not wait in a car for a companion with the engine running and the doors unlocked. A 28-year-old off-duty police officer went into a restaurant to order pizza; his wife waited in their car. He came to her aid when she was approached by a carjacker. Bullets were exchanged, and the officer was shot in the chest. A Canadian couple was looking for a hotel in Manhattan. The man went into a hotel as his companion waited in the car. She was pushed out of the vehicle; then the carjacker sped off with their car.

To avoid attracting thieves, keep your purse or other valuables out of sight, in the glove compartment or under the seat. Avoid wearing expensive jewelry, especially when driving alone or late at night.

Other Guidelines

Don't stop your car merely because someone asks you to, especially in a remote location. If someone appears to need assistance, don't be reckless or foolhardy. You might stop, roll down the window slightly, and ask if you can send help. Don't allow yourself to be talked into giving assistance. Go for help.

If someone other than a uniformed or plainclothes police officer in a squad car or in another clearly identifiable department vehicle attempts to force you to the curb, try to get away, even if it means a collision. Sound the horn, and drive to a service station, a lighted house, or anywhere else you might reasonably expect to find assistance, and from there report the matter to the police.

If someone attempts to enter your car at a stop sign or a stoplight, drive away. Run the light. Risk a collision if you must, but drive on. If you turn to the right, you probably will be heading in the same direction as the traffic, which will minimize the damage of any resulting collision. Since someone attempting to force his or her way into your car will most likely approach you from the curb side, the movement of your car to the right will also tend to force the intruder away from you. Sound your horn, activate your hazard lights, and attract as much attention as possible. If there is an accident, drive to a service station or to any open public business. You aren't leaving the scene; you're merely going to the nearest phone to report an accident.

To whatever extent possible, avoid traveling alone. One woman we know keeps a department store mannequin's head and upper torso in her automobile. This gives the impression that she is not a woman traveling alone. Two unmarried sisters carry a man's hat in their car. When they travel together, one of them wears the hat to convey the impression that a male is aboard.

If you must travel alone on a regular basis, consider these two rules: First, learn the location of all police stations, precinct houses, or other locations that police tend to frequent. All-night restaurants, especially those near the station house, may be favored spots for coffee breaks. Second, travel familiar streets, and make it a point to find out as much as possible about the areas through which you pass. Shopping occasionally in these places may enable merchants to recognize you as a customer. If so, they would much more likely go out of their way to be of assistance when you really need it.

Here are some additional guidelines that should be followed to reduce the chances of your being carjacked:

❖ Invest in a CB radio or cellular telephone for your car. When you're in trouble, you will be able to summon assistance quickly.

❖ Park in well-lit, busy, and open areas. Parking lots with attendants or security patrols are best.

❖ Leave enough room in a parallel parking space between the car in front of you and your car so that you can drive away if threatened.

❖ When approaching a red light on an isolated street, proceed slowly, so that by the time you reach the intersection, the traffic light will be about to change. This way you will not be a "sitting duck" while waiting for the light to change.

❖ Keep your car well maintained, with plenty of gasoline in your tank.

❖ Never leave your registration or any item with your address in the vehicle. Keep a separate record of your vehicle identification number and other information that will help you identify your vehicle.

❖ Keep your vehicle keys on a different key chain from your housekeys, and keep your housekeys in your pocket. If your automobile keys are stolen, the thief will not have access to your home, and you will still have your housekeys even if your purse is stolen. However, in the event your housekeys are stolen, change the locks immediately.

❖ In cold weather, stay in your vehicle as it warms up. Don't leave the engine running while you remain in your house.

❖ Do not leave children and babies alone in your car, even for only a moment. If you absolutely must do so, do not leave your keys in the ignition, and lock all doors.

❖ Avoid driving a car that may be identified as rented. Carjackers are especially tempted by tourists.

❖ Be wary if someone tries to sell you merchandise while you are in your car. They may be distracting you from an accomplice approaching from another direction.

❖ Stay calm while driving. Suppress your need to tell off other drivers or to gesture to them. Such behavior may provoke an incident.

❖ Most important, always be aware of your surroundings and alert to any emergency.

Statistics show that a weapon was used in 77 percent of all carjackings. Experts say that if you get into the car with an armed carjacker, there is a 98-percent chance you will not survive the incident (just about 100 percent for men!). If you refuse to go with the carjacker and run away, however, there is a 98-percent chance you will not be shot. Distract the carjacker with your credit card, ATM card, or money; throw them out the window, get out, and run. Most likely the carjacker will go after the loot. If you can't run, experts suggest that you lie flat on the ground, because it is too much trouble for the assailant to force you to go with him or her. If your child is in the car when you are attacked, throw your keys and pocketbook out of the car, and tell the assailant that he can have the car but not your child. Grab your child and run.

Try to get a description of the assailant. Report the incident to the police, giving them a description of the carjacker, along with any evidence you have and information about your vehicle. Tell them the direction the carjacker was heading in your car.

PARKING YOUR CAR

Park where passersby, either walking or driving, may serve as a deterrent to someone who might steal, or steal from, your car. If it's daylight, ask yourself if it will still be light when you return. Try to park near a storefront that will be brightly lighted, on a main thoroughfare, under a streetlamp, or somewhere you anticipate heavy traffic (either vehicular or pedestrian). In a driveway, park with the front of your vehicle facing passersby who may witness a thief tampering with your engine. Avoid remote, unlighted areas.

Don't park in the same location at the same time every day. Try not to park at the end of the block. Turn your wheels toward the curb, and put on your emergency brake. If you have automatic transmission, leave it in "park." If it's manual, leave the gear in "first" or "reverse." These precautions make it more difficult for your vehicle to be towed. Ten percent of stolen cars are towed away.

Once you are parked, roll up your windows, and always lock your car, even if you will be away for only a few minutes. Remember, more cars (over 200,000 each year) are stolen because a key was left in the ignition of an unlocked car than from any other cause. The National Insurance Crime Bureau reports that 14 percent of Americans leave keys in the ignition, and 31 percent neglect to lock the doors of their vehicles. Always take your key with you when you exit your automobile, and always double-check to be sure that all car doors are locked and all windows closed.

Be particularly careful when parking in public lots. The chances of your car being stolen from an unattended lot are five times greater than from the street or an attended lot.

CAR KEY SECURITY

Those little magnetic holders with spare ignition keys, attached to the car's frame, are an open invitation to car thieves. That is the first thing they look for.

At an attended garage, leave only your ignition key. One enterprising parking attendant had considerable success as part of a burglary ring. When parking a car, particularly an expensive one, he would search for the identification of the driver. A phone call to the house would determine if anyone was home. If not, an accomplice in a truck nearby would duplicate the house key on a portable key cutter and be quickly on his way to strip the place. Even when the victim returned for his or her car and left the garage, the attendant had ample time to telephone the victim's home and warn the accomplice that it was time to leave.

ASKING FOR TROUBLE

If you're in your car at a time when the motor isn't running—while at a drive-in movie, for example—lock yourself in. Roll the windows up, leaving a crack for fresh air. In a drive-in restaurant, if you are in an isolated area, put the food inside the car; don't leave the window open for a tray table.

If you are parked in a completely isolated area, head your car outward, and keep the doors locked and the windows up. Keep your eyes open. Lovers' lanes are favorite haunts, not only for young lovers but also for robbers and sexual deviates.

OTHER SECURITY CONSIDERATIONS

Motor Homes, Recreational Vehicles, and Vans

You can protect motor homes and recreational vehicles (RVs) by employing the same measures as for automobiles. There are, however, a few areas of particular concern. Motor homes are especially vulnerable at times of seasonal change, when they might be stolen for sale to vacationers or for transportation to another climate.

Elaborately styled and personalized vans are another consideration. The individualized nature of many of these vans makes them less attractive to the local thief but more attractive to the organized career criminal, who has the resources to transport them to another part of the country, where an outlet there sells the vehicle quickly. The operator of such an outlet will have little difficulty, if any, in obtaining titles or other documents to transfer to these stolen vehicles. Totally wrecked autos are often purchased just to acquire the ownership documents, which are then altered for transfer to a stolen car.

Motorcycles, Mopeds, and Bicycles

Motorcycles and mopeds are increasingly popular, offering economy and fun while traveling. This has led to an increase in thefts of these vehicles. No lock is 100-percent theftproof, but there are devices that discourage or delay a thief considerably. Invest in a lock that allows you to link your motorcycle to a pole or street sign when it's not in use. Among the locks available today are krypton U-shaped bars, braided and plastic-covered steel cables, and the old-fashioned chains and padlocks. A beeper that sounds when someone tampers with your motorcycle is also available; it is audible for up to a half-mile. Don't rely on the automatic steering lock built into a motorcycle. This will prevent the wheels from turning but will not keep the motorcycle from being lifted onto a truck and spirited away.

A bicycle is easily stolen and extremely difficult to trace, so bicycle security demands your vigilance. Bicycles have "grown up," in the sense that they are no longer transportation exclusively for kids. You can spend as much today for a good bike as you would for a good used car.

Bicycles are "in" as a means of exercise for young professionals. Because they are trendy, they are desirable items. Wherever items are desired, you may be certain that thieves will try to fill the demand.

One way to discourage bicycle thieves is to buy the bicycle secondhand. There is a legal market for used bikes, which usually represent great buys, as bike riders trade up. Since your "like-new" transportation will not have the resale potential of the pacesetting models, you're less likely to be ripped off.

Regardless of whether your bike is state-of-the-art or more sedate, you need to protect it from theft. A good padlock is the most important security protection for your bicycle. Many bicycle locks are available: heavy shackle locks, chain-and-key padlocks, horseshoe-shaped clamps, and cable combination locks. Kryptonite cable or U-shaped locks and the superheated steel chain are considered best bets; but perhaps more important is the way the bike is secured and the object to which it is secured. Secure the bike through the frame or through both the frame and tire, rather than just the tire. Secure it to a lamppost, tree, or other object that is large enough to prevent the object from being removed along with the bike. The object should be tall enough so that the whole assembly—bike, chain, lock, and all—cannot be slipped off the top.

You can further safeguard against bicycle theft by recording your bike's serial number and registering it with your local police department. When you are not riding the bicycle, put it in a locked room, basement, or garage, not in your backyard or driveway where it can be seen from the street. And remember to lock the bike, even if it's in the locked garage. If a thief can get into the garage, your bike will still be out of harm's way, if you remembered to take the approximately 5 seconds required to lock it further.

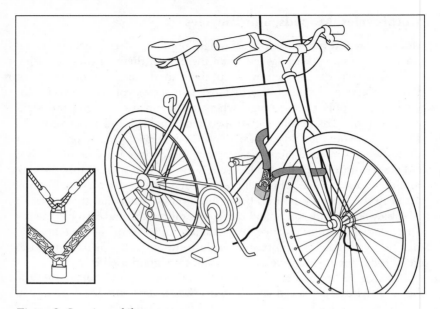

Figure 9. Securing a bike.

PROTECTING BOATS

Protecting a boat is, in many ways, similar to protecting your home. Often your boat *is* your home away from home. You would be well advised to reread the protective principles in Chapter 1. You will require good dead-bolt locks, quality protective lighting, and alarm systems, including local alarms for all hatches, to protect your property. You will need to maintain up-to-date inventory lists (see Chapter 2), and you should etch or otherwise identify items that are part of your maritime home. Compasses, sextants, depth-sounding gear, radar, radios, and life-preserving equipment should all bear your identification marks.

Secure your boat to a mooring with a steel chain in addition to a line. Be certain to moor or anchor your boat, in a secure marina, especially during summer months when anchorages are crowded.

You should cooperate with your neighbors at marinas or anchorages for common security. Ideally, you should make use of continuously staffed mooring facilities. Never leave gasoline in your outboard engine, and remove all portable tanks when your water craft is in the marina.

When you leave your craft, employ the maximum available protections. Secure outboard motors with excellent padlocks and chains. Installing a secret ignition cutoff switch might easily prevent your craft from being stolen. Removing the screw or hiding the distributor rotor could foil thieves. Most importantly, when you leave the boat, make absolutely certain that you don't leave the registration papers behind. You certainly wouldn't want your deck to be sold out from under you.

You may be required to display craft registration numbers on your hull. Though not required, you should also place this identifier on the vessel's structural members in remote locations. Certain boats are exempt from craft registration requirements. If you are permitted to register your boat, even if not required to do so, by all means add this protection.

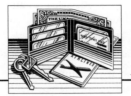

VEHICLE SECURITY AND CARJACKING: A CHECKLIST

1 Automobiles with exterior hood releases require additional precautions.

2 Before getting into your vehicle, check around it, and have your keys ready beforehand.

3 Check inside the car before unlocking it.

4 Lock your doors as soon as you get inside your vehicle, and keep windows rolled up.

5 Don't display accessories such as tape or CD players, CB radios, or radar detectors where they will attract a thief's attention.

6 Consider installing an alarm system or some other security device if you must carry valuable items in your car, and also as a safeguard against car theft.

7 If your car won't start, either get assistance or get away, especially if you are in unfamiliar territory. Your car may have been disabled deliberately.

8 Do not accept unsolicited offers of assistance.

9 Do not unlock the door to admit a stranger.

10 Sound your horn and continue to do so if a stranger remains around your locked car and appears to be a menace.

---

11 Beware of carjacking scams, such as the "bump and rob," false valet parking, and impersonation of a police officer.

12 Be especially cautious at times and places where carjackings are likely to occur.

13 Try to travel through familiar areas, and stay out of high-crime areas. Always map out the safest route.

14 Lock your car if you must abandon it to go for assistance, and exercise prudence while walking away.

15 If someone appears to need assistance, drive to a phone and call for assistance; do not stop.

16 If someone attempts to force you to stop, do not— even if it means a collision. Sound the horn, and drive toward lights or wherever you may find assistance.

17 Take evasive action if you are being followed, and drive in the center lane. If your follower persists, drive to some occupied location, and phone for assistance.

18 If someone attempts to enter your car at a stoplight or a stop sign, drive away, sounding your horn, even if it means running a red light. In general, turn to the right when driving away.

19 Don't get out of your car in a dark, remote location, even if you've been involved in an accident. If possible, drive to an open service station or business, and report the accident to the police.

20 Learn the location of police stations, precinct houses, and other places where police tend to gather. This knowledge may save your life in an emergency.

21 Distract a would-be carjacker by throwing your credit cards, money, purse, or wallet—even your car keys—out of the car, then getting out and running away.

22 Avoid getting into your car with a carjacker. Chances are you'll never return.

23 Report all incidents to the police, and provide evidence and information about your assailant.

24 Park only in lighted, populous locations.

25 Never leave your keys in the ignition.

26 Exercise caution when parked in areas like drive-ins or lovers' lanes. Be ready to leave on short notice.

27 If parked at an attended lot, leave only your ignition key behind.

28 Motorcycles, mopeds, and bicycles left in the street should be secured to lampposts or street signs.

29 Motorcycle steering locks do not offer protection against the vehicle's being stolen by being lifted onto a truck.

30 Bicycle serial numbers should be recorded with the police department.

31 The oversize shackle lock is considered best for security of bicycles, motorcycles, and mopeds.

32 Apply to boat security all principles for protection of your home.

13

SECURITY IN THE STREETS

"I was just standing there," said William Redd, "minding my own business and waiting for the bus. This great big dude walked up, and pow, he knocked me right over. I still don't know what I ever did to that guy, but the next time I'm in the Tenderloin at that time of night, I'm taking a taxi home!"

BASIC PRECAUTIONS

More crimes against people are committed on the streets than in any other place. In a widely publicized case, a New York City woman was attacked and killed in broad daylight as she and her son were going to church, by a stranger wielding a 2-by-4. The police said the assault was "totally unexpected and appeared to be totally unprovoked." A few precautions will greatly reduce your chances of being victimized.

Don't Carry a Great Deal of Money

The first rule is to limit your losses. Don't carry more than you can easily afford to lose. A famous woman was once quoted as saying that she never carried more than $25 with her at any time. She said she carried that amount because she knew that it was the going rate for a heroin fix at that time. Many street robberies are committed solely to finance drug addictions. If you carry little cash, the robber's take won't break you, but it should be enough to satisfy him or her. If frustrated, the robbers may give vent to their rage by a physical assault, especially if they are strung out on drugs.

Sometimes, though, it may be necessary to carry more cash than you feel comfortable with. In that event, carry the money in a stamped, self-addressed envelope, and if you feel the least bit threatened, drop it in the corner mailbox. Obviously, for this tactic to be effective, you must know the exact location of the nearest mail drop. As Chapter 12 advised, make stops at businesses that are along frequently traveled routes. In time, you will be recognized by the merchants, which might stand you in good stead if you are attacked on the street.

Vary the route you travel in making these trips. Vary the time of day, too. You might even wear a disguise of some sort—anything to confuse the crook who is lying in ambush.

When you pick up the cash you are to transport to a destination, ask that someone accompany you to your auto or taxi. Do not carry cash in your handbag. Purses are too easily stolen. A coat pocket (particularly an inside one) is more secure.

Surrender Your Valuables

The second rule is simple. Remain calm and obey all commands. Surrender your valuables, and do so quickly. A tourist was robbed on the streets of a large city he was visiting. He surrendered his cash but claimed that he was unable to remove a ring from his finger. His assailant offered to remove it, finger and all, with the switchblade knife he was carrying.

Try to avoid letting your attacker move you into an alley, doorway, or other secluded place. Explain that there's no need to do that, that you are perfectly willing to cooperate. But don't let your eagerness to cooperate lead you into making any sudden moves. Tell your assailant that you're reaching for your wallet, then do it very slowly. You may be risking a fair amount of money (the average street robbery yield is about $840), but the robber, who is risking a minimum of 10 years in jail, will be as nervous as you are.

Regardless of how accommodating you are, there is still the distinct possibility that you will be attacked. A robber may have emotional needs that can be served only by beating someone—meaning that all the money in the world won't be able to satisfy the robber. In this case, you have little choice but to defend yourself. Your best defenses are screaming for help and running away, not fighting. Chances are the robber is better equipped for combat than you are—that's one criterion in the robber's selection of victims. Moreover, your assailant is likely to be armed with a gun or knife.

Being Followed?

A third protective rule is: Walk in the middle of the sidewalk facing oncoming traffic. This eliminates the possibility of someone's sneaking up behind you in an auto. If you should be accosted, an oncoming motorist might be a witness and send assistance.

If you are being followed on a well-traveled street, slow down, speed up, reverse directions—in other words, indicate to your pursuer that you are aware you are being followed. Then go straight for help. If you are being followed on a deserted street, don't play games. Walk as fast as you can to the nearest police officer or telephone, and report it. Look ahead for other people or a mailbox. The presence of other people will deter a purse snatcher. A mailbox is a relatively safe place to deposit your purse or wallet to avoid its theft. Technically you are in violation of the law by placing something other than mail in a postal box, but this is something that postal authorities are accustomed to handling.

If you're being followed, don't run straight for home, especially if no one is there to assist you. You are safer on the street than you are inside your home or in an elevator alone with your assailant. If your "shadow" is after you, rather than your property, running straight home reveals where you can be found later, at the assailant's convenience.

DEFENSIVE WEAPONS AND PROCEDURES

Many so-called weapons—small handguns, tear gas guns, Mace devices—aren't much help. They may be grabbed and used against you, or, more likely, the devices will still be in your purse when it is taken from you. Nevertheless, the devices are still popular.

Self-Defense Sprays

Over 18 million canisters of defensive sprays have been purchased by the security conscious. Self-defense sprays can provide an option for protection, unless outlawed in your state. Pepper sprays and tear gas are legal in most states, although some restrictions may apply. Florida and New Jersey have size restrictions on canisters. Massachusetts and California require a permit, and according to California law, an individual must successfully complete a state-certified course in the use of Mace. Tear gas, including Mace, allows you to spray an irritant onto the face of your attacker, causing extreme pain and burning the eyes and skin. Mace can be sprayed from a distance of up to 10 feet. This type of spray may be ineffective against a psychotic or intoxicated assailant, who may not respond normally to pain. A red-pepper (capsicum) spray is more effective with abnormal assailants, as it disables mucous membranes. It also works faster than tear gas or Mace and can be used to ward off attacking animals or bees. However, a pepper spray has a shorter range because it is a mist. Certain types of pepper sprays are combined with Mace, offering the advantages of both in a single spray. These sprays incapacitate an attacker for as long as 20 minutes, but the sprays may take anywhere from 3 seconds to a minute to take effect. Some sprays are equipped with an ultraviolet or orange-red dye that can mark an attacker for up to a week, aiding in detection and identification. These sprays are also fairly inexpensive, ranging anywhere from $10 to $50.

A more expensive alternative is a stun gun. It transmits a high-voltage electric shock that can incapacitate an assailant for as long as 5 minutes. However, some types of stun guns require physical contact with an attacker and must be applied for several seconds to be effective. Momentary contact may only result in causing enough pain to provoke your assailant toward even greater violence. Also, it is virtually ineffective if the attacker is wearing thick clothing or if the battery is weak.

A few words of caution concerning these devices: The sprays are ineffectual beyond their expiration date and may be ruined by extreme hot or cold temperatures. Do not leave them in your car in direct sunlight, especially during the summer months, as the canisters will explode at temperatures above 130 degrees. Self-defense weapons are effective only if carried in your hand or in an easily accessible place, such as a pocket or on your belt. They are completely useless at the bottom of your purse. When driving alone, place your weapon on the passenger seat next to you. If you are attacked, your weapon may be grabbed and used against you, or the wind could blow the chemicals in your face instead. Unfortunately, this is especially true of mist sprays, the most powerful type. A stream spray is less likely to do this, but it takes a longer period to be effective.

The effects of the spray could linger for up to a few days. Avoid contact with areas or objects that have been affected. In case of inadvertent contact, remain outdoors (or get there) and flush mucous membranes with water. Medical attention is advisable. A safety latch on the device is a guard against accidental discharge, but it must be disengaged before use. Practice using your weapon or spray before you need it, instead of trying to figure it out at the moment of attack. Test it outdoors every month with a short blast. Replace sprays every year. In addition, the use of a spray is advisable only against an unarmed attacker. If attacked, use your spray or stun gun only as a means of escape; don't attempt to battle your opponent. Run away immediately and seek assistance.

Never buy sprays or weapons from the street. Your local law enforcement agency can refer you to a legitimate dealer.

Other Devices and Precautions

One good protection is a whistle with a piercing sound, like a traffic officer's, worn strapped to the wrist, not carried in the purse. A whistle on a bracelet slipped over the fingers, like the one football officials carry, is also useful if it is worn rather than carried in the purse. But never wear a whistle on a chain around your neck; in an effort to discourage you from sounding it, the robber may well strangle you with your chain.

More sophisticated than whistles are personal alarms. You can purchase a handheld shrieker for under $25. When squeezed, the device activates an ear-shattering and disorienting 120–decibel distress signal. It can be turned off simply by entering a code. Another personal alarm clips on like a pager and is activated by pulling a pin that triggers a blasting, shrieking siren. It can be purchased for under $30. Or you can acquire a battery-powered or pressurized-gas alarm that emits a screeching sound; this type of alarm costs anywhere from a few dollars to over a $100.

Personal alarms might distract the attacker for the second or two needed for escape. They are easy to conceal and carry; they do not involve contact with the criminal; and, unlike a weapon, they can't be turned against you. However, if you live in a large city, don't expect help when the alarm goes off, because people seem oblivious to the many false alarms (car, house, etc.) that are constantly going off. Also, personal alarms offer virtually no help in secluded areas. Besides, there is always a danger that the alarm might enrage the attacker.

You can cut your losses by "spreading the wealth." For years, women who have had to carry money have been hiding it in their lingerie, and old-fashioned money belts are also recommended.

Your keys may also serve as a weapon. While walking alone at night, carry your keys with one key protruding through each knuckle. If someone tries to assault you, punch him in the eye or another vulnerable area. A pen or pencil clenched in your fist would work as well. If at all possible, don't carry keys in your purse along with identification. You might lose your purse and then find that your home has been robbed before you have even finished filing the initial police report.

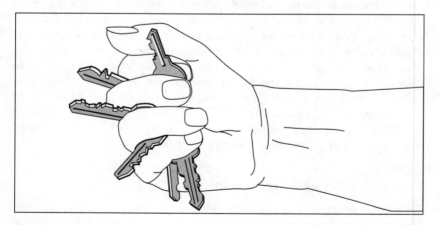

Figure 10. Carrying keys as protection.

Carry only credit cards that you think you are likely to need. (See Chapter 14 for more information on credit card security.)

If you have to make frequent bank deposits in connection with your work, don't carry deposits in your own bag along with your personal valuables. Use a deposit bag that can be slipped loosely over the wrist. The use of armored-car services is recommended for large deposits.

BEWARE OF PURSE SNATCHERS AND PICKPOCKETS

The most frequent type of street robbery is probably the snatching of a briefcase or a purse. Your best defense against the purse snatcher is to walk some distance from the curb, with your purse or briefcase in the hand away from the street.

A purse should be carried with the strap over one shoulder, with the bag suspended between your arm and body. If your handbag strap is too short to carry this way, put your arm through the strap, and cradle the purse in your arm like a halfback carrying a football. A strapless bag also should be carried like a football. Many women carry bags with the shoulder straps crossed over their bodies. This can increase the chances of serious injury, because the purse snatcher's usual method of attack is to yank a purse hard enough to break the strap, at the same time shoving the victim the other way.

Another defensive tactic you might try is to flatten yourself against the side of a building when you hear rapidly approaching footsteps behind you. If you are the intended victim, this might prevent your handbag from being taken. If you aren't, it may keep you from being trampled. But try to avoid flattening yourself against a plate glass window, because if it is the older type of plate glass, you could suffer severe cuts should the assailant give you the customary shove.

A pickpocket works best in a crowd. A subway at rush hour is the milieu of the "dip" (another term for pickpocket). An extremely light touch is the stock-in-trade of these thieves. Your only awareness of anything out of the ordinary will be the feel of a slight pressure. When exerting that pressure, the pickpocket is removing your billfold from your purse or your inside coat pocket.

One method of dealing with the dip is to speak up loudly. "Somebody's pushing on me, and I don't like it" is a phrase that should affect the thief's concentration and warn all others within earshot. If someone does say that, be sure to resist the impulse to check the pockets or purses where valuables are kept. This could tell the pickpocket exactly where to look.

A purse snatching, on the average, nets the thief about $290. Pickpockets do better: about $430 for each theft.

WALKING AT NIGHT

If you must walk at night, avoid the curb, whether or not vehicles are parked on the street. Someone could hide between two parked cars and ambush you. Or someone driving by could reach through the car window and snatch your purse or briefcase. Don't walk too far from the curb either. Be especially guarded about doorways or shrubbery abutting the sidewalk, either of which can afford an excellent ambush point.

If the route to your destination is filled both with parked cars and with doorways or shrubbery adjacent to the sidewalk, then walk in the street (obviously keeping a sharp eye out for traffic).

If your late-night walks are regular and predictable, vary your route, particularly on paydays, Social Security check days, or other times when you might be suspected of carrying more than your usual amount of cash.

Keep a line of communication with others. For example, ask friends or relatives to give you a call when they reach their destination so that you know they have arrived safely. In turn, call them when you arrive at your destination. Keep tabs on each other.

JOGGING AND IN-LINE SKATING

While jogging or running, you may feel invigorated and confident, but be aware: The female runner in particular is a prime target for a criminal. Awareness of crimes against joggers has increased since the 1989 attack on the Central Park jogger in New York City. The 28-year-old investment banker was raped and brutally assaulted by a gang of youths. Recently, another gang of teenagers beat, mugged, and raped a 43-year-old woman at Coney Island after dragging her under the boardwalk. This doesn't happen only in large cities. Across the country, about 7,000 crimes a year are reported involving women who were jogging. These attacks range from muggings and indecent exposure to more violent crimes, including rapes and murders.

You are most at risk when jogging alone, after dark, and on deserted paths. Run with a companion, a friend, or a trained dog. Runners organizations, such as the Road Runners Club of America (RRCA), which has several hundred chapters in the United States, can introduce you to a fellow runner and provide safety tips for running in your area. Stay on well-traveled routes you are familiar with, and avoid trails with shrubbery or alleyways where attackers can hide. Know places along the way you can go to for assistance in the event of an attack. Vary the routes you take and the time you run, and try to let a friend or relative know the path you will be taking.

As with the prevention of other crimes, awareness is key. Even though music makes your workout more enjoyable, wearing headphones is extremely dangerous. As their use has become more widespread, attacks on joggers have greatly increased. Take note of your surroundings, and run in the direction opposite oncoming traffic. Be aware that an apparently friendly fellow jogger may be a criminal in disguise. If someone asks you for directions or the time, don't stop. Ignore lewd comments; the old adage "sticks and stones . . ." applies here.

Avoid wearing jewelry or expensive watches, but do carry identification, and bring change to make a telephone call. Bring a whistle, or a handheld alarm, and don't be afraid to scream if you are attacked. If Mace or self-defense sprays are not illegal in your area, take these along. Keep these items in an easily accessible place, such as in your hand or on your waistband, and be prepared to use them.

Learn self-defense tactics and practice them. If you're an experienced runner, you have a great amount of power in your legs, so kicking sensitive areas can be an excellent way to escape an attacker. If your assailant is unarmed, do everything you can to flee. If he is armed, surrender any money or valuables at his request. Never get into a car—you're unlikely to return.

Much the same applies to in-line skating, the hugely popular variation on the traditional roller skate. Don't let the great speeds you can reach on in-line skates lull you into a false sense of security. While you may have greater speed than an assailant who is on foot, it only takes one blow to knock an unsuspecting in-line skater off balance. And once you've lost your stride, your in-line skates will actually become a hindrance; it will be extremely hard for you to get up, keep your balance, and/or use any self-defense techniques with in-line skates on your feet. In-line skating can be tremendous fun and an invigorating workout; follow the basic guidelines listed above for jogging to achieve the greatest enjoyment with a maximum of security.

A special word of caution: Whether you are in-line skating, jogging, or walking, be careful crossing bridges. Recently, a 23-year-old woman walking on the pedestrian path of the Brooklyn Bridge was sexually attacked, threatened with a knife, robbed, beaten, and choked into unconsciousness. According to the New York City police, there were 42 robberies, 3 grand larcenies, and 1 assault on the Brooklyn Bridge in 1992.

When alone at night, never use a bridge pedestrian walk; have a friend accompany you. Try to take your walks during daylight hours when other pedestrians use the walkway. Make sure the bridge pathway is well lighted and that it is frequently patrolled by the police.

OUTSIDE PHONE BOOTHS

You are especially vulnerable when using an outside public phone booth. Engrossed in conversation, you become a prime target for pickpockets, muggers, and rapists. In the United States, about 27,000 crimes a year occur at pay telephones. While crime takes place at all hours in any location, 80 percent of abductions and rapes occur late at night and/or in isolated areas. Be certain that the telephone booth is adequately illuminated, and if it is not, find one that is. Keep your purse, briefcase, or other personal belongings within grasp. Never stand with your back to the street and facing the phone. Hold the receiver in your hand, and face the street or sidewalk with your back to the dialing mechanism. This way you can observe any suspicious-looking characters who may approach you.

When using a pay telephone, especially an older one, you may experience the exasperation of your coins not being returned to you when they should be. This may be an equipment malfunction or a rip-off. Your loss might be the result of a thief's blocking the coin return chute in order to capture the coins and hold them for recovery later. If this happens to you, notify the operator. Not only will the operator see to it that your loss is reimbursed, but more important, your call will set in motion the restoration of the phone to proper working order, and perhaps the apprehension of the thief. Newer telephone instruments have built-in guards, that thwart this type of nuisance theft.

MASS TRANSPORTATION

Public transportation can be an economical and quick way of getting around in some parts of the world. However, transit crimes—robbery, rape, purse snatching, pickpocketing, indecent exposure, assault, and even homicide—have made public transportation risky. The New York City Transit Authority reported 6,724 felonies in 1995. This figure stresses the need for awareness when using transit systems. Nevertheless, it reflects a 63-percent decrease since 1990.

A few years ago, a family visiting from Utah was attacked and robbed on a Manhattan subway platform by a vicious youth gang. The teenage son was stabbed to death defending his mother from the assault. The youths, apprehended in a dance hall, confessed that they used the stolen money for admission to the club. Late in 1993, a lone gunman, Colin Ferguson, entered a Long Island Railroad train and randomly fired at least 30 shots, killing 6 and injuring 19. Less-sensational crimes occur every day. For example, in April 1994, a 16-year-old student was shot to death on a subway platform after an argument and a "staredown" with two other youths. The slain youth was shot in the back while returning home 20 minutes before the midnight curfew set by his mother. Although a recent study indicates that a person using public transportation has substantially lower exposure to crime than he or she would have on the street, it is still of the utmost importance to be alert and take steps to protect yourself.

Be sure to know where you're going and the safest way to get there before leaving home. Call the place you are going or your local transit company for directions. It is a good idea to travel with a companion when using mass transportation in more dangerous locales. Naturally, this isn't always possible. Have your fare or token in your hand when you leave your home. This way, you won't have to open your wallet or purse. This will go a long way toward thwarting a pickpocket.

Do not carry more cash or credit cards than you need; you should, however, carry a little extra cash in case of an emergency. Separate your money, keeping portions in your purse, pockets, and on your person. This way, if you are the victim of a purse snatcher or pickpocket, your losses will be minimized. Be alert to anyone who bumps into you for no reason. It's a good idea to look around and take note of who is beside and in back of you. If there is no place to sit, try to stand where you are not crowded by other people. Keep your arms close to your body. Thieves can snatch a wristwatch, particularly one held by an expansion band, right off your arm.

Sit as close as possible to the bus driver or, in a subway car, with the conductor, and avoid empty sections. Don't sit near an exit. A purse snatcher could grab your belongings and be gone before you get out of your seat. Similarly, if you are seated next to an open window, consider the possibility of someone reaching through the window to steal your purse. The best way to protect your belongings is to place them on the seat between you and the wall of the bus or car, or protect them by holding them in your lap. Carry your purse like a football, but hold it in the arm up against the wall of the vehicle. You may wish to loop your arm loosely through the bag's strap, but be prepared to let it go. Do not leave bags unattended as you tie your shoe or look for a train or bus.

Leave as soon as possible if trouble starts or if a fight breaks out. If someone harasses or insults you, remain calm and ignore the insult. If the person persists, tell the driver or conductor and move to another seat.

While waiting for a bus, stand back from the curb until you are ready to board. Never stand near the edge of a train platform. Commuters have been pushed off platforms into the paths of oncoming trains. A young woman coming home from work was waiting near the edge of the platform as a subway train pulled away. A man standing between two cars grabbed her purse strap and pulled her along with the train when she refused to let go. Many robberies take place on isolated or poorly lit platforms. It is best to avoid these stops, especially at night. Try to stand near the token booth attendant while waiting for a subway train. If your train or bus runs on a schedule, plan to arrive just a few minutes before. If there is a delay, wait in a local, well-frequented business or restaurant until departure. During the off-hour period, many stations have signals that indicate when a train is arriving in the station. These allow you to wait in the safest area and proceed to the platform as your train is pulling into the station. Numerous stations also have mirrors that enable you to see around corners and determine whether anyone is loitering. If you observe a suspicious-looking person, go back and alert an attendant or police officer.

During summer months, chain snatchings reach epidemic proportions. The best way to protect yourself is to avoid wearing a chain. Turn your rings around, so that the stones don't show. Dress as modestly as possible. Needless to say, don't take out your wallet or display money. Although panhandling on mass transportation is usually illegal, if you wish to give money to a homeless person, have spare change in a pocket separate from your wallet.

Make sure nobody follows you out of the station or from the bus stop. If you suspect you're being followed, don't get off at a deserted stop, and *never* go home. Ride on, to a busy stop, and take a taxi or call for help. Remember, subways and buses are equipped with two-way radios. In an emergency situation, go to the driver, motorman, conductor, or to a police officer.

Be aware of your surroundings. Books, magazines, and personal headphones are distracting. Never become so engrossed that you do not realize who and what are around you. "Don't Sleep in the Subway, Darling" is more than the title of a once-popular song—it's excellent security advice. The alternative could literally be a "rude awakening." Even closing your eyes to relax will signal a lack of awareness. Keep your eyes open, and remain alert throughout your entire trip.

EXCITEMENT IN THE STREETS

Another possible—if uncommon—street hazard is becoming an innocent victim of an incident not directed at you, such as a riot, fire, brawl, demonstration, or some similar chance mishap. More than one innocent bystander has been killed while a desperado shot it out with the law; more than one bystander has been run in by police along with demonstrators. Recently, on the Upper West Side of Manhattan, a shoot-out between a fleeing bank robber and the police resulted in the killing of an innocent bystander. The investigation revealed that the woman, a New York City Board of Education employee, was cut down in a hail of bullets aimed at the criminal. If you find yourself at such a scene, seek a vantage point as far away as possible from the action, one that offers maximum cover between you and the activity.

Incidents Involving the Police

Recently, there has been a series of shootings by police of young kids playing with toy guns mistakenly thought to be real. In one incident, a 16-year-old youth was shot in the stomach by a plainclothes officer who stated that the youth had displayed what later was found to be a toy replica of a 9-millimeter pistol. The teenager was taken to the city hospital in critical condition.

Police officers perceive gun-related calls as extremely serious. They become particularly cautious and taut if they believe you to be armed. If you are stopped by officers, cooperate fully and follow all instructions immediately. Don't argue with the officers. There will be plenty of time for explanations after the officers feel they have the situation under control. The Crime Prevention Unit of the Los Angeles Police Department suggests the following procedures if you are confronted by a police officer:

❖ Don't make sudden movements.

❖ Never reach into your pockets unless ordered to do so by the officers.

❖ Your hands should be visible at all times.

❖ If you are carrying a gun, inform the officers. Do not reach for it or point it at anyone, especially the officer.

❖ If you are carrying a weapon, drop it immediately.

If you're a witness to a crime on the streets, don't help by getting immediately involved personally. Send for help by calling the police or an ambulance. Only then should you offer your personal assistance, and even then, do so only if you're positive that there is no danger to you personally.

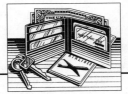

SECURITY IN THE STREETS:
A CHECKLIST

1 Don't carry more money or valuables than you can afford to lose.

2 If approached by a robber, cooperate and remain calm—surrender your valuables.

3 Try to avoid being taken to an alley or other remote location, but if your assailant insists, don't fight back.

4 Don't make any sudden moves—your attacker is probably as nervous as you are.

5 If you are physically attacked, try to get away.

6 Walk on the side of the street facing the oncoming traffic.

7 On a busy street, carry your purse or briefcase on the side of you farthest from the curb, and stay close to the buildings.

8 Carry a shoulder strap purse so that it hangs straight down from your shoulder, suspended between your arm and body. The strap should not cross over your body.

9 Carry handbags with short straps as you would a football, with your arm placed through the strap.

10 If you hear rapidly approaching footsteps behind you, flatten yourself against a building if you think you are the intended victim.

11 If you are being followed on a well-traveled street, slow down, speed up, reverse directions—in other words, indicate to your pursuer that you are aware you are being followed. Then go straight for help.

12 Don't play games if you are followed on a deserted street. Walk briskly either to other people or to a mailbox, preparing to drop your billfold inside to prevent it from being stolen.

13 If followed, don't run straight for home unless help is available there.

14 Self-defense sprays such as Mace or pepper spray are an option for protection, unless outlawed in your state.

15 Running, screaming, and using a loud whistle are recommended defensive tactics. Whistles, however, should not be kept in a purse or around the neck.

16 If you must carry large amounts of money, don't keep it all in one place. Money belts or certain items of women's lingerie are good alternative places for carrying cash.

17 Don't carry keys in the same place as identification that would tell a robber where to find the door that the key fits.

18 Carry credit cards only if there is some likelihood that you will be using them.

19 If you make frequent bank deposits in conjunction with your work, don't carry them with your own valuables. Use armored car services for large deposits.

20 Avoid walking the streets alone after dark. Use taxi-cabs whenever practical.

21 If you must walk alone at night, do not walk near cars parked at the curb or close to doorways or shrubbery, which could conceal an ambusher.

22 If necessary, do not hesitate to walk in the street.

23 If you must regularly walk or go jogging alone at night, vary your route to minimize the possibility of someone's lying in wait to assault you. Let a friend or relative know your route, and call the person when you get home.

24 Be cautious when using outside public phone booths. You become a prime target for pickpockets, muggers, and rapists.

25 When using public transportation, sit near a companion, the motorman, or a conductor. However, take care to avoid the seat nearest an exit door.

26 If seated near an open window, protect your purse or other belongings from being stolen by a thief reaching through the window.

27 Prepare your fare or token before you leave home, in order to avoid opening your handbag or showing your wallet.

28 Be aware of your surroundings, keep your eyes open, and remain alert throughout your entire trip.

29 When you are walking on the street and encounter an arrest, riot, fire, brawl, or other incident, resist the impulse to be a spectator, and shield yourself from the action.

30 If you witness a crime or accident while walking, send for help; don't be of help. Only if qualified help is on the way, and you are positive there is no personal danger to you, should you attempt to be of assistance personally.

14

SECURITY WHILE SHOPPING

Marilyn Bradkowski of Brook River is in guarded condition at Saint Diane's Hospital following an attack that occurred at the Tid-E-Time Washeteria on Locust Street last night. Her assailants, described by passersby as two teenagers, have not been apprehended. No purse was recovered near Mrs. Bradkowski, and police theorize that robbery was the motive for the attack.

Many of the suggestions in the two preceding chapters will enable you to be more secure while shopping, but there are also other factors to keep in mind. During the everyday activity of shopping, you are an especially attractive target because you're likely to be carrying more money than usual. When you shop, you obviously have to pay for your purchases. The most secure method of doing so is to charge your purchases, not with a credit card but through the use of an old-fashioned charge account. The next most secure method of payment is by check, followed by credit card payment. Payment with cash, except for very small purchases, should be avoided.

Don't wear your best jewelry when shopping, and don't wear extravagant clothing—for example, your mink coat. And if, for some reason, you do have to carry a large amount of cash, take care to dress in a modest, inexpensive outfit so as to call minimum attention to yourself.

PARKING WHILE SHOPPING

In a busy store or shop, there is little chance of being assaulted physically, but there is sometimes danger if you are parked in an out-of-the-way location.

Most lots are huge, have inadequate lighting, and lack reliable security. They are perfect places to commit a crime. They are usually outdoor lots set off from main buildings, or multilevel garages connected to an indoor mall or department store and reached by a tightly winding circular ramp. Many hidden spots between and underneath vehicles provide excellent hiding places for criminals. It is easy to be accosted in a wide-open outside area where there are few people and help is far away, or in the more confined isolated space of a multilevel garage. Customers who may be confused about their car's location, loaded down with packages, and concentrating on the search for their car keys are perfect crime victims.

Choose your parking place with care. In a downtown area, for example, try to use an attended parking garage, but remember to remove any personal-identification items from the car and to leave only your ignition key with the attendant. If you're parking in a shopping center lot, select a spot near the mainstream of traffic—the end of the row is ideal. You should choose a space near an entrance or elevator if you decide to park in a multilevel garage connected to a store or mall. If your shopping excursion is likely to extend through sundown, be sure to park near a source of light. Avoid parking near extensive shrubbery, as it provides a perfect cover for a criminal. Do not park next to an occupied car or near suspicious-looking individuals. (For more guidelines on parking, see Chapter 12.)

Never expose cash or valuables in a lot (or, for that matter, at any time while shopping), and never leave valuables visible inside your car. Never leave an animal or, especially, a child inside your car, no matter how short the time you expect to be away from the vehicle. Stay alert as you walk through the parking lot, and walk confidently to communicate that message.

When reentering the parking area, try not to be weighed down with many packages. Have your car keys ready, and do not walk through a lot by yourself, especially after dark. If you feel uncomfortable or see suspicious people, ask a security officer to accompany you to your vehicle. If you think you are being followed, go quickly to a populated area, and find a security or police officer. Report any crime or suspicious incident in the lot. Before you reach your car, look under the vehicle; then check the back seat before getting in, and lock your doors immediately on entry.

Be wary of strangers who approach you in a lot, and never accept their help should your vehicle fail to start. If anyone informs you that there is something wrong with your car, go to the closest building, preferably in a populated area, and find a phone or a security officer. Call the police if you are suspicious.

Follow the regular locking and checking procedures when you park your car and when you return to it. One particularly vicious rapist in a large city preyed exclusively on women at shopping centers. His method of operation was exceedingly simple. He would follow a potential victim, inevitably a lone woman, to her car. Once she was in the car, he would enter through the unlocked passenger door, threaten her with a knife, and direct her to a lonely spot.

If all shoppers took the split second required to lock all doors when leaving and entering cars, a great deal of crime could be avoided.

PROTECTION OF YOUR PURCHASES

If at all possible, arrange to have your parcels delivered. That will prevent your being assaulted by someone trying to snatch your shopping bag. It will also keep a small package from being pilfered out of your shopping bag while you walk down the street or ride on an elevator or subway.

When you do carry packages home, have a small table right inside the door on which you place your parcels. Then close and lock the door. This may help prevent someone from following you right into the house—and even doing so undetected while you're carrying your purchases into another room.

If your shopping jaunt will take you to more than one store and you must carry your parcels home yourself, store them in the trunk of your car, not on the back seat. Remember, though, that while the trunk of your car is considerably more secure than the passenger section, it is by no means impregnable. Therefore, arrange your shopping itinerary so that you acquire the most expensive items last.

It is certainly more pleasant to shop with a friend than by yourself. It is also more secure. In any event, it is a tiring chore, and most dedicated shoppers will occasionally take a short break. We've all enjoyed a cup of coffee or a soft drink, perhaps kicking off our shoes and stretching. But if your packages disappear while you are relaxing, you will find, if you report the incident to the police or to security personnel, that there is little chance of recovering your newly acquired and newly lost property. Larceny/theft is the most common of the eight crimes that the FBI includes in its list of serious crimes, occurring every 4 seconds—15 times a minute, 900 times an hour. The odds are that every man, woman, and child in the country will be victimized by larceny or theft at least once during his or her lifetime.

Don't think only that your property is at risk while you are shopping or when you visit a coffee shop or restaurant; you must also be concerned about your personal safety. In one recent incident, a woman shopping for a wedding gown was killed when armed robbers entered the store. Another woman, dining in an upscale Manhattan restaurant, was robbed by a man who held a gun to her head and demanded money and jewelry. In four other incidents, two well-dressed men followed women leaving expensive restaurants and brazenly robbed them at gunpoint. The police estimated the total cost of the stolen jewelry at over $500,000. Make sure that on leaving a restaurant or store, your guard is up. Relaxation and friendly conversation are fine while dining and perhaps even when shopping; vigilance is called for once you are outside the premises.

MALL SECURITY

According to the International Council of Shopping Centers, there are 39,633 shopping centers in the United States, serving 181 million customers per month: 94 percent of the adult population shop at shopping centers or malls. Malls, then, have become the preferred place to shop.

Attractive as they are, however, malls can be dangerous. In addition to the shoppers' state of unawareness, the wide variety of potential victims and the larger-than-usual amount of cash carried by shoppers attract criminals to shopping malls. Pretending to assist with packages or the car, they pull a weapon and drive away with a hostage. About 95 percent of mall crime is directed against women, the most frequent mall patrons.

Recently, two women were sitting in a car in midafternoon in a Memphis mall when an intruder poked the barrel of a gun through a small opening in the window of the car. He fired twice, killing one of the women and wounding her friend. In one mall parking lot in California, several women were abducted by criminals posing as helpful passersby. In New York City, the body of a woman who had been stabbed to death was found in the back of her car at a shopping center.

While most crimes at malls—like auto theft, abduction, and rape— occur in parking areas, shoppers should also be aware of swindlers and pickpockets. Most importantly, always pay attention to what and who is around you. If you are daydreaming, distracted, or intensely focused on store windows, you are a prime target for criminals. In addition, before entering a store, check to see who's inside. Don't go in if you see a crowd of shoppers together or other "shoppers" staring at you, or if cash registers are left unstaffed. Trust your instincts. If you feel uncomfortable, leave the store immediately.

Always be aware of your purse or bag. Straps are easily cut, and you may not feel your purse being stolen. Keep your bag or purse tucked under your arm. When paying for a purchase, do not place your purse or other purchases on a counter. Alert to the moment of your distraction, thieves take advantage of the opportunity. In the dressing rooms of a store, try not to place purchases or bags on the floor, especially near a door, where they may be easily snatched. Be sure not to leave your purse or bags if you leave a dressing room, even for a moment—a moment is all a thief needs.

Carry as little cash as possible, and don't let anyone see how much money you have. It's better to use credit cards and checks, as these may be canceled if stolen. Never place your wallet where it is visible or easily accessible in your purse or pockets. The pickpocket often bumps into a shopper, seemingly by accident, while deftly lifting a wallet. If anyone brushes against you, check for your purse and wallet immediately. Try to see who bumped you. The criminal may not always be conspicuous, least of all in a crowded mall. Pickpockets usually pass a wallet to a confederate, so you will have to move quickly to catch one.

Always check your purchases before leaving a store to be certain that you got what you paid for. Beware of a "deal" that seems too good to be true. Criminals posing as store employees can offer you a break on a stereo or VCR. When you get home, you may find that your fantastic purchase is a piece of wood in a box.

Crimes at malls are also perpetrated by teenagers and younger children at arcades and restaurants. Groups of teens often menace shoppers, or are disruptive, or are drinking or selling drugs. Report immediately to a guard or police officer any teen causing trouble or engaging in illegal activities. Do not allow your own youngsters to spend excessive time "hanging out." They may be influenced by the negative environment and may even participate in the menacing done by the group.

Malls are the perfect place to abduct a young child. Crowds of people provide cover for the kidnapper, who often targets and accosts children who have strayed from their parents. Know where your children are at all times, and do not leave them unattended in stores, arcades, theaters, or restrooms. Instruct your children to go to a security officer or a store clerk to ask for help if you become separated. Many child molesters wait in public restrooms for children who enter alone. It takes only a second for someone to grab your child. (For more discussion of child abduction, see Chapter 19.)

THE SUPERMARKET

Supermarkets, the most frequent shopping destinations, are often high-crime locations where thieves can easily steal purses or remove wallets from inside purses. Never set your purse on a shopping cart. Keep it on your arm. Many shoppers have had their wallets "pinched" while they were engrossed in pinching tomatoes. Many others have had purses snatched by juveniles running past the cart and right out through an open door or emergency exit.

If you do lose a purse or wallet in a supermarket, report it at once, and demand that store personnel help you try to find it. A supermarket robber, to avoid keeping incriminating evidence on his or her person, will remove the cash and perhaps the credit cards and then discard the wallet, so it is worth looking for.

If your purse is nabbed and it contains keys to your home and identification, change the locks on your home and car.

Many supermarkets will cash checks for the amount of purchase only. The checks must be cashed at a special cashier's window, with the customer returning to the checkout station to exchange the cash for the groceries. If you shop and pay by check at such a store, don't depend on checkout personnel to guard your groceries while you cash your check. Examine exposed items in your bag before you go to cash your check. If any are missing on your return, insist on a recheck before you pay for them. Also, be sure to protect your money by wadding it up in your clenched fist, while transporting it from the cashier's station to the checkout station. This will prevent someone from snatching it from your fingers.

RESTROOM RIP-OFFS

Several years ago, a pair of robbers devised an unusual method for committing their crimes. They simply stationed themselves inside a public restroom and robbed each person who entered. When the crowd was nearing unmanageable proportions, they forced their victims at gunpoint to undress and lie on the floor. Then they left. By the time the victims recovered their composure and their clothes, the robbers were long gone.

It is difficult to see how anyone could have guarded against this bizarre rip-off, but if any of these victims had been shopping with a friend, it is at least possible that the friend, concerned that it was taking too long for the co-shopper to return, might have sounded an alarm.

A much more frequent restroom theft involves women's purses. A thief will wait until she or he sees a purse on the floor inside a cubicle, then reach underneath the partial wall, snatch the purse, and flee. You can prevent this from happening simply by keeping your purse off the floor of the cubicle or placing it on a shelf, if the stall has one. Do not hang it on the clothes hook mounted on the cubicle door. Brazen thieves can reach over and lift coats, jackets, and pocketbooks off the hooks. Looping your handbag over your arm provides a great deal of protection and a minimum of inconvenience, or if you are with someone, ask that person to hold the handbag for you. When using a washbasin, do not select the one nearest the door. A thief could easily snatch the bag and be out the door before you could react effectively.

CREDIT CARDS

The impact of credit cards on the nation's economy staggers the imagination. Over 50 percent of purchases are paid for by credit card. The available purchasing power is enormous. Total credit limits are more than twice as great as the nation's entire amount of money in circulation.

Along with the popularity of the credit card, there has been an increase in credit card fraud. It has become a way for criminals to make billions of dollars worldwide. For example, one credit card company lost over $6 billion, 1.6 percent of all transactions in a single year. The three regions in the United States that have the highest credit card fraud rates, according to the United States Postal Inspector's Service, are Northern New Jersey and Southern New York, Los Angeles, California, and Dallas and Fort Worth in Texas.

Three elements of credit card fraud directly affect you: the use of counterfeit credit cards, the use of stolen cards, and the fraudulent use of valid credit card numbers without the physical presence of the card.

Much of the impact of counterfeit cards has been countered by technological advances. Those birds and monogrammed globes you find on credit cards are not there to amuse your children. They are laser-generated holograms, which are incredibly complicated and relatively expensive to produce, but the card companies realize that the cost of unrestricted counterfeiting would be many times greater. While frauds with fake credit cards may be stymied at present, you may be certain that the cheats are working hard to separate you and your money one way or another.

A less-expensive way for a credit card thief to rip you off is the simple tactic of stealing your cards. For the high-volume thief desiring a larger take, vendors sell lists of valid credit card numbers. These are obtained in a number of ways by various thieves: pickpockets, robbers, burglars, prostitutes, addicts, light-fingered juvenile delinquents, and dishonest bank employees (who may have access to the account numbers of every holder of the bank's credit cards).

Most of the activity on a fraudulently obtained credit card occurs during the first 3 days of a thief's possession. After this time, the "hot" card will be sold to another thief or switched, perhaps by an accomplice, for a "clean" card. Then the whole operation repeats itself.

As you might expect, Fridays are the big days for credit card frauds. Not only is the legitimate cardholder filled with the "thank God it's Friday" spirit, but also the card abuser has two extra weekend days of grace to cheat and steal before Monday's "business as usual" stems the tide of weekend theft.

Merchants and/or their employees may sometimes abet the frauds. Their contribution is primarily apathy and carelessness rather than duplicity. Ask yourself this question: When was the last time that your signature on a credit card was compared with that on the credit card voucher you just signed? Merchants also fail to check the list of canceled credit cards or the card pickup bulletins that the credit firms issue.

In other cases, merchants are cheats. They may cheat by printing extra billing sets using your card or by violating no-authorization limits imposed on certain transactions. Still other merchants are outright crooks. They will buy stolen cards, borrow or steal lists of valid credit card numbers, and run them through as legitimate transactions, often splitting the take with the list vendor.

Make sure that the clerk validates only your charges with your card. It isn't uncommon for a salesclerk to validate two or more charge tickets, then trace your signature through one of the very thin copies of the document set, and fill in some additional items later. This is a particular hazard in a service station, where you might remain in your car while the attendant takes your card inside to complete the paperwork. Try always to stay with your card, and thereby avoid the effort of having to prove forgery later.

Although most stores have eliminated use of carbon paper in credit card receipts, some may not have. Make sure that the clerk returns all of the carbons to you along with your receipt. The numbers on the carbon may be easily read, and this information in the hands of a card "booster" could result in an expensive experience for you. Take all receipts with you, and tear them up before throwing them away.

Avoid revealing personal information such as your address and telephone number on credit card receipts. And if you are using your credit card as identification for cashing a check, make sure the clerk does not write your credit card number on the check. Merchants are prohibited from charging your account if your account is not valid according to operating rules of Visa, Mastercard, and American Express.

Organized-crime rings steal and sell credit cards. There is usually a time lag of several weeks before the numbers of stolen credit cards are distributed widely, allowing the credit card criminal considerable time to use a stolen card. When the card does get listed as missing, however, a thief may try to switch cards with you, exchanging his hot card for your clean one. Get into the habit of checking the name on your card each time it is returned to you. If you are victimized by a switch and you discover it immediately, take it up with a manager, not the salesperson or waiter involved. The clerk or waiter could simply claim an error and hurry to retrieve your card.

Con-artists may attempt to steal from you by representing themselves as "security officers" checking into illegal use of credit cards. They will ask you for your credit card number in order to "verify" it. *Do not give your credit card number to anyone.* And needless to say, if anyone calls and asks for your credit card number, hang up. Even a representative from your issuing bank or company will not request this information. Call the issuing company immediately.

Many cardholders themselves are credit card criminals. They have only $50 to lose—the maximum liability for any illegal charges on a card reported lost or stolen—so they think they can get away with reporting the loss of their card, and then going on a spending spree. If they report the loss early enough, they will probably not be charged the $50 fee.

Of course, it may be their bad luck to attempt a charge through one of the so-called point-of-sale terminals. These are tied into a central computer that updates customers' balances as transactions occur. These smart "real-time" systems, which are increasingly replacing the slower manual systems, make things tougher for the credit card sharpie, as any such charges would not be honored.

Protection of Your Credit Cards

Some banks offer to imprint your picture and signature on your credit card. Provided the store checks, picture and signature offer extra protection against the use of the card by an unauthorized person. The best recourse, though, is to leave your credit cards at home; take them with you only if you plan to use them.

Keep credit cards in one secure place. That way, if they are lost or stolen you will know right away. To protect yourself, compile the following information for each credit card in your possession:

❖ Card name (American Express, Visa, Mastercard, etc.).
❖ Issuing organization (such as a bank or other financial institution).
❖ Your account number. (This is usually the longest number on the card. There may be a four-digit number elsewhere on the face of the card; include this number, too.)
❖ Telephone number for reporting lost or stolen cards. (The number may be displayed on the card.)
❖ Street address for sending a telegram to confirm card loss. (The operator responding to your telephone call may advise you that this is an unnecessary expense; on the other hand, your copy of the confirming telegrams could be worth a great deal of money. Should you decide not to confirm in writing, at least get the name of the person to whom you made your last report.)

If You Lose a Credit Card

Report the loss as soon you realize it has occurred. Follow religiously the instructions you receive from the issuing firm. File a report with the police within 24 hours of the loss or theft. You will probably be issued a new card by your credit card company. In many instances, you will find that you haven't lost your card at all but merely misplaced it. In this event, you need only to destroy the old one and begin using the new one. You may be contacted by the security department of the issuer, particularly if a number of bogus charges are made to your card. Of course, you should cooperate.

Finally, when you get your bill, it may include some unfamiliar charges. You should call these to your company's attention, but at the same time pay only the charges you legally owe. Federal law allows you to challenge charges for which you are not responsible, but the law will not exempt you from paying your just debts.

Even your reports of a lost or stolen card to the issuing bank, the credit card company, and the police may not be enough to protect you from a rapidly increasing type of fraud known as "true-name fraud." This is when a criminal uses the information from your credit cards and/or identification to impersonate you in order to open lines of credit. To prevent this, call all three major credit agencies and ask them to add a fraud statement to your file immediately. This statement will prevent anyone from using your lost or stolen card to open a new line of credit. The companies following this request should send you a free credit report, and you should keep checking your credit reports regularly for any fraudulent activity. Telephone numbers of the three major credit agencies are:

Experian Consumer Assistance (800) 422-4879
Trans Union (714) 870-5565
Equifax (800) 685-1111

When you wish to obtain credit in the future, tell the credit issuer why the fraud statement is in your file.

Credit Card User's Responsibilities

You have probably been screened by the issuing company, and they have determined that you are a responsible person. As such, you are morally, if not legally, required to do certain things:

❖ Examine all charge tickets before you sign them. In this way, you can prevent errors or fraud before they become fact.

❖ Personally destroy all carbons of your billing sets. Do not allow the clerk to do this for you.

❖ Retain your copies of billing sets, and compare them to charges on your statement to protect yourself from charges that appear on the statement but aren't yours.

❖ Hang on to your billing copy until you pay it. There is a time lag, often a considerable one, from the time of the charge until it finally appears on your statement. Don't make the mistake of feeling you have met all your financial obligations merely because you have paid your current statement in full.

❖ Don't leave your credit cards lying around your home, office, or, especially, your car.

❖ Don't carry your credit cards in your billfold along with your cash and driver's license. In this way, you won't risk losing everything at once.

❖ An essential safety precaution is to destroy any unneeded duplicate cards. You are liable for the first $50 of illegal charges made before you report the theft or loss of a card. Insurance is available for reimbursing losses stemming from credit card theft or loss.

Services that will register all your credit cards are available. Should your cards be stolen, you call a 24-hour toll-free number, and the service will immediately notify all issuers of your credit cards. All liability is ended as soon as you report the loss, including the $50 of illegal charges. Related services are also available, including emergency cash and prepaid airline tickets for a stranded traveler, requests for replacements of stolen cards, and warning labels to affix to each credit card. There is no limit on the number of cards covered by these services, so the more cards you carry, the more advantageous the service is to you.

NIGHTTIME SHOPPING

Today nearly half the workforce is female, and for many the most convenient time for shopping is after work, at night. All elements of concern during daytime shopping are also present at night, when there are a few additional causes for alarm. Darkness is the ally of the thief, because visibility is impaired at night. You must be more alert at night. If you are on foot, you will be less able to discern someone approaching you. An intruder crouched in the backseat of your car will be more difficult to spot, and a thief who took your belongings will find it easier to disappear under the cover of darkness. Moreover, the composition of nighttime crowds is different—more muggers, pickpockets, and robbers are cruising the streets at night. Most retail establishments have fewer personnel on the job at night, so you will be less protected in the places where you do shop. At night there also tend to be more intoxicated shoppers, who are subject to irrational behavior that might be directed at you.

Self-service laundries—or, for that matter, self-service anythings—are especially dangerous at night, so dangerous that you should never go to such places alone at night. If you can't arrange to have someone accompany you, don't go.

24-HOUR BANKING

The computer-operated, 24-hour banking establishments that have proliferated throughout the country can be extremely hazardous. One hears of victims being forced at gunpoint to withdraw money or having their money taken after withdrawal. Some thieves watch as you enter your Personal Identification Number (PIN); then they steal your card and take the money out themselves.

A 34-year-old man was withdrawing $100 from a cash machine when two youths entered the facility. They robbed him at gunpoint and fled in a waiting car. Many victims lose much more than their money. Some have been raped, kidnapped, and murdered. Off-duty New York City police sergeant Keith Levine came to the aid of someone being mugged by two thieves. The police sergeant was shot and killed after an exchange of gunfire. Ironically, the man who was robbed had been trying to use a stolen bank card. A young woman was withdrawing money when a mugger grabbed her from behind, put a gun to her head, and demanded she withdraw $400. After this, he abducted and eventually murdered her.

The media has also reported incidents of fraud at Automatic Teller Machines (ATMs). Two men rigged a fake ATM machine in a Connecticut mall and made illegal withdrawals along the East Coast totaling over $100,000. The fake machine copied people's PINs, and the men proceeded to make counterfeit cards using these secret codes. Each of the men was sentenced to 2½ years in federal prison.

Crimes such as these have focused on the need for legislation to ensure customer security. In 1990, California was the first state to establish mandatory security standards for ATMs. Since then, other states have followed suit.

Surveys of the Bank Administration Institute (BAI) report that more than half the crimes committed in banks involved ATMs. Approximately half the incidents take place between 7:00 p.m. and midnight. Almost two-thirds of the victims are women. You are most vulnerable when by yourself. Nearly all attacks, 96 percent, involve a single victim. Try to bring a friend along to watch your back while you are at the machine.

The number of muggings at cash points are lower than you might expect, with a national average of one mugging out of every 3 million transactions. However, this rate fluctuates according to region. In New York, for example, your chances of victimization are three times higher. Moreover, about 14 percent of ATM crimes result in injury of the victim. In about 13 percent of these episodes, the victims denied their assailants requests or fought back. A weapon, most frequently a gun, was involved in almost 50 percent of the incidents.

In providing a service, the bank is responsible for ensuring personal safety. Nevertheless, always seek bank machines with good security. A few simple yet practical guidelines to watch for include:

❖ Untinted glass doors so passersby can see inside and call for assistance in the event of an attack
❖ Entry limited to ATM cardholders, with a door that locks behind you
❖ Well-lit and populous locations in a safe neighborhood
❖ Surveillance cameras
❖ A screen and data entry pad that can be viewed only by you, as a customer, so that others may not learn your access code
❖ Mirrors at the terminal allowing you to see who's behind you
❖ Telephones with an operator, not a recording, who will answer when you pick up the receiver or push a "panic button" to summon assistance
❖ A security officer

Use a machine you are familiar with. Avoid ATMs on the street. If you have a choice, choose an indoor machine in which the door locks behind you over an outdoor machine, especially a location with security officer and cameras. Never let a stranger in! Steer clear of facilities with panhandlers operating as ATM doormen. Even if they are harmless, they might let in somebody behind you who is not. Stay away from cash points that have available hiding places or bushes. In addition, don't use the same cash point at the same time every day. Criminals are on the lookout for routines.

Safe locations for using bank machines after the banks close are located in 24-hour stores, like an all-night supermarket. Many supermarkets allow you to pay with your ATM card. The purchase price is deducted automatically from your account, so you don't have to worry about carrying cash. The cashier will give you a handheld entry pad to enter your PIN. Do *not* give your PIN to the cashier, and make sure nobody watches you enter it.

Perhaps the safest location of all is the recent installation of ATMs in police station lobbies. One is already in place in the Englewood section of Chicago, and the Los Angeles City Council has approved the installation of 30 new ATMs in various local police stations.

If you feel you are being menaced while operating an ATM, you can protect yourself somewhat by entering an incorrect number three times in succession. If you do this, many machines not only will fail to deliver money to you but will also keep your card; that might avert a robbery. However, not all computerized banking devices work this way. Still better protection is to do your banking during daylight hours.

If, however, you must go to the bank at night and cannot arrange for someone to accompany you, be cautious. Look around for suspicious people loitering outside the bank or waiting in a nearby car. Check for loiterers inside the banking area as well. Have your card ready so that you don't have to fumble for it, and don't waste time. Complete your transaction, and leave as quickly as possible. Don't leave your receipt behind. (Follow the same guidelines for terminals located outside a building.) Put the money and your bank card into your pocket, wallet, or handbag quickly; take the time to arrange everything later. Check to see if anyone is following you; if someone is, go directly to a police station or any public place to ask for assistance. Some banks in Tucson, Arizona, and Oakland, California, have installed red panic buttons that can be used to summon emergency assistance.

If you drive to the cash machine, park as close to it as possible. Do *not* leave your keys in the car with the engine running, and lock all your doors. Many have run to the machine for "just a second," only to find their vehicles gone when they return.

When using drive-up teller machines, be certain to lock all doors and keep all windows rolled up, except the driver's. Keep your engine running and remain observant. As with walk-up machines, don't use those in isolated and poorly lit locations. In 5 percent of muggings at drive-up ATMs, the victim's vehicle was also stolen. Remember, your best ATM protection is increased awareness.

Treat your bank card like cash. If it is lost or stolen, report that fact immediately. Your loss is limited to $50 if it is reported within 2 days; beyond that your loss limit is $500. Similarly, check your monthly statement for unauthorized usage. If you report an unauthorized use of your card within 60 days, you will be held accountable for only $50. Send a letter to your bank via certified mail, so that you will have a receipt of when the notification was mailed.

Never lend your card to anyone or use it to help someone else with a transaction. Do not accept assistance from anyone on the use of your card. Never disclose your PIN. Be wary of con-artists who try to persuade you to hand over your card. A common scheme is to pose as a bank security officer attempting to repair a malfunctioning machine. The crook will ask for your card and PIN to try and test if the machine is operating correctly.

No bank employee should ever request your PIN. A thief who has stolen your purse or wallet may call you and impersonate a police officer or bank employee. The caller will claim to have caught your purse snatcher and will request your PIN to determine if any cash has been withdrawn from your bank account. Don't fall for these scams! Report suspicious events to the bank security office or the police.

If you must record your PIN, store the record securely. Better still, memorize the number. In selecting an identification number, do not use a sequence of numbers from your phone number, date of birth, Social Security number, street address, or any other numbers found among identification papers you carry. If a dishonest person should come into possession of your bank card, you want to deny him or her an easy guess of your identification number. If you carry several such cards, select different ID numbers for each. Thus, if someone guesses (or observes) one number, you may limit your losses to assets available through the use of that one compromised card.

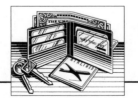

SECURITY WHILE SHOPPING: A CHECKLIST:

1. Don't carry cash while shopping, if you can avoid it.
2. Use a charge account, followed by—in order of preference—check, credit card, or cash.
3. Do not overdress while shopping, and avoid wearing jewelry.

4 Select a secure parking spot, especially if your shopping is likely to extend through sundown.

5 Deliberately park close to the building you will be entering, or park near the main flow of traffic; avoid the edges of a lot. In a multilevel garage, choose a space near an entrance or elevator.

6 At night, park in a well-lit area or under a light. Avoid bushes that provide cover for a criminal.

7 When choosing a spot, avoid suspicious-looking persons, and do not park next to occupied vehicles.

8 Lock all doors when exiting your vehicle. If you are in an attended garage, leave only your ignition key with the attendant.

9 Never expose valuables or personal identification in the car.

10 Never leave a pet or, especially, a child unattended in a vehicle.

11 Walk purposefully through the lot to communicate confidence.

12 Avoid overloading yourself with bags when returning to your vehicle, and have your keys ready before entering the lot.

13 Do not walk alone in a lot, especially at night. If you feel uncomfortable, ask a guard to escort you to your vehicle.

14 If you suspect someone is following you, go to the nearest populated area, and find a security or law enforcement officer.

15 Report any crime in the parking lot.

16 Check your backseat before getting in your vehicle, and once inside lock all doors immediately.

17 If you have car trouble, never accept a stranger's help. Return to a populated area, and find a phone or security officer.

18 Arrange for delivery of parcels, if possible.

19 Locate a small table near the front door of your home on which to place parcels while you lock the door.

20 Use the car trunk, not the passenger compartment, for storing parcels.

21 Arrange to purchase expensive items last, to minimize the time you will be required to safeguard them.

22 Shop with a friend whenever possible.

23 Keep an eye on your purse, bag, and other packages. Hold purses under your arm, and never put them on a store counter or on the floor or near a door in a dressing area.

24 Do not place your wallet on top of your bag or in a pocket where it is visible and accessible. Be extra alert if someone brushes against you, and identify who it was in case you have been pickpocketed.

25 Be wary of "bargains" offered by "store employees"; they may be criminals attempting to swindle you.

26 Do not permit your children to spend extended time at malls, and report any disruptive or illegal teenage behavior that you experience or witness.

27 Never leave young children unattended in a mall, especially in crowded areas or restrooms.

28 Do not leave a purse unattended in a supermarket cart.

29 Search for a purse or billfold that has been lost in a store. Thieves usually discard all but money and, in some instances, credit cards.

30 If your stolen purse contains keys and IDs, change your locks.

31 If you must transport money from a supermarket cashier's cage to a checkout station, protect it.

32 Keep your purse off the floor when using a public restroom. Be cautious about hanging your purse on a hook on the cubicle door.

33 Be sure that only your own credit card charge has been validated. Personally destroy all carbons of the billing set.

34 Beware the switch of a stolen credit card for your own.

35 Plan your course of action in the event that your credit cards are lost or stolen. Destroy unneeded duplicate cards.

36 Always examine your monthly credit card billings for fraudulent charges or errors, particularly if a card was lost or stolen.

37 Take extra precautions when shopping after dark. At night there are more muggers, pickpockets, robbers, and drunks, and fewer store clerks, all of which works to the shopper's disadvantage.

38 Do not go to self-service laundries or unattended merchandise or service outlets alone at night.

39 Be cautious when using 24-hour banking equipment. If you notice suspicious-looking people hanging out, wait until they leave, or visit another branch.

40 Select random, difficult-to-guess identification numbers for use with your ATM bank cards. Don't use a Social Security number or phone number, a street address, or any other numbers on identification papers you carry.

41 If you utilize several different bank cards, select different ID numbers for each.

15

SECURITY IN THE
WORKPLACE

A third-grade teacher had her purse stolen from a desk drawer in her classroom. The thief was never caught. The teacher had only a few dollars and no credit cards with her that day, and a relative was able to bring her a spare set of keys, so she was inconvenienced very little. Still, after she had changed the locks in her home and car and replaced her lost purse, wallet, glasses, driver's license, and other documents, the theft had cost her well over $200. She never recovered her loss from her insurance carrier, nor was she able to establish it with the Internal Revenue Service, simply because the desk drawer was not locked.

SECURITY ON THE JOB

The workplace, once an oasis of security, has evolved into a dangerous site. Don't view company security policies as an expression of your firm's lack of trust in you, but rather as a proactive shield for you and your job. Company security really can mean protection for your job as well as your person. If you or anyone you worked with experienced, while on the job, an assault, stabbing, shooting, an act of arson, or a suicide, then you were the victim of violence in the workplace. Crime and violence on the job not only diminishes your productivity; it also could result in loss of your property, in bodily injury, or possibly even in death. Workplace security encompasses more than protection from bodily harm, however. A multitude of property crimes plague offices regardless of the type of company for which you work. Most of us spend about one-third of our time on the job—not counting the time it takes us to get there and back—so it's worth taking steps to protect yourself during what is actually most of your waking hours. Every company—ranging from the one-person shop with a special hiding place for accumulations of cash to the giant defense contractor with a security department numbering thousands of employees—has some sort of security program.

Protecting Your Property

Don't leave billfolds or keys in your jacket or coat at work. Put your purse in a desk drawer, and lock it. Take nothing for granted. One excellent rule for protecting a handbag is this: If you are not in physical contact with your bag—actually *touching* it—then it must be locked away.

A purse is not all you might lose at the office. Other favorite targets are cash, small calculators, diskettes, typewriters, clothing, pen and pencil sets, cameras, radios, color television sets, and computer equipment. If you work in a building with many tenants who are strangers to each other, you are much more likely to suffer a loss than if you work in a place where everyone knows everyone else, at least by sight.

When leaving your office, put calculators or other small valuable items in your desk, and lock it. Few desks have adequate locks, but you might at least prevent random pilferage this way.

Protecting Your Company's Property and Information

You can secure large equipment such as computers, faxes, slide projectors, and adding machines with special desktop equipment locks, using bolts or adhesive pads. Some adhesive pads resist a pull of 3 tons, yet do not require the drilling of any holes in the desk.

If you encounter strangers passing through your office, a friendly "May I help you, please?" is an excellent deterrent. If the stranger is in need of assistance, he or she will be grateful. If not, he or she will probably go away. Of course, this could backfire. We know of one instance when a buyer in a major midwestern department store asked that question of a man in coveralls holding an appliance dolly. "Yes, sir, I'm supposed to pick up that television set for the window display at the [so-and-so] suburban store," came the reply. The buyer not only let him take the set but even helped him load it into a truck. No one saw the driver or the TV set again.

The protection of a company's information is often more critical than the security of a company's property. A switchboard operator who says "I'm sorry, Mr. Smith is out of the country and won't return until the twenty-seventh" might be responsible for a burglary at the Smith residence, maybe even the kidnapping of the Smith children or an assault on a member of the family, without ever realizing it.

An engineer might make a remark like "If we don't get that boron in we'll never have the new condensers ready for the 1998 models" and thereby place millions of dollars' worth of research and development expenditures at the disposal of a competitor. A secretary might be careless in disposing of an extra photocopy (or carbon copy, for that matter) of a highly confidential memo and cost the company millions. A casual remark by a lawyer's or physician's clerk-typist could cause a large loss in an invasion-of-privacy suit.

The list of things that can go wrong through the inadvertent release of confidential or personal information is endless. So lock up all important reports and memos when you leave the office, even if only for a few minutes. And don't be in such a hurry at quitting time that you fail to lock filing cabinets. In short, leave a clean, orderly desk when you're away from it. This way, you are doing all you can to guard against the use of confidential information against your company and thus indirectly against you.

PROTECTION AGAINST COMMON BUSINESS CRIMES

Here are just a few of the things that you, as an employee, can do to protect yourself and your company against the most common types of crimes committed against business.

Bad Checks, Counterfeit Money, Forgeries

Bad checks probably account for between 10 and 15 percent of crime-related business losses. If your work involves handling checks, you must guard against this type of loss. Follow all your company's procedures, and insist on adequate identification before you cash a check for anyone. If there is any doubt in your mind, or if the person offering the check cannot provide satisfactory identification, don't cash it.

If you handle cash on the job, you may come into contact with *counterfeit money*. The government will not reimburse a businessperson who accepts a counterfeit bill. If he or she accepts a counterfeit bill and attempts to pass it on, knowing it to be a bogus bill, the person might well be in violation of federal laws. The easiest way to spot a counterfeit bill is to look at it and feel it. The paper on which legitimate bills are printed is of a special manufacture, available only to the government. It has a distinctive enough feel that a side-by-side touch comparison will enable you to determine the difference. The authentic paper is made from fibers, and its red and blue fibers are visible even to the naked eye. The engraving reproduction quality of a bogus bill will be noticeably inferior to that of an authentic bill. The background behind the pictures on genuine bills is composed of many small dots or finely etched lines. Even if the counterfeiters use a photographic process in their reproduction, counterfeit backgrounds will tend to "close in" and be considerably darker than those on legitimate bills. The same is true of the fine weblike filigree work around the borders of genuine bills.

The difference between most counterfeit bills and the genuine article is so striking that there is really no excuse for accepting a fake. When in doubt, make a side-by-side comparison, and refuse to accept a questionable bill. The person offering it will be outraged, but by holding your ground, you can avoid loss to your company.

Forgeries, especially forged checks, are another problem you may encounter. If you can't adequately identify an endorser, and the endorser can't adequately identify him- or herself, don't cash the check. Satisfactory identification consists of at least two items that bear the person's signature—for example, a driver's license and a credit card. Strictly enforced limits on the amount for which a check may be cashed are especially recommended.

Don't assume that a check is good just because it is drawn on the federal, state, or local government. If you cash such a check, and the signature of the rightful recipient has been forged by someone who stole it from a mailbox, you and your firm will suffer the loss. This is especially hazardous in the late spring or early summer, when income tax refund checks are abundant, and also at those times when welfare, Social Security, or other assistance checks are in the mails.

Shoplifting

The National Coalition to Prevent Shoplifting estimates the cost of shoplifting to be $26 billion a year, raising consumer prices 5 to 7 percent. Another study indicates that the estimated loss of profits resulting from shoplifting ranges from 0.5 percent to a full 5 percent, depending on the business. This may not sound like a large amount, but in most businesses a loss of 1 percent can cause heavy damage; higher losses can be crippling.

While anybody fitting any description can be a shoplifter, the great majority of shoplifting is done on impulse by amateurs, compared to planned theft by professionals. Juveniles are often involved as part of a dare, peer pressure, gang initiation, or just for "kicks." Occasionally it is a cry for help; troubled children will attempt to steal, subconsciously hoping to get caught to create attention for themselves.

After juveniles, housewives are the next most likely group to shoplift; in fact, the majority of all shoplifting incidents, 59 percent, involves females.

While accounting for a small number of shoplifting incidents, "professional" shoplifters do a great deal of damage. They will go into a store, often searching for a designated item, steal it, and resell it at a much cheaper price.

The most likely target items for all shoplifters are the following: For women, it's cosmetics, women's clothing, and jewelry. For men, it's alcohol and cigarettes.

If you work in a place that may be victimized by a shoplifter, keep your eyes open, and don't forget to ask "May I help you?" The last thing a shoplifter wants is a lot of attention. Often, especially when the thief is a nonprofessional, the suspected shoplifter will appear nervous and jumpy, with a flushed face. Usually he or she will try to distract you by requesting additional merchandise or by dropping items on the floor. Actions such as repeatedly comparing two different samples of the same item, the frequent opening and closing of a purse, or erratic movement around the store are possible indicators that something is wrong. Keep an eye out for people wearing bulky clothing (especially in warm weather) or carrying large shopping bags, partially opened umbrellas, folded newspapers, or schoolbooks.

Shoplifters often work in teams. One person may take a position to block your view of the other's theft. An accomplice may create a distraction while the partner steals. Small children, accompanied by their parents, can be unwitting accomplices or may even have been trained to steal. Pay attention to people who try on merchandise in open view of store personnel. Professional shoplifters may don sweaters, gloves, hats, and scarves and walk casually out of the store as if the merchandise were theirs.

It is estimated that only 1 in 49 shoplifting incidents ends with the apprehension of the suspect. While these data may urge you to be overzealous, be careful; stay alert and be concerned, but follow your company's policies concerning the apprehension and detention of shoplifters. No matter how well intentioned it may be, an overzealous reaction on your part could result in losses to you personally and to your company in the event of false arrest.

A number of actions can minimize shoplifting losses. Practically no one steals when store personnel are looking. It is advisable to lower displays and shelving to no more than 5 feet in height, enabling employees to see much of the store. Wider aisles and open spaces add to the visibility and make theft more difficult. This economy is achieved, however, at the expense of space that otherwise could contain merchandise. Some trade-offs will be necessary to achieve optimum use of space. Obviously, adequate lighting is recommended.

You can also extend your employees' range of vision by judiciously placing mirrors (especially two-way and convex mirrors) throughout the store. A reward program for employees who turn in shoplifters can be effective (and could curtail employee theft, as well).

Security officers and/or floorwalkers are also deterrents to theft, especially when they (especially near exits) are clearly visible. Floorwalkers, as plain-clothes officers roaming the store as customers, are used to nab shoplifters after they've done the deed.

Electronic surveillance devices, such as removable tags and disposable labels, are currently used more often than not as preventative measures. Unless removed or demagnetized, the devices will sound an alarm as the shoplifter attempts to leave the store. These are not foolproof, however;

anyone determined enough (i.e., the professional) will find ways to render these devices useless. Some stores actually plant subliminal antitheft messages in the Muzak that's played over the loudspeakers.

There is a debate over the effectiveness of fake deterrents, such as simulated video cameras or phony loudspeaker statements asking for security. While they may deter some shoplifters from giving in to temptation, there is the risk that word will get out about the authenticity of these "dummies," leading to an *upswing* in shoplifting.

Remember, some of your merchandise is more expensive than other merchandise. The most expensive items should be protected with locked showcases. Another protection for your better goods is to locate them as far from the exit doors as is practical. Doing so will require the thief to negotiate a longer escape route.

Just as it is practical to increase sales help during the holiday season due to the heavy volume of sales, it is wise to increase security help as well, as 45 percent of *all* shoplifting crimes are committed during the holidays.

Spread the word that you're tough on shoplifters. Post signs in the store: "Shoplifters Will Be Prosecuted." And mean it.

Employee Theft

Employee theft is a more serious threat to business than shoplifting, burglary, or bookkeeping errors combined. Mark Lipman, one of the world's foremost experts on security, wrote: "The average company thief is a married man, has two or three children, lives in a fairly good community, plays bridge with his neighbors, goes to church regularly, and is well thought of by his boss. He is highly trusted and a good worker, one of the best in the plant. That's why he can steal so much over such long periods and why it's so hard to discover his identity." (New York: Harper's Magazine Press, 1973, p. 160).

Despite the millions spent on security devices, employee theft continues. According to the National Retail Merchants Association, large retailers (those selling more than $100 million of merchandise per year) lose a national total of $20 million a day through *internal* theft.

Thefts often occur after business hours. Preparing to steal, employees put merchandise into their cars or hide it in garbage cans or empty boxes for later removal. Other common methods of employee theft include under-adding merchandise at cash registers and changing inventory counts and accounting books.

The best way you as an employee can help fight theft is to abide by and respect company rules. The most dedicated scofflaw might well be stealing—while attempting to make you an unwitting accomplice by undermining employee respect for antitheft rules. Such rules are necessary because some of your co-workers are undeserving of trust, and it is your obligation to do whatever you can to get rid of them.

Discovering that a co-worker is stealing is a tough problem, leading to the question of how many pencils one must steal before it becomes serious. Knowledge of an obviously serious theft might place you in actual physical danger. Yet failure to do anything about it would make you a morally, if not legally, culpable accessory. Your obligation to your employer should outweigh any loyalty that you might have to a thief who also happens to be a friend.

Experts estimate that stealing by employees accounts for two-thirds of retail theft. In addition to as much as the $13-billion annual take of employee thieves, there are other losses impossible to quantify. How much, for example, does it cost the basically honest employee, in terms of lost self-respect, when he or she takes things "because everybody else does"? What does it cost a harried manager to receive a financial statement that shows sudden and unexplainable losses? How much time is lost pondering these imponderable questions?

Employee Screening

Companies should thoroughly screen all applicants, in order to determine character and integrity as well as technical qualifications. Fingerprinting, background checks, and indepth interviews are valuable tools for selecting employees who will have access to confidential data or software.

WORKPLACE VIOLENCE

According to the National Institute for Occupational Safety and Health (NIOSH), homicides are the third leading cause of death in the workplace for all workers, after deaths from motor vehicles and machines. Homicide is the leading cause of death among women in the workplace, accounting for 42 percent of such deaths. On average, 15 people are murdered each week in the United States.

Assaults on workers occur much more frequently than occupational homicides. These are no longer isolated events. Assault and harassment can occur at anytime. The National Safe Workplace Institute estimates that workplace violence costs American businesses at least $4.2 billion in employer medical/legal expenses and lost worktime.

Victim and Attacker Patterns

Nearly half the victims of on-the-job homicide were 25 to 44 years of age, but the most vulnerable group were workers 65 and older who experienced the highest rate of homicide: 2.0 per 100,000. A gun was the weapon of choice in at least three-quarters of occupational homicides. Only 14 percent of murders were inflicted by knives or other sharp-edged or pointed instruments.

Research has determined that the typical workplace killer is a male loner, 36 years of age, with few friends, low self-esteem, scarcely any interests outside the job, an affinity for guns, a fascination with the military, a vicious temper, and a history of family problems. He holds extremist attitudes and grudges and is likely to abuse alcohol and drugs. Additionally, the workplace attacker is likely to have an unstable family life, a migratory job history, few healthy outlets for anger and resentment, and an obsession with media reports of violence, especially in the workplace. Often, the killer is depressed or suicidal, acts paranoid, and files unreasonable grievances and lawsuits. In perpetual denial, the killer tends to assign to others responsibility for his personal and on-the-job problems.

Factors that may precipitate workplace violence include inadequate security, stress, alcohol or drug abuse, loss of job, being passed over for promotion, arguments with a boss or co-worker, disagreement over a new policy or procedure, refusal of worker's compensation claims, disputes over pay, a bitter divorce, and personal conflicts with a spouse, ex-spouse, or girl- or boyfriend.

Hazardous Activities

Be especially aware and alert if you engage in the following activities identified by NIOSH as high-risk factors for on-the-job homicides:

❖ Exchanging money with the public

❖ Working by yourself or with few people

❖ Work that requires late night or early morning hours

❖ A job in a high-crime area

❖ Protecting valuable property or merchandise

❖ Working outside, often in isolated locations

No wonder taxicab drivers, police officers, and store clerks are among job holders suffering the highest rates of occupational murder.

A Tense Situation

If you are confronted with a volatile situation on the job that appears to be heading towards physical violence, don't take a confrontational stance; try to walk or run away. Say you have to go to the washroom, or to retrieve a file, or to get a cup of coffee. If you are unable to leave at that moment, try to position yourself near an exit, and if that's not possible, try to avoid being blocked in an area you can't easily get out of. If an employee becomes hostile towards you, try to divert him or her by redirecting the conversation, using calming words and a reasonable tone of voice. If this doesn't work, agree with the individual's point of view or complaint and explain that you share similar feelings. Lower your voice, and talk slowly and politely. Never, ever, argue or humiliate the aggravated person.

Take Action to Prevent Homicides

Environmental designs incorporating up-to-date security and risk control concepts that build in safety and exclude hazards are among the best ways for an employer to provide security. Several procedures and actions recommended by NIOSH and other experts which you and your employer can take to minimize the hazards of occupational homicide include:

❖ Never resist during a robbery.

❖ Do not overly antagonize co-workers.

❖ Do not get involved in a heated dispute with co-workers, especially when they have a weapon.

❖ Avoid working in isolated locations; choose areas visible to others.

❖ Avoid carrying large amounts of cash.

❖ Try to work with other people.

❖ Read books or take training courses on conflict resolution and nonviolent mediation.

❖ Insist on bullet-resistant barriers or enclosures if you constantly handle money in high-crime areas.

❖ Request that your local police check on you periodically.

❖ Try to avoid working late-night and early-morning hours, especially when alone.

❖ Try to avoid hazardous workplaces and high-risk occupations.

❖ Insist on security officers during hazardous late hours.

❖ Install good external lighting.

❖ Use drop safes to reduce cash on hand.

❖ Post signs indicating that little or no cash is at hand.

❖ Have access to a beeper, a silent alarm, and a panic button.

❖ Invest in magnetic-card access systems.

❖ Install surveillance cameras.

❖ Thoroughly screen job applicants.

❖ Identify risk factors particular to your workplace, and develop a plan to deal with an emergency. Even better, engage in activities that help minimize or reduce the risks.

Danger Off the Premises

On Long Island, several gunmen hijacked an overnight delivery truck in a secluded residential neighborhood in broad daylight. They left the driver bound and gagged in the woods after rifling through the packages inside the truck. In Brooklyn, a man entered a rented van and then shot and killed the driver after robbing the passengers.

A company obviously has less control of their security once employees leave its facilities to perform work off premises. Even a company with state-of-the-art security systems, highly trained security officers, and best intentions is at a definite disadvantage to provide proper protection from dangers lurking outside. A company's employees, like all citizens, may become the victims of crime or violence in a split second. And you can expect the problem to balloon, because most workers today are employed in service industries and perform the majority of their tasks off company property. These employees include delivery persons, tourist guides, repair personnel, consultants, computer specialists, gardeners, home-care workers, traveling salespersons, case workers, law enforcement personnel, exterminators, and company meter readers.

The company can do little to provide protection on the "outside," but you can employ a few simple rules that will increase your personal safety. Avoid street crowds; don't let curiosity get the best of you. Stay away from arguments over parking spaces and people who push ahead in line. Ignore discourteous remarks or behavior. Stay away from abandoned packages; steer clear of armed guards transporting money; and do not stop to view police actions no matter how interesting. Each of these situations can spell trouble, including getting hit by stray bullets.

Two-way radios or cellular phones are important security devices that can summon assistance in an emergency. Arrange with your employer to call in every hour or after each service call. Try to work in pairs or in threes in high-risk areas, and avoid these neighborhoods after dark. Wear a company uniform or jacket and cap so that you will not be mistaken for an intruder. Make sure the name of your company is visible on your vehicle or uniform. Avoid carrying cash on the job. Always lock your vehicle, and never leave in it anything of value, especially if it is visible. Have painted a large, clearly discernible number on top of your company vehicle so that it can be easily identified and followed in the event of an emergency. Most important, when outside the company perimeter, remain attentive and very alert.

SECURING THE WORKPLACE INSIDE

It is unfortunate that the specter of crime threatens us in our offices as well as in our homes and on the streets. Merchants and cab drivers are used to on-the-job assault; secretaries, executives, and the steno pool are rapidly rising on the risk scale.

Today's office is much more sophisticated than in days past, and the equipment used is much more expensive. A generation ago, a steno pad and a typewriter were the tools of the trade for secretaries and typists. Today's equipment can command much higher prices. The wonder computers of the 1960s, which revolutionized our banking industry, had less computing power than the PC sitting on the secretarial desk of today.

Among many truisms about crime is this: If you have something both valuable and small, someone will try to steal it. That is why security officers have replaced elevator operators in most office buildings. Even if your office has no other easily portable and valuable equipment, a thief may steal your telephone in a second or two.

An intruder in your building may be looking for a physicians' office and drugs; on the way out, the thief may take your purse. At lunchtime, most office personnel take a break, leaving one person to take care of the office. If safeguards are ignored, much mischief may follow.

A building guard, a strong deterrent to the would-be thief, is good protection against stealing. Designated areas where valuable items, including the personal property of those working in the building, can be kept under lock and key are additional protection. Installing your cash register as near to the front of the store as possible will allow passersby to note an in-progress robbery or an after-hours burglary.

Cooperate with neighborhood merchants for your mutual self-protection. In one of the toughest areas of the South Bronx, a group of merchants banded together. They installed buzzers that sounded in the buildings next to their own. It was thus relatively easy for an in-progress crime to be reported to the police, without a confrontation with the thieves. These "buddy buzzers" proved to be excellent security weapons, at the cost of only a few dollars.

SECURING THE WORKPLACE OUTSIDE

A determined thief will exploit every weakness that you fail to remedy adequately. Your place of business should be as secure as your home, if not more so. According to one source, the typical losses of a small business are 25 times greater than those of large businesses.

Obviously, your protection must begin outside the workplace, for that's where you want to contain an intruder. You should avoid leaving ladders or stacks of pallets outside the building. Either of these could provide above-ground-level entry into your business. Parking up against the building should be discouraged, because an auto not only can be used as a stepladder to the second story but also because it is a convenient method of removing the loot.

The very best protection, however, is to be found in alert and caring employee groups. Employees should be reminded regularly that they devote about 30 percent of their lives to their jobs, and with that sort of commitment, they need to do everything they can to protect the environ-ment in which they spend so much of their time. Much of what is stolen is their property. And what is stolen from the employer affects them as well, since their job security and prosperity depend on the employer's continued survival.

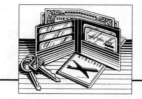

SECURITY IN THE WORKPLACE: A CHECKLIST

1 Comply with and support your company's safety and security program and regulations, and insist that oth-ers do the same.

2 Protect billfolds, keys, purses, and other personal valuables on the job.

3 Challenge strangers in restricted areas.

4 Do not discuss company affairs off the job.

5 When leaving the office, even for a short period of time, clean up and secure your workspace, with spe-cial attention to confidential documents, and secure company equipment assigned to you.

6 If you handle money as part of your job, insist on positive identification before you cash any checks, and refuse to accept counterfeit or questionable currency.

7 If you work in a retail establishment or in any other business, guard against shoplifting and employee theft within the framework of the law.

8 To deter shoplifting, speak to all customers in your area. Be wary of bulky coats, large shopping bags, partially opened umbrellas, and folded newspapers.

9 Know your company's policy on dealing with shoplifters, and adhere to it.

10 Retain security officers, because they are substantial deterrents to criminals.

11 Be especially aware and alert if your job involves ex-changing money with the public.

12   Be cautious if your job is in a high-crime area, if you work alone, work late-night or early-morning hours, or work outside in an isolated area.

13   Be certain the company you work for thoroughly screens all applicants to determine character and integrity as well as technical qualifications.

14   Always respect co-workers. Avoid volatile confrontations that appear to be heading towards violence.

15   Never argue or humiliate a person who appears hostile, aggravated, or angry. Try your best to calm the employee.

16   If you hear gunshots, run from the scene or lock yourself in a closet.

17   Never challenge a killer's instructions.

18   Learn the warning signs of potential mass murderers, including sudden changes in personality, demeanor, attitude, mental health, marital situation, work behavior, or chemical dependency.

19   Encourage troubled individuals to seek counseling, whether from your company's employee assistance program or from counselors or private therapists.

20   If you work off the company's premises, avoid unnecessary risks, including spontaneous street crowds, arguments, and police activity.

21   When you perform work away from the company facility, always carry a cellular phone or two-way radio to summon assistance in an emergency.

22   Try to work with partners, especially if you must perform your activities in high-crime areas.

23   When you leave the company perimeter, remain attentive and in high alert.

16

VACATIONS, BUSINESS TRIPS, AND TRAVELING

Travel usually imposes an entirely different regimen on a person. The traveler may suffer from jet lag. He or she almost certainly dines differently, does different things, perhaps keeps different hours, may drink more, and in general attempts to cram as much of the new and different as is possible into a limited space of time.

The traveler also is probably carrying more money than usual, feels less self-confident, has fewer places to turn to for assistance (and is less able to find the assistance that is available). And, because of their dress or speech, travelers may be easily identifiable as being out of their element. In other words, travelers are often easy "marks," and everybody knows it—unless, of course, the traveler takes the trouble to dress to blend into the surroundings, to behave in a manner that doesn't attract attention, to avoid overindulgence in drink, to confine his or her activities to the wholesome, and to leave dens of iniquity to the more daring.

GETTING THERE BY PUBLIC TRANSPORTATION

At the Airport

If you're traveling by air, it is best to have a friend or relative drive you to the airport. If this is not possible, it is preferable to take a taxi or use an airport limousine service. If, however, you do end up leaving your car at the airport, consider what time you'll be returning when deciding where to park. For example, if you're arriving late at night, park under a streetlamp and avoid isolated areas.

Leave yourself plenty of time before departure, and take as little luggage as possible. About 6 of every 1,000 pieces of luggage were lost, stolen, misrouted, or damaged by 10 of the largest U.S. air carriers in 1992. In 1994, there were 2,902 incidents of luggage theft at New York City's Kennedy Airport.

Safeguarding Your Luggage

Don't pack your luggage too full, and be sure to lock it. An overpacked bag will often pop open if dropped. Dishonest baggage handlers may drop bags deliberately and rifle their contents, or may open unlocked bags. Of course, even a locked bag can be broken into with little effort, so cash, jewelry, and other expensive items should always be packed in carry-on luggage. Be careful, though. Avoid expensive luggage, and label your bags with your name and address. However, instead of your home address, use a work address or the place where you'll be staying, so thieves will not know the location of your empty home. Make your luggage distinctive, so that you or another well-meaning traveler will not accidentally take the wrong luggage. Pick up your luggage as soon as you arrive at your destination. Watch out for thieves hanging around security screening checkpoints looking for purses or briefcases to steal. Keep yours in sight and close to you. If your luggage is lost or stolen, report it and fill out a certificate of loss immediately. If you have a homeowner's insurance policy, check to see if it covers valuables stolen during your trip.

Be careful about safeguarding your airline ticket. Not only are unused tickets redeemable for cash, but also organized rings of thieves steal and re-sell valid tickets. Some particularly brazen thieves have even been known to approach passengers seated in waiting areas and ask to see their tickets, whereupon they take the valid tickets from the passengers' flight coupon books and then hand them boarding passes picked out of a trash container.

If you have several packages or pieces of luggage, and if you have a long layover in an air terminal, use one of the coin-operated lockers, preferably near your departure gate, to store your belongings. When storing or retrieving your packages, be extremely careful about accepting offers of assistance from anyone other than air carrier station personnel or skycaps.

Taxis and Drivers

Try to establish in advance taxi fares from the airport to your destination. Unscrupulous drivers in communities with few or no regulations will often overcharge an unwitting visitor. Before you enter a cab, ask the dispatcher or driver how much the ride will cost. If you feel you are being taken to your destination in a roundabout way, let the driver know immediately, and tell him you will not pay for the extra traveling. If the actual fare is more than originally stated, and an argument ensues when you protest, note the cab number, the driver's name, and the time. Do not give a tip, of course. Ask for a receipt, and report the incident to the company and/or taxi commission and the police. Find out about shuttles to and from the airport before you leave. These cost much less.

If you have bags or luggage with you, be certain the driver puts *all* your baggage into the trunk and takes *all* your belongings out when you are dropped off. The driver's leaving your suitcase behind may not be an accident; it may be a scheme with an accomplice waiting to grab the loot.

Be sure the cab you are using has a legitimate medallion and that the driver identification is clearly visible. Do not ride in unlicensed cabs. They are dangerous and illegal, and are not covered by insurance in the event of an accident.

If the driver is operating the vehicle recklessly, tell him so and threaten to file a report. Never sit in the front seat next to the driver if you are alone. Do not respond to personal questions or offer information about yourself, and never accept any food or candy a driver offers you. If you are uncomfortable with the driver's knowing where you live or work, have him drop you off a block away.

A STRANGER IN TOWN

You are considerably more likely to encounter crimes against your person, especially assault and robbery, when you're away from home. Particularly on the increase are thefts, which the robber is reasonably certain will never be reported. A classic example of this involves the big-spending visitor who asks a taxi driver or bellhop to find him an after-hours bottle of bourbon or a supply of marijuana. Even if he receives colored water or a small packet of oregano, he will, in all likelihood, take no action. To do so would be to implicate himself in a crime.

A variation on this theme involves a prostitute and her accomplice. She lures her victim to a hotel room, where he is rewarded not with rapture but with robbery by an accomplice. Rarely will the visiting "john" report the crime, even if he has no wife or family at home, simply because he does not wish to return to the city to testify at a trial. He may chalk it up to experience, even though he will probably have suffered a greater-than-average loss.

Choosing a Hotel or Motel

Although budget motels may be enticing for their low prices, many are not as secure as their higher priced counterparts. The lower price may attract an undesirable element and the surrounding areas may be dangerous.

Survey the hotel or motel during daylight hours. Make sure it is not a "hang out" and that people are not loitering in the parking lot. It is best to avoid hotels that have outside entrances to rooms from the parking lot. A criminal can wait in a car and attack you as you are about to enter your room. Use hotels that have indoor entrances in which access is strictly limited to guests and hotel employees. Hotel employees and/or security officers should be visible throughout the facility. Criminals are less likely to flock to secure hotels for fear of being seen and challenged. Some experts also suggest smaller hotels or motels because strangers can be more readily detected.

You may wish to request a room near places of activity, such as the front desk, hotel offices, or room service stations. Rooms near the elevator are much safer than those at the end of the corridor. The extra noise is well worth the added security. The room you stay in should be equipped with a peephole on the door and double-bolt locks. Electronic card locks provide even better security.

Although many women's sections in hotels have been eliminated, there are some hotels that are test-marketing designated women's areas. Another alternative is to make reservations in a hotel that caters exclusively to women. More and more hotels and motels are addressing the needs of women, because, by the turn of the century, women are expected to comprise the majority of business travelers.

The staff of the hotel—particularly at night—is as important as the clientele. The staff should be large enough to provide a modicum of protection, and the composition and capability of the hotel's security staff—as well as the screening procedures for prospective employees—are characteristics you should try to determine in advance.

Most important, consider the construction of the building. The section of bedroom floors should be protected. Fire escapes should let you out but no one else in, and doors and windows should be secure against undesired entry. Ideally, you should select a hotel room on the fourth through seventh floors. In all likelihood, this would put you high enough to avoid most of the street noise. A more important consideration is your safety. In the event of fire, your only means of escape could be out the window of your bedroom. The aerial ladders used by fire departments rarely reach heights higher than the seventh floor of a new hotel. In older structures with high ceilings, the fifth or sixth floor might be safer for you.

Security in Your Hotel Room

Perhaps you have concluded that the best way to avoid being victimized in a big, unfamiliar city is to avoid the hostile environment outside by retreating to the safety and security of your hotel room. However, thousands of travelers are victims of crimes that take place inside their hotels.

When you check into a hotel or motel, make sure the desk clerk does not loudly announce your room number. If this happens, request another room, and tell the clerk to write down the number and show it to you. You may not be the only person interested in learning your room number. Check in using your last name and only your first initial, and tell the clerk not to disclose it to anyone. Request that you be notified if someone asks for it.

The key or magnetized key card you are given when you check in isn't, unfortunately, the only one that will open your door. Most hotel rooms provide some backup device, such as a door chain or a deadbolt that is operated by a turn knob, by the additional turn of a key, or by a button that, when pushed, "excludes all keys." Use all locks and devices when you are in the room. Never leave your door open, even if you're just running out for ice or a soda.

Because there are ways that these added features may be defeated, you should consider improvising certain protective measures of your own. For example, a chair wedged under a doorknob can be an effective additional "lock," as can a furniture barricade. Inserting a simple rubber wedge in the crack between the door and floor will always prevent the door from being opened. There are doorstops that emit an alarm when the door is opened, and there's an alarm that can be hung from the doorknob that will sound if the knob is turned *before* the door is opened. You might opt for an inexpensive personal beeper-sized motion alarm for detecting intruders. And as a last resort, you might even want to consider carrying your own portable travel lock; when this lock is attached, it is very difficult to open the door without breaking it down.

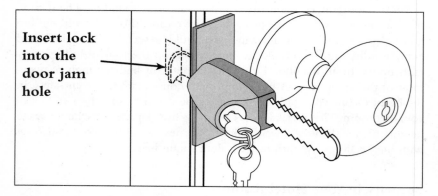

Insert lock into the door jam hole

Figure 11. Portable travel lock.

Windows or balconies accessible from the outside should be locked, and don't open your room door unless you determine the identity of the caller. Call the front desk if you are in doubt about room service, a bellhop, a housekeeper, or other hotel personnel.

If you are a woman traveling alone, you should request that a bellhop escort you to your room to check for intruders before you enter. Don't be embarrassed to request this service when returning by yourself, especially at night. Use only the main entrance. Be on the lookout for suspicious people loitering in the hallway, and look out the peephole before exiting your room. Needless to say, never invite strangers to your room, even for business purposes.

Do not leave valuables in plain view. Use the safe in your room or the hotel safe. The amount the hotel is responsible for varies and can be quite low. The best policy is to secure your valuables before you travel. If you do leave your valuables in the hotel safe, seal them in a manila envelope as if they were business documents, and be sure to get a detailed receipt. You may also purchase portable "safes" that look just like toiletry cans and are indistinguishable from them. Or you can make your own book safe by cutting out a square in the inside pages of a thick paperback. Put valuables inside and place this book among other similar ones. As you put your belongings in drawers or closets, arrange them so that you will notice if something is missing. Do not leave keys, money, or valuables in your room, and have your key in hand before you get to your room.

Park only in well-lit areas, or try to frequent hotels with valet parking services, but give the attendant your ignition key only. Never leave anything behind in the trunk, even if you are only staying for one night.

If you pay in cash on checking out, but the clerk made an imprint of your credit card, make sure the imprint is destroyed. Employees have been known to put the bill on your credit card and keep the cash.

A Hotel Fire

There are more than 6,000 hotel fires in the United States each year. In 1992, hotel fires caused 30 deaths and 250 injuries. Review carefully all fire instructions provided by the hotel. These are usually posted on your room door; if not, request a set of instructions from the front desk. Determine whether the fire signal is a bell or other audible signal, and ascertain what to do if the alarm is activated.

Before retiring for the night, you should perform this life-saving exercise: Step into the corridor outside your room, and locate the nearest fire exit. Usually, it will be easy to find, because it will probably be illuminated and should bear the word *EXIT*. Next, count the number of doors between your room and the emergency exit. If smoke should engulf the floor on which you are staying, you should be able to locate the fire exit even if your vision is completely obscured. Having counted the doors could lead you to safety.

In the event of fire, try to leave as soon as you see or smell smoke. First, however, carefully touch your room door. Only if it is not hot should you slowly open it, just a little, and while holding your breath, examine the passageway. If all appears in order, return to your room, get your key and a wet towel, and fill your lungs with air. Make for the emergency exit, either upright or on all fours, depending on air quality. The wet towel can, literally, be a life saver. It may be used for many things. Use it to wipe your face and eyes, to cool and filter the air you breathe, and to cool and protect exposed skin surfaces. If you encounter smoke outside your room, drop to your knees, since the air near the floor is less likely to be filled with volatile, toxic substances. Do not use the elevator; elevator shafts usually fill with smoke during a fire. Proceed to the nearest fire exit, and determine the location of the fire. If it is above you, go down the stairs; if it is below, go up the stairs to the roof.

It is possible that you will not be able to escape a fire that has spread to a number of floors. You may be forced to return to your room to wait out the fire. In this event, close the door. It offers protection against the spread of the fire into your room. Fill the tub with water—immersing yourself may save you from serious burns. Put dampened towels around the door to help prevent the spread of noxious gases into the room. Try to maintain an attitude of optimism. Most occupants survive hotel fires, and the responding fire-fighting units will muster every available resource to combat such fires.

Above all, do not panic. Your chances of surviving are greater if you maintain your composure.

ON CAR TRIPS

If you are traveling by automobile, make special efforts to travel securely. The trunk of your car is more secure than the passenger compartment but is still no formidable obstacle to a burglar. If you are stopping for the night, take all your bags and packages into your room with you. They are much more likely to be there when you look for them the next morning.

Consult a service such as the American Automobile Association (AAA) or a travel agency for travel advice about such matters as speed traps or other hazards, things to do, things not to do, recommended motels, and so forth. Remember, your out-of-state (or out-of-country) license plates brand you as a stranger and hence as an easy, potential victim.

Take time to learn the local traffic rules and regulations, and be certain that you are adequately covered by your insurance company.

SOUVENIR SHOPPING

Shopping is almost invariably a part of any trip. It is unlikely that you will be shopping in a place where you have a charge account, and little more likely that you will be able to pay by check. However, traveler's checks are almost always a suitable substitute for cash, and many stores worldwide accept credit cards. When souvenir shopping, you can anticipate walking the streets with your packages. Carry your purse or briefcase in the same hand as your parcels, with the purse or briefcase—and your most valuable purchase—close to your body.

CAMPING OR WILDERNESS VACATIONING

If you are taking a vacation trip using a camper or motor home, be sure all the doors and windows are locked while you're on the road. It is relatively easy for you to avoid picking up a hitchhiker, and it is also in your best interest to avoid harboring a stowaway.

Maybe your vacation is going to involve a return to nature. You're going to backpack through the high country and commune with the earth and sky. Fine—but watch yourself. A bear rummaging through your food isn't the only hazard you might encounter. A far more serious threat to your safety and security is your fellow camper. Every year, there are many reports of rapes, assaults, robberies, and other crimes in isolated camping areas. You can best protect yourself by checking in with ranger stations or park police and by camping at sites they suggest. At least let them know where you plan to be. Take the time to find out how to reach help on foot, just in the unlikely event that you might need to. Introduce yourself to any seemingly friendly campers near you; you *could* need their assistance.

If you are threatened and your car is nearby, your horn will carry a long distance in still mountain air, or carry an air horn.

RESORT AREAS

Your taste in vacation spots may run more to the bright lights and activity of the resort than the isolation of the campsite. At resorts, marauding bears may be a rarity on the beach, but human wolves and jackals are not. Pimps, hustlers, deviates, robbers, organized criminals, con-artists, addicts, shakedown artists, pickpockets, and all types of plain and fancy hoodlums haunt these areas. Always ask yourself why any stranger is going out of his or her way to be friendly and accommodating. If you can't come up with a nonthreatening answer, beware.

If you are going to devote an evening to a round of nightclubbing or a day to shopping, take the suggestions of the hotel manager or desk clerk rather than those of a taxi driver or the local cocktail waitress in a bar. If at all possible, go with a crowd of your choosing. It is usually the lone, lost sheep that falls victim to the wolf pack. Stay on the beaten path, especially at night. See the quaint out-of-the-way places during the day, when the light is better, preferably in the company of a reliable guide.

PRECAUTIONS FOR OVERSEAS TRAVEL

The U.S. Travel and Tourism Administration estimates that over 47 million Americans venture abroad each year. Travel abroad is not what it used to be. These days you may be greeted in some countries with shouting, jeering, anti-Yankee slogans, and verbal and physical harassment, even threats on your life. Increases in terrorism, violence, and crime dictate that you must be prepared for any contingency. About 1 of every 2,000 American tourists has her or his passport stolen. Careful preparation and common sense are your most important weapons.

The ordinary traveler should avoid known trouble spots and be familiar with any problems in a particular region. Consular information sheets and travel warnings published by the U.S. Department of State contain useful information for travelers, including names of countries dangerous for Americans, the location of the U.S. Embassy or Consulate in the subject country, crime, security, drug penalties, minor political disturbances, passports, currency, medicines, and what to do if you get into trouble in a foreign country.

This information may be obtained by writing and sending a self-addressed envelope to:

Citizens Emergency Center
Bureau of Consular Affairs
Room 4811
U.S. Department of State
Washington, DC 20520

or

Call (202) 647-5225
Fax (202) 647-3000

Another State Department publication that includes useful tips on safety and security is *A Safe Trip Abroad*. It is available from:

The Superintendent of Documents
U.S. Government Printing Office
Washington, DC 20402

A travel agency or airline can provide additional information, but it may not be precise or up-to-date.

Information you should try to gather includes the frequency of terrorist acts against U.S. installations or businesses, whether American travelers have been attacked or threatened, and whether an active propaganda campaign exists in the underground press. Talk to travelers who have recently returned from the area, and ask about such events as demonstrations, strikes, and threats.

Record your passport number and store it separately, and bring along a copy of your birth certificate.

Language Problems

Don't assume that wherever you travel someone will be able to communicate with you in your own language. Learn at least enough of the local language to be able to ask for assistance, report a crime, and find out if your language is spoken. Portable dual-language dictionaries can be helpful. If you need help with the language, be sure you get it from a trustworthy individual.

Some of the people you encounter, though quite fluent in your language, will act as if they have no idea what you are saying. Some do this simply to be difficult. For reasons of their own, they dislike Americans, and they are merely being contrary. Others, though, practicing their own language skills, want you to speak English very much, particularly if you are with another who is speaking your language. Still others pretend not to comprehend in order to lull you into falsely believing that when you speak English you won't be understood. If you are bargaining with a foreign shopkeeper and at the same time discussing prices in English with a companion, you may be undermining your bargaining position. You almost certainly will end up paying more than you should.

Automobiles and Driving Regulations

Driving regulations and traffic laws in other countries often differ substantially from those in the United States. One American tourist was involved in a routine accident in Mexico and was detained in jail for months while an investigation and proceedings were completed.

Find out as much as possible about local traffic rules and regulations, and make sure you are adequately insured and have the correct papers. Personnel managing border-crossing points can be particularly helpful regarding this kind of information.

Choose an inconspicuous car, and do not display any identifying information such as corporate names or distinctive license plates.

Money

Whenever you travel, and especially when going overseas, you are faced with the necessity of carrying more cash than you feel comfortable with. Be sure to use traveler's checks or credit cards, and don't keep all your money in one place. It's a good idea to keep your funds and important papers in at least a couple of safe places, so that if one stash is wiped out, you are not completely helpless. When you have to carry cash on your person, a money belt worn under your clothes is a good way to thwart a pickpocket.

A large safety pin can be used to secure money inside your clothing or pockets. Also, a nylon wallet with a velcro closure is more secure and less attractive to thieves than leather. Be aware that pickpockets can slice your purse, purse strap, or pocket with a knife and remove its contents. Wear straps under a coat or jacket, always keep bags and fanny packs in front of you, and wear sweaters or overshirt over your purse or fanny pack. Remove extra credit cards and membership and business cards from your purse before departing on your trip. Make a copy of all credit cards and identification and personal papers, and keep these separate from the originals. Avoid carrying any political items with you. You might also carry a handheld shrill alarm to sound in case of attack or in an emergency.

Be familiar with the exchange rates and the appearance of all foreign money you are likely to handle. Also, don't exchange your money for local currency on the street or at your hotel. Go to a bank for this purpose.

The Business Traveler

Business travelers, especially executives, must be careful, because they are particularly vulnerable to acts of terrorism. The business executive must practice all the general tips for the typical overseas traveler; in addition, special precautions must be taken because corporate officers are special targets for terrorists.

The first precaution is to maintain a low profile. Do not broadcast your travel plans and itinerary. Provide information about your schedule only on a need-to-know basis. Some executives visiting a hostile country may even travel under assumed or modified names and make reservations in several hotels. Try to avoid repetitious patterns, and vary the days and hours of travel and the routes you take. Plan your trip carefully to minimize the time you actually spend in a foreign country. Prepare your itinerary carefully, and give it to a trusted colleague or to a member of your family. In case of an emergency, this information will be helpful in locating you, and it may even save your life.

Avoid seedy establishments, including hotels and restaurants. Do not leave valuable papers in your hotel room; check them for deposit in the hotel safe or a safe-deposit box. Avoid rooms on the first floor or those easily accessible from the outside. Try your best not to be paged. Avoid traveling alone, especially at nighttime, unless absolutely necessary; try to travel in a group. Your luggage should not display your name, home address, or company logo, although the company address is usually all right. Finally, do not display large sums of money or expensive jewelry.

In a Foreign Land

Your hotel can be a citadel when you're away from home, or it can be a trap. Look for accommodations in the middle of things, where you can blend into your surroundings, particularly when you are in a foreign country. The availability and response time of police services are necessary considerations. The size of a hotel is important—in general, bigger is better, certainly for anonymity.

Once you have settled in, try to befriend local residents who can apprise you of the political situation and its dangers. Register with the nearest American Consulate or Mission. If there is no American representation, contact the embassy or consulate of the country designated to handle U.S. interests. In the event of an emergency, such as a sudden evacuation or riot, these contacts could be more vital; more usual assistance includes replacement of lost passports, a telegram home in case of illness, and resolution of minor communication problems.

Ordinarily, American government representatives will not make travel arrangements, replace airline tickets, lend funds to stranded travelers, or, more significantly, intervene with local law enforcement officials. You must abide by the laws of the host country, and if you get into trouble, you will be judged according to local law. Your U.S. representatives will be limited in power and influence, but they can arrange for representation by a local attorney, and they will notify your family of your plight.

Beware of Drugs and Other Criminal Activity

Obviously, it is imperative to uphold the law wherever you are. Doing so is absolutely essential, however, in foreign countries, where penalties for committing a crime can be extremely severe, especially for American citizens, who are often picked on to make an example. One problem you might encounter in an unfamiliar place is being able to recognize a law enforcement officer when you see one. Uniforms vary widely from country to country, and even within a single community.

Drug laws are particularly severe in many foreign countries. Avoid drugs, addicts, or pushers at all costs. It is estimated that about 2,600 Americans are in foreign jails, about one-third on drug charges. Most are males under 30. Many have been detained for long periods without trials, in primitive and unsanitary facilities. A conviction on charges of drug use or trafficking abroad could result in a long prison term and even a death sentence. Recently, a 26-year-old disk jockey, Christopher Lavinger, was arrested in Osaka, Japan, for possession of 3.5 grams of cocaine, 1.5 grams of marijuana, and some psychedelic drugs. After spending a month in the Osaka House of Detention, he was sentenced to 22 months in Tokyo's Fuchu prison, Japan's largest maximum-security institution. Lavinger had to work in silence and eat in silence, and he was forbidden to turn his head. Crying was an infraction of the disciplinary code, and prisoners had to sleep in a set position on their backs.

Stories of mistreatment in foreign jails abound, such as the story of Billy Hayes, Jr., the American arrested for narcotics in Turkey several years ago and whose escape from prison was portrayed in the film and book

Midnight Express. Drug infractions aren't the only crimes dealt with harshly in foreign lands. Attracting equally wide attention was the case of an 18-year-old American, Michael Fay, who was sentenced in Singapore to 4 months in jail and a "caning" for acts of vandalism, including the spray-painting of cars. The caning consisted of four strokes with a 4-foot rattan cane moistened with water to prevent fraying. This instrument causes excruciating pain by cutting into the victim's skin. In addition, the rattan cane often results in bleeding and permanent scarring. The best way to stay out of situations like these is to *not break the law.*

Special Considerations in Third World Countries

Third World countries can be especially difficult for the traveler. There may be customs officials or local police who like to throw their weight around. The best advice is to be careful and use common sense. Be aware of the proud nationalism of most Third World officials, and assume that they are going to be more sensitive than many Americans would be in similar circumstances.

Shopping Overseas

While overseas, avoid shops in airports and train stations because of high prices. Haggling is not only acceptable but is expected in certain regions. In most of the Caribbean and in some of Europe—such as Spain, Portugal, and Greece—it is virtually unheard of to pay the ticketed price. Be extremely careful in native marketplaces. What is professed to be genuine gold or silver, an antique, or an artifact is often not. In addition, if you pay by credit card, the conversion value used is the one in effect at the time of billing, not when your original purchase was made. Further, card issuers will increase the exchange rate in their favor when computing your bill.

In most countries in Europe and the Orient, you may be reimbursed for a value-added tax (VAT). Ask the merchant about local tax rules. If you are eligible, you can get a VAT form that can be submitted to a U.S. customs official at the airport. A check will arrive after a few months for as much as 25 percent of the purchase price. Of course, allow yourself extra time at the airport.

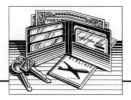

VACATIONS, BUSINESS TRIPS, AND TRAVELING: A CHECKLIST

1 Use traveler's checks or credit cards, rather than carrying large amounts of cash.

2 Lock your baggage, and take only what you need on a trip.

3 Guard your transportation tickets.

4 Store luggage in a coin-operated locker during a layover at an airport, train, or bus station.

5 Use only skycaps or other authorized baggage-handling personnel for assistance with your luggage.

6 Determine taxi fares before you use taxi service.

7 Don't ride in unlicensed cabs that do not have driver identification notices.

8 Select a hotel with adequate security, and avoid rooms easily accessible from the outside.

9 Request a room near places of activity, such as hotel offices, elevators, or room service stations.

10 Don't depend on the door of your hotel room to safeguard you and your valuables. For extra protection use a chair, a drawer, a rubber wedge, or a portable travel lock.

11 Do not leave important papers or other valuables in your room. Use the hotel safe.

12 Lock balcony doors and windows accessible from the outside.

13 Locate fire exits; be able to recognize the fire alarm signal, and plan your actions in the event of a hotel fire.

14 If escape during a fire is not possible, fill the bathtub with water, and immerse yourself to lessen danger of serious burns.

15　In selecting a hotel room, avoid any above the seventh floor. Most aerial fire ladders do not reach higher than that.

16　On a car trip, use your trunk for carrying luggage, and bring all your luggage into the hotel room at night.

17　Use the AAA, travel agencies, or other reliable sources for information about where you're going and what you should do or avoid doing while there.

18　Be careful when shopping, because you probably won't have the convenience of charge accounts, check cashing, or package delivery that you have at home. Take precautions against pickpockets in a crowd.

19　Lock camper or motor home doors, even if driving.

20　Notify rangers, park police, or nearby campers of your camping location.

21　While camping, use your car horn or portable air horn as a security alarm.

22　Be especially dubious of unwarranted attention or offers of friendship from strangers at resorts.

23　Go sightseeing with a group of your own choosing, and be wary of suggestions about places to see and things to do.

24　When traveling overseas, avoid known trouble spots.

25　Gather full information and prepare all necessary precautionary measures before you travel to an area.

26　Be sure to have a valid passport; record its number and store it in a separate place, and take along a copy of your birth certificate.

27　Be particularly cautious and aware of local customs in Third World countries.

28 Learn enough of the local language to be able to ask for assistance or report a crime.

29 Be familiar with local exchange rates and the appearance of foreign currency. Do not exchange money on the street.

30 Register with the American Consulate or Mission.

31 Abide by all laws of the host country. Be sure to avoid drugs, drug abusers, and drug sellers.

32 Learn local traffic laws before driving in a foreign country.

33 The business executive should be aware of special vulnerabilities while traveling abroad. Dress inconspicuously, maintain a low profile, and do not display large sums of money or expensive jewelry.

34 Avoid seedy establishments, including hotels and restaurants.

35 Avoid being paged.

36 If you are famous or a top-level executive, your luggage should not reveal your name, home address, or company logo. A corporate address should suffice.

37 Travel in a car with no identifying signs or logos.

38 Do not advertise your itinerary and schedule. Avoid taking the same route each day.

39 Leave your itinerary with a relative or trusted colleague.

40 Try not to travel alone at night.

41 Be cautious shopping in native marketplaces. Avoid airport shops where prices tend to be unusually high.

17

~

MOVING TO
ANOTHER COMMUNITY

The Blake family moved to another city because of a job change. One week later, their house was burglarized, the family car was stolen, and someone tried to sell their children marijuana. Unlike the place where they had lived before, their new neighborhood and school were in a high-crime area, where the children were assaulted by young toughs in school.

Over 42 million Americans change their residences each year, and, according to the latest Census Bureau analysis, 2 in 10 of the nation's households move every 15 months, evidence that the United States exhibits the highest mobility among developed nations. Anyone who has moved can tell you that this complicated process requires careful planning. A high priority on your moving list should be protection from crime. Nothing is more disheartening than moving from a stable low-crime area to a neighborhood high in crime and where drugs abound.

The first item on your agenda should be to determine the incidence of crime, including the levels of violence and theft, in your new neighborhood. Go to the library and look up the *Uniform Crime Reports* published annually by the FBI. If you are unable to find it, ask your reference librarian for assistance. This publication contains useful and interesting information on the levels of crime and the number of police officers for most cities and towns in the United States. For your city or town, look up how many homicides, rapes, aggravated assaults, robberies, burglaries, and auto thefts occurred during the last year. Then compare the numbers with similar crimes in cities nearby of comparable size. For your convenience, population figures are provided for each city.

You can also determine how many officers your new city's police department has, compared with other cities in the same category. This effort should not last more than half an hour. The effort is well worthwhile, because you may be able to protect yourself and your family from danger for many years to come. You might as well choose a location close to your job that has a low, rather than a high, incidence of crime.

FIELDWORK

Before you sign a lease or buy a house, walk or drive around your prospective new neighborhood, especially at night or on weekends, and look for signs of crime. These signs include such undesirables as young toughs, youth gangs, drug addicts, prostitutes, panhandlers, and derelicts. Beware of outdoor gambling, like three-card monte or other forms of street betting. Also, determine if there are bars, saloons, drug dens, "smoke shops," or similar crime hazards in your new neighborhood.

Try to determine whether people routinely use the streets during the day and night or if they are afraid to venture outside. Are the streets deserted and isolated? Ask the same questions about nearby parks. Next, check the lighting in the neighborhood. Is it adequate for the nighttime? Is there sufficient lighting outside your new home? Also, examine the exterior of your new house or apartment building to see whether it is surrounded by untrimmed shrubbery or foliage, excellent hiding places for criminals.

Make sure there is convenient and efficient transportation. You or your family do not want to have to walk a mile through deserted streets to the bus stop and then wait an hour for the bus, especially late at night or very early in the morning.

Schools

Familiarize your children with the safest and shortest route to the new school. Have them review the bus or subway routes several times, until they are thoroughly knowledgeable and can avoid getting lost or ending up in a dangerous area. Instruct your loved ones never to get off at an unfamiliar stop, or to explore strange neighborhoods.

Check the level of safety in your youngsters' new school, including any statistics on the presence of weapons. (For more information, see Chapter 24.) Discuss with your family the security and safety measures needed to ensure maximum protection. Be certain also to check the incidence of racial and religious hate crimes on school property and in your new city. Newspaper accounts and the annual report by the local police often provide this information. You might even contact the public-relations unit of the local police for information on this highly dangerous crime.

MOVING TIME

You also need to plan properly your actual move. A reliable moving company is of critical importance, because of the hazards of thievery when movers and packers roam around your house. Also, reliable companies are less likely to experience robberies from moving-vans. Remember, all agreements must be in writing.

If you move within the same city or state, make sure your moving company is authorized by the appropriate *state* regulatory agency, usually in the public utilities commission. Don't forget to notify your post office, banks, relatives, friends, business acquaintances, and credit card companies of your change in address. The U.S. Postal Service provides cards designed specifically for this purpose.

Security experts recommend the following simple rules when moving. Never leave valuable items exposed. Pack your computer, printer, CD player, VCR and stereo in their original packaging, but mask identifying icons and words so that the boxes become nondescript and noninformational. This way, the curious will not know you have expensive electronic equipment. Some people clearly label all contents after they're packed. Mark your boxes "fragile" and add a code number; indicate in which room they belong, so that bystanders will not be aware of their contents. Enlist the help of friends or family members to watch your possessions while you load or unload. Also, if you live alone, a friend should be with you when utilities are connected in your new home, so that no one is aware that you reside by yourself. Remember, moving is a team effort, and family members and friends are an important asset.

Make certain your previous landlord or anyone else does not give out your new address unless it is specifically authorized by you in writing. On the day you move, arrange to have new locks installed in your new residence so that anyone with access to the old locks will be out of luck. Make sure you install a high-quality deadbolt on all your doors. Also, cover all windows immediately with curtains, shades, or blinds. If you haven't had a chance to order coverings, block your windows with blankets or sheets. These devices will prevent the unwanted from observing anything of value, eliminating an opportunity for crime.

On moving day, carry in a backpack your purse, wallet, jewelry, checkbooks, cash, change, keys, important telephone numbers, and anything else that may aggravate you if lost, like special family photographs. This effort also will help ensure timely and safe arrival at your new address.

ESSENTIAL INFORMATION

As soon as possible, obtain the following emergency, information, and referral phone numbers. They may save your life or the life of a loved one. If you can't obtain these numbers before you move, make sure they are recorded as soon as you arrive at your destination. You might photocopy this page and use the space to enter the proper telephone numbers. Post the information so it is easy to access.

Police Department ....
Fire Department ....
Poison Center ....
Suicide-Crisis Hotline...
Emergency Medical Service or Ambulance...
Rape Hotline...
Arson Hotline ....
Child Abuse or Neglect Hotline..
Elderly Abuse or Neglect Hotline...
Spousal Abuse Crisis Center ....
Runaway House ....
Drug Abuse Referral ....
Alcoholics Anonymous..
Alcohol and Drug Council...
Toxic Waste Hotline ....
FBI ....
Physician...

MOVING OVERSEAS

You have to deal with your home here in the United States. First, discuss with your company the possibility of financial help in selling your home, although such opportunities are rapidly fading. Many companies are tightening their belts and are reluctant to participate in the high costs associated with selling a residence. Still, the best strategy may be to sell your residence. As an absentee landlord, you are much more likely to experience problems than one who is on the scene. Also, rental management programs are expensive and may be unreliable. The worse thing you can do is leave the house empty. Word quickly spreads about an empty house, not only to neighbors but also to burglars, vandals, squatters, and/or arsonists.

If you decide to rent after all, make certain your lawn and shrubbery are neatly maintained and that all repairs are conducted immediately. Properties with shabby appearance have a way of catching the attention of criminals. If feasible, you might consider retaining a professional lawn mowing service, landscaping company, or gardener. Also, make certain your tenant or property manager has the phone numbers of reliable repair services before you move. Otherwise, you may be the victim of a repair rip-off while you are abroad and not in a position to protect your property.

After you have planned carefully and completed all the steps outlined here, you are ready to move. Best of luck and success in your new home, whether here or abroad.

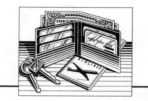

MOVING TO ANOTHER COMMUNITY: A CHECKLIST

1 Determine the expected incidence of crime, including the extent of violence and theft, in the city or town to which you intend to move. Compare these numbers to places nearby with a similar population.

2 Determine the amount of police coverage at your final destination, compared with nearby cities of similar size.

3 Spend several hours walking around the neighborhood to which you intend to move, and observe such indicators of crime as drug addicts, prostitutes, derelicts, street gamblers, youth gangs, and neighborhood toughs. Also, note area crime hazards like bars and drug dens.

4 Observe how neighborhood sidewalks and streets are utilized. They will usually be deserted in high-crime areas, except for criminals, street people, and young neighborhood toughs. Employ similar criteria to determine safety in nearby parks.

5 Be sure lighting is adequate on your neighborhood streets and outside your home.

6 Make certain that your new destination is near safe, reliable, and convenient transportation.

7 Check the level of safety in the schools your children will attend.

8 Notify your post office, relatives, friends, business associates, bank, and credit card companies of your new address.

9 Select a reliable moving company, and be sure to put all conditions involving your move in writing.

10 Pack expensive electronic equipment in original cartons. Mask any type and logos that advertise what is inside.

11 Arrange to have new locks installed in your new residence on the day you move in.

12 If moving overseas, try to sell your present residence rather than become an absentee landlord. The worst thing you can do is leave the house empty.

13 Obtain emergency and essential phone numbers before you move to a new community.

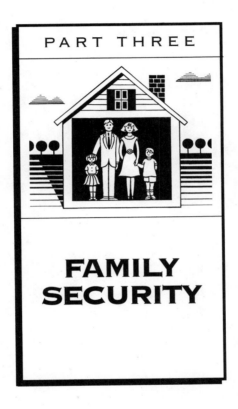

PART THREE

FAMILY SECURITY

18

~

FAMILY VIOLENCE

Family violence, one of the most underreported crimes, includes child abuse, spousal abuse, and elderly abuse. According to a recent report by the U.S. Department of Justice, 16 percent of homicides are intrafamilial. The most frequent victims are wives; the second most frequent, children murdered by their parents.

SPOUSAL ABUSE

Spousal abuse involves physical, emotional, and/or sexual abuse. The majority of the victims of spousal abuse are female, commonly referred to as "battered women."

Certain circumstances or certain jurisdictions may preclude an arrest, but frequently spousal abuse is a criminal assault that can be diligently prosecuted—if it's reported to the police. However, spousal abuse, like child abuse, is an underreported crime.

Over 1 million women a year require medical assistance as a result of physical abuse; it is the number-one cause of injury to women in America. According to studies conducted by the American Medical Association, more women are injured by the men in their lives than in automobile accidents, rapes, and muggings combined. A woman is more likely to be killed as a result of family violence than on the streets, and family violence has more long-term effects than any other crime.

Spouse battering tends to occur more often on Sundays and during vacations or holiday seasons. In addition to the emotional stress that holidays and vacations can bring, spouses are together more frequently during these times (and on weekends), which can result in attacks of "cabin fever." Most domestic violence occurs between 8:00 p.m. and midnight, partly for the same reasons.

It is a myth that battered women are only young, poor, and uneducated. Battering is not limited to any age bracket, race, religious background, or educational or income level. Don't let the fear of being alone keep you with a man who abuses you; there are millions of nonabusive men out there. Do not marry an abusive man no matter how much he promises to change. He almost certainly won't. You will become more isolated and dependent, and it will be much harder for you to escape.

Cycle of Violence

The cycle of violence, according to experts, begins with a buildup of tension and anxiety where the woman strives frantically to calm and placate her potentially violent partner. Then, violence erupts and continues either sporadically or steadily over a period of several months or years. As the violence escalates, the woman may seek help from friends or relatives or call the police. Although many men are enraged further by a police response, most will become contrite and beg forgiveness for their behavior. During this phase, the batterer is kind, compassionate, attentive, loving, and totally cooperative. Flowers, dinner out, and nonviolent sexual activity often are part of this phase of extreme contrition. But soon the violent behavior returns. During this phase, the woman decides to leave or seek out a new partner for support. These events, leaving or finding a new partner, infuriate the angry and jealous batterer more than anything else, because he feels he cannot exist without control over his spouse. It is during this highly volatile and dangerous phase that a woman is at highest risk of critical injury or even murder.

Characteristics of the Batterer

Psychologist Amy Holtzworth-Munroe classified batterers as three types. The first type rarely assaults his partner, and his violent behavior does not escalate over time. These abusers always are contrite and become violent because of a perceived breakdown in communication. The second category of batterer fears abandonment and is dependent on his partner. He feels an urgent need to control her. The final and most dangerous type is the "sociopathic" man possessed by an antisocial personality. Spousal violence is a symptom and consequence of this underlying sociopathic personality, as is a pattern of frequent violations of the law, including violence against others. All types of abusers deny responsibility for their violent acts and blame the victim.

Men who attack and beat women tend to be insecure, frustrated, possessive, and extremely jealous, and do not know how to handle anger in a nonviolent way. Unable to manage these feelings, abusers use violence as a means to control the people in their lives. Abuse is rarely a one-time occurrence. Unless the batterer gets help and learns to express his feelings in an alternative way, he will continue to be violent.

As do their victims, batterers come from all walks of life, and most are not mentally ill. It has been estimated that more than 80 percent of batterers were exposed to abuse as children, either having been beaten themselves or having seen one of their parents constantly beaten.

Often there is a predictable progression to a violent relationship. It usually begins with a series of violent acts that may continue for years. At this point, the woman may seek outside assistance, while the male abuser denies responsibility for his behavior. The two factors that contribute most to murder in such a relationship occur when an abuser's partner moves out of a shared residence or starts a relationship with someone new.

Ten risk factors for abuse have been identified by Richard J. Gelles, Regina Lackner, and Glenn D. Wolfner. The occurrence of two or more of these factors makes violence in the home twice as likely. Identifying with *seven or more* increases one's risk by 40 times. These risk factors are:

❖ An unemployed male.
❖ Illicit drug use at least once a year. (One study found chemical abuse in 42 percent of spouse arrest incidents.)
❖ Partners with different religious affiliations.
❖ The male witnessed violence in the home in which he was raised.
❖ Partners share a residence but are not legally married.
❖ If employed, the male has a blue-collar job.
❖ The male does not have a high school diploma.
❖ The male is between the ages of 18 and 30.
❖ Violence is used toward children by either partner.
❖ The family has an income below the poverty line.

Additional warning signs that a husband is or may become abusive include the following:

❖ He is extremely jealous and possessive.
❖ He exhibits hypermasculine behavior, such as declaring where a man's and woman's place is, and makes all household decisions.
❖ He attempts to prevent you from spending time with your family and friends, especially when he is not there.
❖ He tries to control you financially, for example concealing income, preventing you from getting a job, and refusing to give you money.
❖ He is unable to discuss his feelings calmly and rationally.

❖ He is continually critical of the way you look or what you say and do.

❖ He gets angry easily or insults you.

❖ He threatens you with violence, displays weapons, abuses pets, or destroys your property.

❖ The best indicator of all: He has previously hit or injured you in some way.

Domestic violence tends to increase in frequency and intensity with time. The best way to protect yourself is to avoid putting yourself in the position in the first place.

How to Recognize a Battered Woman

Psychologists and sociologists have not been able to pinpoint exact characteristics of battered women. However, most of these abused women seem to be very trusting, have low self-esteem, and have a need for recognition, approval, and affection. Many are nonaggressive, dependent, powerless, and isolated, and have been brought up to accept traditional values, such as the idea that the man is the head of the household, without question. Often, these women exhibit physical symptoms, like headaches, difficulty in sleeping, anxiety, and stomach pains. Being young, unemployed, poor, and having a history of alcohol and drug abuse increase your chances of being abused. Many battered women are pregnant at the time of the abuse.

If a woman you know interrupts her regular routine, such as missing days at work or not attending social functions she used to, be concerned. If a woman has mysterious cuts and bruises, puts on heavy makeup, and often wears out-of-season clothes (for example, long-sleeved shirts during the summer months) be concerned. She may be covering up the evidence of abuse out of fear and embarrassment. Another cause for concern is a woman who seems to fear the man in her life, or if her behavior becomes drastically more inhibited or controlled around him.

If you believe a neighbor or friend is being hurt, do not hesitate to call the police if it's an emergency situation. The battered spouse may be unable to get to the phone. In a nonemergency situation, try to open lines of communication with the battered woman. For instance, give her the phone number of a battered women's shelter, or make the call for her.

Why Don't Battered Women Just Leave?

This is the most commonly asked question about battered women. First, many abused women are emotionally and financially dependent on their male partners and often believe the beatings are their own fault. Second, abused women may not know where to turn for help, because few support systems are available. There are three times as many animal shelters as shelters for battered women in this country. Also, only 5 percent of the 1,500 battered-women's shelters in the United States accept women with children. If a woman walks out on her husband and leaves her children behind, she risks losing custody of them. Many battered women are afraid their abusers will retaliate if they leave them or have them arrested.

If You Are Battered

The very first thing you should do if you are a battered woman is to admit to yourself that you are abused. Many women are so fearful, intimidated, and controlled that they refuse to admit their state of dependence and victimization. But you must plan and then act. Put money, important documents, and car keys in a secure hiding place, so that you will have access to them in a hurry if you need to leave. Find out the location of an emergency shelter, or make arrangements to go to the home of a trusted friend or relative before you are beaten again. Plan how to escape with your children. If you do not manage to escape before the next attack, try to defend yourself to the best of your ability. After the assault, call the police and seek medical help. You should have color photographs taken of cuts and bruises. If the beating results in hospitalization, the names of the doctors, nurses, police officers, and witnesses should be obtained, as should copies of X rays and medical reports. Those listed above can be called to give testimony, and the photos and documents can be used as evidence if the incident results in a court appearance.

Expert Jennifer Baker Fleming urges the victim to develop the following positive attitudes:

❖ You are not the cause of the batterer's violent behavior; *he* is.

❖ You do not enjoy the abuse nor should you tolerate it.

❖ You are a worthwhile and important human being who deserves love and respect.

❖ You can have power and control over your life.

❖ You are not alone; others can be there to help.

❖ You deserve a life of safety, security, and happiness.

As a battered woman, you may find the most immediate and useful help at a woman's shelter. Such shelters can provide a place to stay, food, clothing, financial and legal advice, emotional support, and counseling for you and your children. Staff members, often victims of domestic violence themselves, will accompany you to court if you wish to press charges and will help you with job interviews, apartment hunts, and welfare benefits if you need financial aid. Women's shelters are not exclusively for poor women. They are for any woman who needs help. These shelters are in secret locations, so your abuser will not be able to find you. If you do not know of the nearest women's shelter, call the police to take you there, or call the National Victim Center: (1-800) FYI-CALL.

Some other sources of assistance include the church or synagogue of your faith or a psychological counselor or therapist. If you have to go to the hospital as a result of a beating, tell the doctor or nurse how the injury really occurred. The hospital staff can connect you with a source of assistance. The Salvation Army helps people of all faiths and backgrounds and can refer you to people who can assist you. In addition, you can look up crisis intervention services in the telephone book. Lastly, friends and family can be a great source of help by providing a temporary place to stay or emotional support.

You can also call the National Coalition Against Domestic Violence: (303) 839-1852 for referral to local agencies. Local hotlines are staffed by counselors willing to help. Don't be afraid to tell these people everything. They are specially trained and have heard it all. All information given is strictly confidential.

Do not leave your children behind. This could subject them to violence from the abuser. Furthermore, your leaving may be later interpreted as abandonment and may be held against you in your fight for custody.

Treatment for Batterers

Batterers never learned as children how to manage anger and resentment, and often were abused themselves. As adults they take out their frustrations on their partners by acting on these violent impulses.

Through others, urge your partner to seek therapy to learn how to reroute his anger and resentment without having to act violently. Be aware, however, that many abusers refuse treatment, and only about half who appear for therapy complete the program. This is unfortunate, as those who complete programs are much more likely not to use violence as a means of expression.

CHILD ABUSE

Perhaps the most despicable crimes are the crimes committed against children by adults. The saddest of all may be child abuse, because it is so often inflicted by parents, whom the child loves the most and on whom the child is most dependent for his or her very life. A few years ago, the entire country was traumatized when Susan Smith of Union, South Carolina, confessed to murdering her two boys: Michael, 3, and Alex, 14 months. The police found the car Susan was driving in a lake, with the children securely strapped in, drowned to death. She attempted to throw the police off her trail by alleging that a man stole her car and kidnapped her sons.

The police concentrated the investigation on Susan only after a nation-wide search failed to turn up any evidence to support her false allegations.

What Is Child Abuse?

The law describes a child as a person under age 18. The abused child is one who is assaulted with weapons, but most frequently with the abuser's hands; sexually assaulted; held in close confinement, as when locked in a closet or tied up; emotionally or verbally abused; or otherwise mistreated. Another aspect of child abuse is neglect. A neglected child does not receive necessary care, lacks adequate supervision or medical assistance, and, most importantly, is receiving inadequate nurturing and affection. A parent must provide a safe environment for the child, including taking measures to prevent accidental harm or injury, such as swallowing poison or falling out an open window.

Outside the home, physically challenged or different children, even including those who are especially bright and talented, have high risks of victimization, both sexually and physically. The attacker frequently looks for the child who stands out in a crowd.

Children who have run away from home or children born without homes are particularly vulnerable to attack from pedophiles—adults who are sexually attracted to children. These children may be coerced into becoming prostitutes or taking part in child pornography.

Child abuse is an underreported crime. Most children never tell. Adolescents are less likely to report abuse than younger children. Many adults have forgotten about their abuse when they were children, only to have delayed remembrances later in life.

Profile of a Child Abuser

It would be a lot more comfortable to think that child sexual abuse is perpetrated only by sick strangers, because then one could "see them coming," but this is not always the case. The most frequent abuser is a *male relative*. Indeed, 80 to 90 percent of these cases occur within the family. An estimated 5 million American females have suffered a sexual assault at the hands of a relative at least once in their lives. According to some studies, in 85 to 95 percent of sexual abuse cases the abuser is a person the child knows. Often it is a parent, a brother or sister, a neighbor, a baby-sitter, a day-care employee, a teacher, a coach, a minister, or someone else who is surrounded by children. Molesters usually find ways to spend a large amount of time with children.

Older children may molest younger children. From one-third to one-half of sexual abusers commit their first abuse before they reach 18 years of age. Some sexual abusers are women. Mothers are responsible for about one-third of the cases of child abuse and are themselves often victims of abuse in the same home.

Most child abusers themselves were battered children or witnessed violence in the home in which they were raised. They have been led to believe that this type of interaction is acceptable and are only repeating the violence they experienced while growing up. Many molesters were victims of sexual abuse as children as well. Many people who assault children have a hard time controlling their emotions; they lash out at the child, the one thing they *can* control.

Child abusers do not fit a single profile. They come from all walks of life, from all races, ethnic backgrounds, religions, age brackets, and income levels. Children of wealthy parents are often as abused as children from poor families.

Recognizing an Abused Child

A seriously abused child shows signs of battering and neglect—for example, frequent, unexplained injuries, such as bruises, welts, cuts, burns, and even bites. Some injuries may even appear not to have been accidentally caused, such as a bruise or a welt with the shape of an object like a coat hanger, an iron, or a belt buckle. A neglected child may be left alone for many hours or be outside in cold weather without a coat. A neglected child may be continually tired and listless or constantly hungry. Neglected children have been known, for example, to search for food in garbage cans in school lunchrooms or even to beg for food. The child may roam the streets after dark. He or she may seem excessively fearful of being touched, shying away from a hug or a pat on the head.

Some other warning signs experts recognize include:

❖ Being very withdrawn or clingy to parents or, conversely, very aggressive

❖ Bedwetting, nightmares, tantrums

❖ Age-inappropriate sexual behavior demonstrated through language or acting-out with peers or dolls, or reflected in drawings

❖ Fear of certain people or of going to particular places

❖ Trouble in school

❖ Depression or behavioral problems

❖ Changes in eating or sleeping habits

❖ Poor hygiene

❖ Irritation, pain, bleeding, or itching in the genital area

❖ Excessive anxiety or nervousness

- ❖ Regressive behavior, such as thumb sucking or developmental slowness
- ❖ Feelings of guilt, anger, or shame
- ❖ Short attention span and inability to concentrate
- ❖ Stealing and other forms of delinquency
- ❖ Substance abuse

If only one or two of these signs are present, the signs may not be due to abuse, but if you observe any of these tendencies in a child (whether yours or someone else's)—especially if they represent changes from his or her routine behavior—it is a good idea to investigate them with a therapist or family doctor.

Assisting an Abused Child

Neighbors often know of abuse but are reluctant to report the parents to a child protection agency. This fear of involvement is unfounded. If a child needs immediate medical attention, you can safely phone the police. You do not have to give your name. You can also place a call (anonymously if you wish) to your local child welfare bureau. Do not inform anyone that you have taken action. Abusive parents have been known to coach a child, so that when an investigator shows up, everything seems normal.

If a child comes to you to report abuse, you should believe him or her. Children hardly ever lie about sexual abuse. Tell the child you are glad he or she told you. Make sure the child knows you will protect him or her and that the abuse is not his or her fault.

If there is any physical evidence of abuse, take pictures and make copies of any X rays or medical or psychological reports. Put these away in a safe place, and clearly label each item. The evidence should be given to the police or the child protective agency when you make your report, and you should get a receipt.

Do not confront the person or organization suspected of abuse. Call the police or an appropriate social service agency. The only evidence needed is what the child has told you. It is absolutely essential that you report it immediately to prevent the abuser from victimizing more children. Research has shown that sexual assaulters who molest girls tend to repeat acts of abuse an average of 62 times, and those who molest boys tend to repeat sexual assaults an average of 30 times.

Seek out professional therapists and doctors who specialize in the treatment of child assault cases. Use the help they can provide for you and your child. If you are an abused child, you can call the National Child Abuse Hotline, (1-800) 4A-CHILD or (1-800) 422-4453, to speak to a trained professional.

Protecting Your Children from Abuse

Guidelines are important and should be taught patiently to your child over a reasonable period. Here are some tactics you can use to help protect your child from abuse:

❖ Make certain you warn your child to be wary of strangers.

❖ Make certain your child knows it's important to tell you (or, if at school, a teacher) about any incidents of improper touching by adults, and by older children as well.

❖ Make sure your child knows he or she can tell you anything, even if it makes the child or you feel awkward and uncomfortable. Also tell the child he or she won't get in trouble for telling.

❖ As soon as your child is able, teach him or her to use the telephone. Make sure the child knows how to reach you at home or at work.

❖ Teach your child when to scream for help and run away.

❖ Respect your child's feelings. For example, if the child doesn't want to kiss Grandma now, do not resort to force. Coercion teaches children that they must do what adults ask, even if it makes them uncomfortable.

❖ Teach your child appropriate names for the private parts of the body. Avoid secretive names or euphemisms, as such terms make these areas seem forbidden and may make it more difficult for the child to discuss them with you.

❖ Teach your child that his or her body, especially the genitals, belongs to him or her, and that nobody has the right to touch it.

❖ Play an age-appropriate "what if" game with your child, and see how he or she responds to different scenarios. For example, ask "What if a stranger approaches you?" or "What if somebody touched you in a way you did not like?" Correct the child gently if he or she gives an undesirable answer, and encourage the child to ask questions. Be sure not to scare the child.

❖ Teach your child that it's okay to say No! to adults if he or she does not like what is going on. When children say No and leave immediately, most abusers will not pursue them.

❖ Find out what the school can do to help, not only with programs teaching children about abuse but also with specialists on site who may be able to recognize the signs of child abuse.

❖ Determine the screening procedures under which teachers are hired in your community. Be sure that people with police records and poor character are screened out.

❖ Consider self-defense classes for older children, including karate, and also personal electronic alarms to carry in the event of an assault. These suggestions may result in high costs, but they are definitely worth thinking about.

You don't want to weigh the child down with an endless list of things to do, to avoid, and to think about. This list is short and to the point:

❖ Police officers are your friends; they will help you.
❖ Go to school with your friends; come home with your friends.
❖ Whenever you leave home, tell your parents where you're going.
❖ If you're not at home or at school, and you have to use the restroom, ask a friend to go with you.
❖ Play where other kids play: friends' houses, playgrounds, or at home.
❖ Never play in empty buildings.
❖ Never get in an automobile with anyone you don't know.
❖ Never talk to people you don't know.
❖ When a grown-up does something bad to you, tell your parents, your teacher, or a police officer.

Remember that the consequences of child abuse are lifelong. The best solution is to prevent child assault in the first place.

If You Feel Violent

If you yourself feel violent and are quick to get angry, take time to cool down. Some things you can do that are calming are:

❖ Take a short walk or run.
❖ Take a soothing shower or bath.
❖ Call someone you can talk to.
❖ Listen to music or watch TV.
❖ Leave the room or house for awhile.
❖ Take deep breaths or count slowly until you are calm.
❖ Go for a short drive.
❖ Try something as simple as making yourself a cup of tea or coffee.

After you calm down and no longer feel angry, call your local division of youth and family services. A child will not be removed from the home unless all else has failed. It may be helpful to contact Parents Anonymous, a nationwide group of adults with abuse problems who meet to give mutual support and to learn ways of dealing with their children without resorting to physical violence.

ABUSE OF THE ELDERLY

Less is known about abuse of the elderly than about spousal abuse. While hard statistics are few, one study does provide a clue. This research indicates that slightly more than one-fourth of wives are abused by their husbands, while approximately one-sixth of the elderly are victimized.

A similar study asked people their opinions of the seriousness of certain actions. About two-fifths thought spouse abuse to be serious, while almost two-thirds of the sample considered child abuse to be very serious. Almost as many thought abuse of the elderly was just as serious.

Incidence of Maltreatment

Repugnant cases of mistreatment of the elderly by family members, often by children, unfortunately are not rare events. Victims themselves are often incapable, physically or psychologically, of reporting incidents. Some fear further and more severe punishment or, even worse, abandonment.

Abusive family members will sometimes threaten the aged with nursing homes or hospitalization. If the abuser is imprisoned, no one will be around to provide care. They may endure the abuse rather than plunge into unknown living arrangements, or they may stay out of fear of living alone. Many aged also hope the abuser's behavior will change.

Others are embarrassed, ashamed, or guilty about coming forward. Like battered wives, elderly victims often have a poor self-image and believe they deserve the brutal punishment, thinking, "If I behave myself, nobody will hurt me." Many elderly citizens do not know where or how to find assistance.

Abused and Abusers

Many men in their 70s, 80s, and even 90s are victims of maltreatment by their "loved ones." But the typical victims of abuse are women about 75 years old. While over half of abusers are male, about two-thirds of victims are female. The median age of elderly abuse victims in 1994 was 76.4 years old. Often ill or weak, they are unable to care for themselves, and they make easy targets for the degenerate adult child. Recent research suggests that the aged with health problems are at least three times more likely to be abused than elderly persons in good health. Surveys tell us that six out of seven, or 86 percent, of the abused elderly are mistreated by members of their own families.

As with child and spousal abuse, elderly abuse occurs at all income levels and afflicts the aged of all races, ethnicities, and religions. However, some researchers have suggested that middle-class families suffer greater stress as caregivers than lower- and upper-class families. Affluent families can afford to hire outside help, and lower-class families tend to be more intergenerationally dependent. It is the middle class who, unused to such relationships and without adequate resources to hire outside help, can feel more of the burden in caregiving.

Forms of Abuse

Elderly abuse has many different faces. Perhaps the most horrible is *physical*. This includes beating, punching, slapping, bruising, burning, bone breaking, raping, or even killing. Almost one-sixth of abuse cases in 1994 involved such severe forms of abuse. Physical abuse may comprise more than one form of violence.

Psychological abuse often can be as severe. This mind abuse frequently includes humiliation, subjugation, denigration, degradation, subordination, domination, and control. Verbal abuse is part of this formula. The vulnerable, sometimes entirely defenseless, victims are told they are evil, insane, and unstable. They are handcuffed to their beds, locked in their rooms, and forced to eat out of the dog's dish.

Yet another form of brutality is *financial/material,* in which money or some object, such as a bed, is withheld from the victim. Most instances of financial/material abuse involve taking the victim's money and using it for the caretaker's personal needs. This type of abuse is also the most difficult to detect, especially if it occurs little by little.

Neglect is another form of abuse when food or medication, for example, is withheld, or when the helpless victim suffers bedsores from long periods of confinement. This is the most common form of abuse, occurring in 58.5 percent of elderly abuse cases in 1994. There has been an emergence of incidences of "granny dumping"—when adult children or other caregivers abandon an aged person in their care.

Causes

Care of the elderly is extremely difficult. The average length of time a caregiver will have to care for an elderly person over the age of 70 is between 5 and 6 years. One home-care worker spent 84 hours a week caring for a 90-year-old who was wheelchair bound and suffered many medical problems. Another caregiver spent every night in a small apartment with his elderly ward. He bathed, dressed, and fed the older man. He had to lift his patient from bed to wheelchair without mechanical aid and take him along when he went out to shop or to a movie.

Stress, pressure, persistent responsibilities, and vulnerability of the victims are only partial reasons that caregivers abuse the ones they care for. Adult children who are alcoholics or drug addicts are likely to abuse their parents, especially physically. Troubled, unstable, or mentally ill adult children who are economically and emotionally dependent on their parents may also become abusive. Patterns or cycles of domestic violence from generation to generation, including spouse and child abuse, frequently evolve into patterns of mistreatment by an adult child who "pays back" the parents for childhood suffering and pain.

Solutions

Elderly abuse can be prevented, or at least controlled, by following a few, simple procedures. First, you should be alert for signs of abuse in others, and, on discovery, immediately intervene by notifying the proper authorities. Learn to recognize injuries, bruises, welts, scratches, or bite marks whose origins are unknown. Long periods of isolation, frequent screams and yells for help, self-reports describing abuse, signs of malnutrition, filth in the home, and unwashed clothes and bodies are equally significant danger signs. However, remember that all families argue, complain, and have problems, and that not every disagreement or temper tantrum signals elderly abuse. Many children manage their parents' finances or attend to their personal needs honestly and intelligently.

Finally, before agreeing to take care of an elderly loved one, you must go through a process of self-evaluation. Assess your own abilities and resources; it's okay to realize that you are incapable of effectively dealing with the pressures and responsibilities that go along with caretaking. This does not mean you love the person any less; it means you are concerned about taking on too much and want what is best for your loved one. This is a key aspect of abuse prevention.

If you don't live near an elderly parent, relative, or friend who needs help, call the nationwide toll-free Eldercare Locator telephone number, (800) 677-1116, to find out about services available in their community.

Self-Protection for the Elderly

If you are elderly, maintain contact with other senior citizens in your family and community, especially with those who are isolated and housebound. As a parent, you should do everything to open communication channels with your adult children. You should get together and talk about the increasing requirements for care as you age. The discussions should include sharing responsibilities, budget management, and available community help. You should suggest that your adult children take courses on care for the elderly to help them learn what to expect, what to do if the tasks become intolerable, and how to reach out for help.

If you are being cared for by a friend or relative, make every effort to maintain your independence. Be responsible for your own personal needs, and keep medical, hairdressing, and other personal appointments. Keep your possessions neat and organized, making sure others know that you are aware of where you place your belongings. Have your own telephone line, and open your own mail. Just because someone is helping you does not give them the right to make decisions for you or to invade your privacy.

There are many steps that you can take now to put your finances in order. One of the most important is to prepare a will. Review it annually, but think hard before revising it. Be suspicious of suggestions to deed your house, personal property, or other assets to anyone in exchange for care or other assurances that you will not have to enter a nursing home. Sign nothing before you check with someone you absolutely trust and whose interests are not being served.

Thoroughly familiarize yourself with your financial situation, know how to manage your assets, and determine who will take over for you in an emergency. This is particularly essential for older women who may not have experience in financial management. Don't agree to transfer funds or property to a caregiver in return for assistance without the advice and witness of an advocate, attorney, or other trusted person.

Always have your Social Security checks and other regular payments deposited directly to your bank account. While it is a good idea to have another well-trusted person, such as one of your children, listed on your bank account, this can be extremely risky if you don't know the person well. If at all possible, leave your account in trust for this person, instead of listing her or him on a joint account.

Be sure to cultivate new friends, and maintain old ones of all ages, so that you do not rely only on your family for social activities and for health care. Be very careful about allowing an adult child to return home to live with you, especially one who is troubled or who might have a history of drug addiction, alcoholism, compulsive gambling, violence, mental illness, or criminality. As an alternative, helping to support your adult child in a separate residence is an excellent way of preserving everyone's dignity and at the same time protecting yourself.

Now is the time to make peace with alienated friends or family, not only because you will be cheered by the added companionship but also because it provides a pool of caring people to assist you in time of need. Plan for later periods of vulnerability by having your attorney advise you about the powers of attorney, conservatorships or guardianships, "living wills," and natural-death acts. Appointing several individuals to serve as co-guardians or co-conservators assures that, in case of an emergency, there is always someone responsible and available to manage your affairs.

Remember, not only are you an individual, but you are also a member of the community. You can help diminish mistreatment by joining a community group that educates you about where and how to get assistance and, even more important, emphasizes that it is not shameful or a sign of weakness to seek help. You should have ready access to a hotline for emergencies and any other situations requiring assistance.

Find out about adult protective services in your community where reports of abuse are immediately investigated and where appropriate action can be taken to resolve unbearable situations. Learn about home-care services that will send a companion, practical nurse, or home health aid to look after an aged citizen part-time or at least once a day. If your community has an adult day-care center, visit it and introduce yourself to the people in charge. Don't hesitate to contact professionals who are concerned with elderly abuse, including social workers, nurses, physicians, health-care workers, members of the clergy, and police officers. If you can, join a Neighborhood Watch program, and suggest that it expand its responsibilities to include daily checks on individuals who are housebound, infirm, or otherwise vulnerable to abuse and neglect.

We can only guess the pervasiveness of all these family violence components—spousal abuse, child abuse, and abuse of the elderly—for each of them is highly underreported. But remember, no one deserves to be beaten. Once physical violence occurs, it is more than likely to recur unless measures are taken to stop it. Do not wait for a serious injury to occur before you seek help.

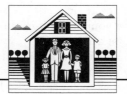

FAMILY VIOLENCE:
A CHECKLIST

1 The first thing a battered woman should do is admit she is being abused. She should look for warning signs; if they are present, she should leave the relationship. It will only get worse, probably much worse.

2 Frequent screaming and sobbing coming from a woman's home strongly indicates that she is being battered. If you believe a neighbor or friend is being hurt, call the police.

3 Be concerned if a woman you know drastically alters her routines, if her behavior changes when her husband is present, and if she makes excuses for cuts, bruises, or injuries.

4 If you yourself are being beaten or threatened, call the police. Arrest and subsequent counseling may be the most effective remedies for the spousal abuser. Make the decision to arrest him in consultation with the responding officers.

5 If you have been previously hit by your spouse, chances are it will happen again. Plan how to escape, then act, and seek help for the problem.

6 Collect evidence after a beating incident, such as pictures of your injuries, hospital reports, and names and addresses of possible witnesses.

7 Call the National Coalition Against Domestic Violence or your local family violence hotline to speak to specially trained counselors who can help.

8 Do not, for the sake of your children, stay with someone who beats you. A violent home is not a happy place for anyone. Do not leave your children behind and risk your chances for custody.

9 Remember, you are a victim and do not deserve bad treatment. You are in a life-threatening situation and must escape.

10 Urge your partner to seek therapy that may teach him to reroute his anger and resentment.

11 Help discover others who are abused. Look for the physical signs of child, spousal, and elderly abuse, such as frequent bruises, cuts, and welts.

12 Know and look out for warning signs of child abuse, especially behavioral problems and trouble in school, that may indicate your child or a child you know has been abused.

13 Be aware of children who act unusually fearful of adults. If a child comes to you to report abuse, believe him or her.

14 If a child is seriously injured or ignored by parents, call the police.

15 Report cases of child abuse to your local child welfare agency. Do not tell anyone, especially the parents, that you are calling the agency.

16 Instruct your children to follow specific safety measures when they are alone.

17 Only a parent or someone delegated by the parent should punish a child.

18 If you yourself feel violent, take time to cool down. Never punish your child so severely that she or he will be harmed.

19 Avoid the use of derogatory terms when instructing your children, and take time out to cool off when angry.

20 If you were a victim of child abuse, it's not too late to get help. Consult a professional with experience in child abuse cases.

21 Learn to recognize the signs of abuse of the elderly and children, including long periods of isolation, malnutrition, and other signs of neglect.

22 If you are abused or are aware of someone else in similar, unfortunate circumstances, notify the authorities immediately.

23 If you are elderly, discuss with your children requirements for your care for a time when you will be unable to take care of yourself.

24 Familiarize yourself with all community support services, including visiting-nurse care, home health aides, household help, senior day-care centers, and adult protective services.

25 Have ready access to an abuse hotline for the aged, and keep a list of emergency numbers by your telephone.

26 Join a Neighborhood Watch program that checks on the housebound, infirm, and other individuals vulnerable to maltreatment.

27 Prepare a will, and put your finances in order now before it is too late.

28 Don't sign anything unless it is reviewed by someone you have good reason to trust.

29 Assign someone you have trusted for a long time to take over your financial matters in an emergency.

30 Learn about powers of attorney, conservatorships or guardianships, "living wills," and natural-death acts.

31 Have all regular payments and Social Security checks deposited directly into your bank account.

32 If your adult child has a history of substance abuse, compulsive gambling, violence, mental illness, or criminality, be certain of total recovery before asking the child to come live with you.

19

SECURITY FOR INFANTS AND YOUNG CHILDREN

Parents must protect little ones at any cost, and that is why it is so important for working parents to find the finest and safest day care for their child.

Only 12 percent of American families fit the classic configuration of father who goes to work each weekday and mother who stays home to care for the children. More typical is the family of the late 20th century—a family in which both parents work and the children are tended by relatives, baby-sitters, or, outside the home, day-care centers. In recent years these centers have been the focus of a great deal of negative publicity.

DAY-CARE CENTERS: A BOOMING INDUSTRY

One would hope that day care is safe and secure. But shocking cases of child abuse and sexual molestation are reported in day-care facilities across the nation. Among the more frightening aspects of this type of abuse are the increasing proliferation of day-care centers, the large number of children at risk, and the long time it takes to detect the incidents.

Of course, some facilities will be better than others, and you will wish to utilize only the best available for your children. If you aren't familiar with the care units in your area, ask the principal of your school, your physician, neighbors, or your priest, rabbi, or minister.

Types of Day Care

It is easy to become confused when attempting to classify the varieties of day care. There are public nonprofit centers that charge on a sliding scale depending on income. Private day care usually is more expensive but may also offer "scholarships" (discounts) based on need. There is highly structured care outside the home, as well as more intimate family-type programs in private homes; there are all-day and half-day programs. Many day-care programs have extended hours for latchkey children, who return from school while their parents are still at work. (See Chapter 20.)

Only you can judge which program is most suitable for you, your child, and your budget. But whatever form of day care you choose, be sure it is effective, safe, and wholesome.

How to Recognize Safe Day Care

Signs of child abuse at day care are not recognized easily by how play activities, toys, games, and equipment are organized. Nor will you detect any indication of child molestation from the quality of food or snacks or the safety precautions against accidents. But several basic signs will alert you to the possibility of danger.

By contacting your local government organization that monitors day-care centers, you can determine if the day-care center is properly licensed, certified, or registered to carry out its activities. Inquire if any background checks were carried out by the center to determine the fitness of personnel, including the custodial and kitchen staff. Were their references checked carefully? Are the caregivers qualified for the work? How long have they been in child care? What procedures are in place if someone other than the parent or designated person comes to pick up the child? Determine whether an adequate staff-to-child ratio exists; experts have recommended a ratio of about one to four for children 3 years old and younger, and about one to seven for children 4 years old and older.

Find out as much as you can about disciplinary procedures, how misconduct is managed. See if the administration is comfortable discussing the subject of child abuse. And don't hesitate to ask the day-care center administrator questions about strategies for preventing sexual molestation or physical abuse. Make sure the children are never the object of physical punishment, especially beatings.

When you visit a prospective center or other day-care facility, do so without an appointment. You'll get a good idea of what goes on there. Then, later, when you sign your child up, make a few occasional spontaneous visits. If you see anything that you don't approve of, you can discuss the problem with the management—or take your child elsewhere. Don't feel strange or embarrassed to visit the center at any time. By observing the children in their routine activities, you will sense what life is really like at the center. No area should be off limits. You will be able to determine whether the children are happy or if there is an air of tension, anxiety, and intimidation.

Be sure that caretakers always receive your written permission to take your child on a trip away from the day-care center. Instruct your children in no uncertain terms that they are prohibited from leaving the day-care center without your permission.

Care You Don't Need

Once you find the best care suitable for your child, you still have to assume an active role to make sure that the care does not deteriorate because of staff turnover, changing policies, shifting organizational structure, or general loss of enthusiasm.

Never allow your child to continue in a program that is poorly evaluated by neighbors, friends, or parents familiar with it. The old adage "where there is smoke, there is fire" certainly is applicable to day-care centers, because infants, toddlers, and preschoolers are virtually defenseless against abuse. Remove your child from a program that does not welcome unannounced visits while the center is open. Be especially on your guard if you are required to call before each visit and then are confined to the office or other administrative areas but not allowed into places where children are at play or engaged in other activities. Be suspicious if, after a reasonable period of adjustment, your little one is afraid of the caregivers or resists returning to the center.

Should you notice a major staff turnover and strange people caring for your child, find out immediately what's going on. Be aware if your child comes home with suspicious injuries or body marks. These are not always signs of abuse, but at least they indicate deteriorating, negligent, and eroding care. Sure signs of impending problems are your child's complaints about long periods of playing or waiting alone. If these occur, you will probably begin to notice poor supervision, indifference, and a lax attitude on part of the caregivers.

Fewer organized activities and outdated or broken toys often signify a diminution in the level of supervision. Another danger signal is harsh, rude, and irrational behavior by the caregivers toward the children and toward you. They may, for example, become defensive, and even angry, when you express your concerns. You will know the program is not for you when you begin to worry about your child, lose confidence in the caregivers, and generally feel uncomfortable with the level of care and organization.

PREEMPTING SEXUAL ABUSE

Several steps can be taken by you and your little one to prevent sexual abuse in day care before it occurs. At home, instruct your children about the body's private parts, and rehearse alternatives for reacting to an unusual situation. Teach your children in advance to say No to adults who threaten them or touch them in places where they feel uncomfortable. Convince them that it's not their fault if an adult touches them in a sensitive area. Instruct them that their body belongs to them, and they have the right to tell adults not to touch it. Tell your children to report to you anyone who touches them where they shouldn't. Small children should be taught to tell you about any pain or punishment or any other dangerous situation they experienced in day care. Explain to your child that you can always provide protection. A child will confide in you if convinced that you have the power to help. (You should review the section on "Child Abuse" in Chapter 18 for additional information.)

Should your child report to you any form of physical abuse, follow through as you promised, and contact the police or a social service agency. For your child's sake, don't procrastinate, since circumstances are likely to deteriorate further. Remember, the abuser is likely to repeat the behavior either with your child or with another youngster. Also, when your child requires medical or psychological assistance, seek it without delay.

The safety, security, and health of your child depends on you, and on the time and energy you spend investigating the best day care and being alert for danger signs. Don't fail to take all necessary steps to ensure protection.

CHILD ABDUCTION AND MISSING CHILDREN

One of the biggest fears parents have is the possibility that their child may be abducted. The abducted and missing include children kidnapped by strangers, relatives, or by parents who do not have custody or legal guardianship.

Abductor Profile

The typical abductor is a white male in his 20s or 30s. The National Institute of Mental Health reports that most molesters begin early, at around 15 years of age, and may attack over 100 children before they are caught. The most frequent motivation is sexual. The National Center for Missing and Exploited Children (NCMEC) has discovered that girls are more likely than boys to be abducted. The average age of abducted children is 10½. Preteens and early teenagers are at the highest risk for victimization. Blacks and Latinos are disproportionately victimized. The FBI is currently trying to develop a psychological profile of a typical abductor.

It is a myth that the majority of abductors are strangers lurking in alley-ways. Most abducted children are taken by a parent or family member during a custody battle. This is usually not done out of love or a strong desire to be with the child but is instead the result of an overwhelming urge for control or revenge aimed at an ex-spouse in a divorce struggle. Studies estimate that these cases number anywhere from 350,000 to 500,000 each year; the growing incidence of such cases is attributed to the increasing divorce rate in America.

Child abductions can occur anytime, but the hours of highest risk are from 3:00 to 6:00 p.m., when children are out of school, playing, and less likely to be supervised. Many abductors ask kids for help to search for a lost puppy or kitten, or to assist them in crossing the street or going to their car. Many act as if they were disabled. A frequent ploy is to tell kids there is an emergency and that they must be escorted home. Others entice children by inviting them to participate in a television show or a beauty contest. Bribery with candy or ice cream is still surprisingly effective.

Protecting Children from Abduction

The most basic rules are to ensure that your child knows his or her full name, your full name, address, telephone number (including area code), your telephone number at work, how to use the telephone, and how to call the operator or 911/emergency assistance. Teach your child these basics as soon as he or she is ready.

The most frequent precaution is "Don't talk to strangers." This is not enough, and many experts agree it is mostly ineffective in preventing abductions. Children don't usually find strangers ugly, frightening, and dangerous. On the contrary, most abductors appear to be warm and friendly and have no trouble getting the child to trust them. The abductor can cease to be a stranger within a very short time. Teach children that all people with whom they are not acquainted or do not know well are strangers, and that they should never go home with them, especially in cars. Your children, of course, should never hitchhike.

However, you must be sure not to induce paranoia when educating your children about the potential danger of strangers. Obviously, most strangers are not harmful and will help in an emergency. Never allow your children's suspicions, diffidence, and apprehension to escalate to the point that they are fearful of all strangers in every situation. Children should be alert and prepared, not in a constant state of terror.

Children are also commonly taught to be polite and respectful to adults. You need to let them know that you would like them to behave this way but that they also have their own space and the right to say No, even to a grown-up, if they are made to feel uncomfortable or if an adult touches them inappropriately. Teach them to report such behavior without delay. Always encourage your children to tell you about strange events, and assure them that you will always protect them.

Basic Guidelines

Here are other guidelines that should be followed to help protect your child from abduction:

❖ Your children should be well supervised. It is important that you know where they are at all times and know how they are going to get to a destination and home again. You must also be familiar with your children's friends and have their telephone numbers and addresses available.

❖ Do not leave children unattended at home, at the playground, in your car, or in any store while you shop, even for a moment. This is the kind of opportunity the abductor looks for. Also, teach your children to play and go places with others. Make sure they know they are much safer when not alone.

❖ Make sure your child knows what to do if the two of you become separated in a store or if he or she is lost; tell your child to go to an employee, security officer, a checkout counter, or some other pre-arranged location. Wandering around makes it more difficult for you to find each other. Some parents avoid separation from toddlers by using expanding cords to tether them.

❖ Avoid personalizing children's clothing or other personal items, so that an offender will not know your child's name; an offender may trick the child into thinking that he or she is a family friend.

❖ If followed or forced to go somewhere, your child should yell or scream for assistance. Hiding is a dangerous tactic.

❖ Be certain your children know that they shouldn't answer the door when alone, or answer the phone if you aren't home. They should know to let the answering machine take a message. Such statements as "My mother can't come to the phone right now. May I take a message for her?" is a signal that the child is alone. Caution the child never to tell his or her name to an unfamiliar caller. If someone delivers a package while you or another adult is not there, the child should ask that the package be left at the door.

❖ Be careful with whom you leave your children. Trust your instincts about caregivers, teachers, or others who are in contact with your child. Do not leave your child in the care of anyone with whom you are not completely comfortable.

❖ Be certain your child's baby-sitter, school, or day-care facility will not release your child unless you have authorized them to do so first, and then only to those whom you have specifically designated. They should also be aware of your child's custody status. If you are divorced, be fully informed of your legal rights. Make arrangements with your baby-sitter, school, or day-care facility for them to alert you if your child fails to arrive.

❖ Make sure your child knows not to go with your ex-spouse without your permission. Also, when your child does leave with a noncustodial parent, make sure the child knows the agreed-upon time of return and is instructed to call you if he or she is going to be late.

❖ Select a secret password that only you and your child know that can be used in case you need to send someone to pick him or her up. Make sure you change the password if you've been separated or divorced. Instruct your children never to get into a car with anyone who doesn't know the password, unless you have told them it's OK.

❖ Play an age-appropriate "What if . . ." game with children. Present them with situations like "What would you say to a grown-up you didn't know who asked you to help find his lost dog?" or "What would you do if a stranger pulled up in a car and wanted to give you toys or candy?" Let the children answer, and gently correct them if the response is not a desirable one. Be sure not to scare them, and let them ask questions. You can even role-play the situations, so that your child can practice yelling No! and running away. You and your child can even take turns.

❖ Abductors frequently tell children that you don't want them or love them anymore. Be certain your children know you will always love them and definitely want them, no matter what.

❖ If you notice an adult paying a lot of attention to your child, be concerned. Teach your children to inform you or their teachers about strangers who want to photograph them.

❖ Teach your children to tell you if someone asks them to keep a secret or offers them presents.

❖ If a grown-up approaches your child to ask for directions, or for help in finding her or his lost child or a lost puppy, teach the child to run away immediately. Adults don't need a kid's help; they should be asking other grown-ups for assistance.

❖ Know what your child is wearing each day, in case you need to provide a description to the police.

Tell these things to your children over a reasonable period of time. Limit what you say to what they need to know at their age, and discuss these issues in a way they can understand. Experts suggest starting when they are old enough to stray away from you. You may also start by asking them what they already know, or if any of their friends have had experiences they would like to talk about with you. It is very important not to scare children when teaching them these things. Also, keep reminding them every so often. Children forget things, so telling them once is never enough.

High-Tech Protection

Keep a current picture or video of your child in a safe place. You should have a good set of fingerprints taken, and keep copies of medical and dental records. These may be kept in a file that could be turned over to the police to aid in search and identification in the event your child is missing. Numerous gadgets are also available, such as an identifying microchip that can be secured to a tooth and which is only visible to a dentist or the police; beepers equipped with alarms that sound if a child goes outside a certain vicinity; and identification bracelets or tags. Of course, fairly extreme measures such as these may not be for every parent, and their constricting nature is more suitable for younger children; as children become older, such devices become related less to security and more to an invasion of privacy. Remember, these gadgets won't prevent an abduction in the first place. They are, however, very helpful in the location and identification of your child should an abduction occur.

New high-technology devices have appeared on the market. These gadgets allow you to "eavesdrop" on your child with a hidden microphone, sound an alarm to scare off potential abductors, or send verbal messages to your child's receiver. However, some researchers are concerned that these products may scare children or reduce the vigilance of a parent or caretaker. Technology can assist, but it will never replace, good old-fashioned parental supervision and common sense.

WHAT TO DO IF YOUR CHILD IS MISSING

If your child is missing or unduly late returning home, first of all it's extremely important to remain calm; there is seldom reason for panic. Most missing children return safe, sound, and unscathed, having been so engrossed in what they were doing that they simply lost track of time. If you have been separated from your child in a store or other public place, alert security immediately. Many facilities will page lost children. If your child has not returned home, call the places where he or she is supposed to be. Call your friends and neighbors. If you still are unable to find your child, call other places that the child is likely to be.

If you still have not located your child, notify the police and give them a complete and detailed description. This should include your child's age, weight, height, hair and eye colors, and unique characteristics, such as birthmarks, moles, eyeglasses, braces, and the clothes he or she was wearing at the time of disappearance. Make sure the police file a report with the

FBI, or do it yourself. The National Child Search Act of 1990 mandates that law enforcement agencies immediately accept and record all reports concerning a missing child. Also, the police must provide a description of the child to the National Crime Information System. The police in another area may have found the lost child, and may be trying to locate the parents.

Look for your child yourself, and enlist friends, relatives, and neighbors, as well as the child's friends (and their parents), to help you. Put up posters in your community, and call various organizations for missing children listed in your telephone directory, such as Child Find or the National Center for Missing and Exploited Children. NCMEC serves as a clearinghouse of information, distributes descriptions and photographs of missing children, does age progressing of the photographs of long-term missing children, and assists police agencies in the search for serial offenders who prey on children. The Federal Parent Locator Service may be used to find an ex-spouse who has abducted your child. If these efforts locate the missing youngster, or if he or she turns up, remember to notify the authorities so that the police search may be terminated. Support groups are also available for parents of missing children.

As a parent, you should educate yourself in ways to protect your children. Consult your local libraries for materials on child protection. Join a victim advocacy group that aims at initiating legislation that addresses the rights of victims. Get involved in action groups and coalitions dedicated to assisting victims and survivors of abductions. One of the most prominent groups is the National Organization for Victim Assistance (NOVA). You may contact them at P.O. Box 11000, Washington, DC 20008, (202) 232-NOVA. For emergencies call (800) TRY-NOVA. You may also contact the National Center for Missing and Exploited Children at 1835 K Street N.W., Suite 700, Washington, DC 20006, hotline (800) 843-5678.

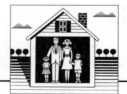

SECURITY FOR INFANTS AND
YOUNG CHILDREN: A CHECKLIST

1 The day-care facility of your choice must be fully licensed or accredited and have an effective system for checking the qualifications and references of its staff.

2 The staff-child ratio must be adequate, about one to four for children 3 years and younger, and one to seven for youngsters 4 and above.

3 The day-care staff must never administer physical or abusive punishment to discipline children.

4 To access the level of care, you should observe the children in their usual routine.

5 Unannounced visits to the day-care center should be permitted at all times, and all areas of the day-care center should be accessible to parents.

6 The staff should be prohibited from taking children away from the day-care center without written permission from parents.

7 Your children should be instructed never to leave the day-care center without your permission.

8 The day-care center's policies for preventing child abuse by the staff should be discussed openly.

9 An active interest in the day-care center will allow you to learn about deteriorating care. Also, note any major shifts in the staff.

10 Negative reports by friends, neighbors, or parents familiar with a specific day-care center should be heeded.

11 Children who are afraid of returning to a day-care center after a reasonable period of adjustment should be removed from the program.

12 Immediately investigate injuries or bruises of unknown origin.

13 Investigate any complaints by your child of long periods of playing alone, and be alert for any rude, harsh, or otherwise discourteous behavior by care-givers.

14 Instruct children at home on the signs of child abuse, and rehearse alternatives for reacting to an uncomfortable situation.

15 Teach children to say No! to adults who threaten them or touch them in sensitive places, and urge them to report any such incidents.

16 Encourage your children to tell you about all punishment received at the child-care center.

17 Any incident of child abuse should be reported to the proper authorities.

18 Telling your child "Don't talk to strangers!" is not enough to protect against abduction. Most abductors are people the child knows—or soon feels comfortable with.

19 Make sure your children know they can say "No!" to grown-ups whose actions or manner makes them feel uncomfortable.

20 Be sure your children know their full name, your full name, and telephone numbers at work and at home, and how to call the operator or 911 for emergency assistance.

21 Be certain your children know people and places they can go to for help when they are lost or feel threatened.

22 Teach children safety guidelines over a reasonable period of time, and periodically remind them. Children forget.

23 Determine whether new technological devices suit you and your child's needs, but realize that these are no substitute for your continued supervision.

24 If your child is missing, don't panic. Notify the police and try to locate the child on your own. Most children return home safe and sound.

25 Keep a file of current photos and information about your child that can be given to the authorities if your child is missing.

26 Educate yourself as a parent. Read materials on child protection, or join an advocacy group, action group, or coalition.

20

SECURITY FOR OLDER CHILDREN AND TEENAGERS

Our school-age children and our teenagers are special individuals with special problems that must be faced. The youngest of them are the most vulnerable. Without adequate experience or judgment and totally without guile, they can become both victims of and accomplices to many security incidents. And young people continue to be at risk during all the years they are growing up.

SECURITY EDUCATION AND PROTECTION FOR CHILDREN

Children should be taught certain ways of life, such as to avoid unnecessary contact with strangers and to withhold all personal information from strangers. By age 5, a child should be able to use a telephone and know how to dial the operator for assistance. Children should also be able to recite their full name, address, and telephone number, and where their parents work. (See Chapter 19.) They should learn which neighbor to go to if they are threatened and be reminded to be extra careful in opening doors to anyone they don't know.

In addition, the FBI makes these suggestions for the self-protection of children:

❖ Travel in groups or pairs.
❖ Walk along heavily traveled streets, and avoid isolated areas when possible.
❖ Refuse automobile rides from strangers, and refuse to accompany strangers anywhere on foot.
❖ Use city-approved play areas where recreational activities are supervised by responsible adults and where police protection is readily available.
❖ Immediately report to the nearest person of authority anyone who molests or annoys you.
❖ Never leave home without telling your parents where you will be and who will accompany you.

Your child's school maintains certain information about him or her as a matter of course. This information should include photographs, personal and medical history, and descriptive information. If any of these items are not included in the school's files, give them to the principal, and request that they be placed in your child's records.

Inform the school of those individuals authorized to pick up your children at the end of the day. If you are divorced or separated, provide the school with a copy of the applicable court order. Likewise, inform your children that they should leave school only with people you designate. Make certain that each child knows exactly who has your approval. Here are other matters to consider:

❖ Alert the school if the safety or life of a family member has been threatened.
❖ Advise the school of the details of your children's before- and after-school care.
❖ Inform the school when the child will not be present.
❖ Advise schools of the names, addresses, and telephone numbers of people to contact in emergencies. Also, explain the relationship of the emergency contact.

Protecting Latchkey Children

A recent phenomenon or, to be more precise, a label for an older phenomenon is occupying a great deal of media attention. That phenomenon is latchkey children. These are children who have working parents who leave them alone after school without adult supervision. To cite one example, many working parents find it convenient or necessary, according to librarians, for their youngsters to roam the library stacks for hours.

Estimates of the number of latchkey children vary considerably. In a survey conducted by a respected public-opinion sampling firm, it was determined that 12 percent of elementary school children are left alone after school each day. Latchkey children are at three times greater risk of being victims of crime, accidents, or involvement in delinquency than are children who are well supervised.

There are a number of things that parents can do to increase the safety margins for their children. They should, for example, investigate organized after-school care centers for at least the younger children (grades 1 to 4). Parents associations or community centers may have after-school programs, or you can suggest that they start one in your community. Also:

❖ Have a clear understanding with your children of the route they should follow when going to or coming from school. Do not permit your children to walk to or from school alone, and tell them to call you or a trusted friend or neighbor when they return home. Designate a person who lives nearby to whom your child can go in the event of an emergency.

❖ Make sure your child knows how to carry the key to your home securely, so it will not get lost and will remain out of view. A chain with the key worn around the child's neck under his or her shirt, or the key pinned to the inside of clothing are two good suggestions.

❖ Teach your children how to handle callers at the door or on the telephone when they are home alone, and tell them never to let a stranger in. Make sure they don't reveal that you or another adult is not with them. Remind them that a stranger is anyone who is not a friend of yours or a guardian.

❖ Know who are your children's friends; that way you can anticipate where they might be at any given time.

❖ Work with your neighbors toward the establishment of safe houses or other havens for a child who is frightened or in some real or imagined trouble.

❖ Above all, listen to your children. Even more important, take what they say seriously. What they tell you may be the wildest flight of fancy imaginable, or it could be a veiled recitation of a dire physical threat, in which case your belief in your child could avert tragedy. If threats prove baseless, you could allay the child's fears.

Halloween Hazards

Halloween should be a fun time for you and your children. Unfortunately, what used to be scary fantasy has now too often turned into a night of unusual fear. Every year, incidents occur, often tragic ones. Some include children who bite into apples or candy laced with psychedelic drugs or containing razor blades, hard-to-see, dark-costumed children who are struck by motorists, and small children who stray too far from home and are unable to find their way back. Also, older teenagers now use Halloween as an excuse to vandalize and terrorize. People stay behind locked doors and do not answer doorbells.

To help ensure that this day is safe, take precautions. Do not let children go trick-or-treating alone. Make sure there is a responsible person with the group.

Check your child's costume. It should be flame retardant and have adequate holes for your child's eyes, nose, and mouth. In addition, it should be light enough in color to be seen at night. Pin your name, address, and phone number on the costume of a very young child.

Know where your child is going. Instruct him or her to stay in the neighborhood. Warn your child not to ring the doorbells of any houses where the lights are out. Keep your own house well lighted, and make sure that someone is home.

Set and enforce a curfew for your child, and make certain a responsible person is at home at this prearranged time. Inspect all candy, fruit, or other goodies that a child brings home. Throw out anything that is unwrapped or looks suspicious.

VIOLENCE AND THE MEDIA

Parents, researchers, and politicians have long expressed a concern over violence in the media: How is it affecting children and their perceptions of the world? Research has shown that 79 percent of voters believe violence on television and in the movies is a serious problem, and 91 percent think that violence presented through media outlets contributes to real-life violence. In many forms of entertainment today—including television, motion pictures, music videos, and video games—violence is commonplace. Often the more graphic the violent scenes in a program, the more it is sought after. In recent years, movies such as *Terminator 2, Lethal Weapon,* and *Demolition Man,* all focused on physical and firearm violence, became huge box office hits. Ultimate success in one video game depends on a player's ability to rip the spinal column out of his or her opponent's back. Music videos have long flaunted acts of violence, particularly violence against women.

Television reaches a huge viewer audience and has become the center of attention in many American homes. Children watch a disproportionate amount: Nearly 40-million viewers between the ages of 2 and 11 watch approximately 3½ hours a day, that is, almost 1,300 hours a year. The National Coalition on Television Violence says that by age 18, the average American child will have seen 200,000 violent acts on television, including 40,000 murders. And many daytime and weekend children's programs, especially cartoons, contain even more violence than prime-time programming.

As children begin to accept the persistent images of violence as a standard form of behavior, they become desensitized. Even though they understand that what they see on TV and the movie screen is made up, they may nevertheless believe it. Children may view violence as an acceptable way to solve problems. They may imitate what happens around them, and violence on the screen may serve as a model. Children exposed to violence in cartoons have shown an increase in loss of temper, in fighting, kicking, selfishness, and cruelty to animals. On television, more and more "reality-based" programs document the exploits of true-life criminals, turning them into celebrities.

But these are not the only ways children are exposed to violence through the media. Movies that were once off limits to children in the theaters are now readily available in the video store. Cable television is expanding, leading to an increase in violent programming. Arcade and home video games have grown increasingly more violent.

Some parents, ignoring the negative effects of violence in the media, argue that they see no obvious difference in their children's behavior. Perhaps they do not understand that desensitization is a gradual process. Or, more likely, they simply do not welcome the prospect of monitoring their children's viewing and enforcing decisions about television viewing. Much of what a child is exposed to, and in what context, is up to you, the parent. Parents can't complain about the violent content of television their children watch if they use TV as a baby-sitting tool.

The most important thing you can do as a parent is to supervise program selection. In cartoons, videos, and other programs, it is important to limit the viewing of role models that you would not want your children to imitate. Be consistent in this monitoring, and do not hesitate to enforce the viewing rules you set down. Giving in to arguments only proves to children that they can have their own way if they apply enough pressure. Discussing characters and their actions in the shows your children watch may help them make sense of what happens, and may provide an opportunity to discover how they see the world.

Of course, parents should try to expose their children to other, more productive ways to spend time. If a child lives in a household where the television is an occasional diversion, and not something to plan the day around, they will be much more likely to treat TV as such themselves.

Parents should also express their views to their government representative and, especially, to other parents. Putting pressure on local TV stations, movie theaters, and cable and national networks will advertise that parents are concerned about what their children are watching and that they will not accept violence as the norm. Voicing a desire to see more constructive children's programming may encourage the replacement of violence as a main attraction.

These concerns are given more attention when delivered by a group of parents acting as a coalition. Many parent groups, calling for a national violence rating system for all television programs, advocate a compromise with networks, rather than strict censorship of programs. Over the past several years, responding to such views, the major networks have gradually reduced the amount of violence in the shows they present and have agreed to run a warning notice before programming that does contain violence. A possible alternative is the V-chip or other sort of "blocking system" that would allow parents to block out shows they feel are inappropriate for their children. Parents should also be aware of the wide variety of material that is accessible via the internet. Some internet providers offer a filter that can block out material that is unsuitable for children.

TEENAGERS AND CRIME

Children are probably never so troublesome as when they are in their teens. When a child reaches puberty, the changes that alter his or her body often proceed too fast for the child to make proper adjustments. Awkward, clumsy, or gawky describe the not-quite-adult adolescents. As the body changes from childlike to adult, it does not progress in orderly fashion. "Fits and starts" is more descriptive.

Children under 18 may be responsible for offenses that the general society considers unacceptable. Some of them may be general violations of the law; other actions may be criminal only when committed by the young. A college student may cut class and be guilty of no crime. A junior high student cutting class could be charged with truancy. The only difference is that the junior high student is a few years younger. Besides truancy, these status violations, as they are called, include curfew violations, tobacco or alcohol violations, loitering, and being a runaway. These young offenders may also be called unmanageable, incorrigible, or "in need of supervision."

As many as 90 percent of all young people, male and female, have committed at least one offense for which they could have been brought to juvenile court—although few are. Only one in nine (one in six if you consider only males) is referred to juvenile court for nontraffic offenses prior to her or his 18th birthday.

According to FBI statistics, those under 18 account for 35 percent of the arrests for larceny and burglary, and they account also for 24 percent of motor vehicle thefts and arson committed in the United States during 1994. Another quarter of such crimes involved those 18 to 24 years old. Arrest rates were higher for the 15- to 17-year-old group than for any other group, and this group also had the highest incidence of arrest for "property" crimes: larceny, burglary, and vehicle theft. The 16- to 20-year-old group led all others in being arrested for the personal crimes of murder, rape, robbery, and aggravated assault.

For a parent, all this leads to a first, and most important, recommendation when it comes to protecting your teenager from crime, either as victim or criminal: Know where your children are, what they are doing, and with whom. Your child is just as likely to be bad company as to be in bad company, and if you are too quick to spring to your offspring's defense, you may be an unwitting accomplice. Admit that your child could run afoul of the law, and plan for this possibility with your teenager.

If possible, take one or more teenagers to visit a jail. Let them see what goes on inside those walls. If you can convince them that they could be incarcerated, they may be deterred from the temptation to commit a crime. At least keep the lines of communication open. Doing so may help to head off a teenager's problems before they get too serious.

Teenage crime is often spawned in an atmosphere of poverty, hopelessness, drunkenness, squalor, frustration, idleness, and adult crime. It is a function of nobody-giving-a-damn, especially not parents; of school absenteeism and dropping out; and of peer group pressure. Juvenile delinquency is not the exclusive province of the ghetto. The greatest growth in the crime rate is found in the suburbs. Rates of increase in the commission of serious crimes are much greater for females than for males, especially for juvenile females.

Of the ingredients for spawning crime, only poverty seems to be an exclusive characteristic of the ghetto. The suburban juvenile delinquent is less deterred by possible consequences, because he or she is much more likely to get off scot-free, or at least to draw a suspended sentence, than is the ghetto offender. Idleness is a problem as common in suburbia as in the city. A part-time job is excellent for combating idleness and for building self-confidence.

Open lines of communication between parents and children are wonderful, and although the teenage years are probably too late to start to establish these, you have nothing to lose and much to gain by trying. You need to make a teenager belong. Teenagers who don't feel a sense of belonging at home will surely look for places and groups where they can have that feeling.

CULTS

The unhappy teenager may be attracted to cults. The formation of a cult is not in itself a violation of the law, but the way many cults conduct their activities is. There is evidence, verified by police and medical authorities, of child abuse, neglect, beatings, and other acts of violence. Former cult members have reported being slapped, being forced to make public confessions, having their food spat on, and being forced to eat pet food off the floor. Members of some cults have engaged in prostitution and have encouraged both incest and sexual abuse of children. Cults may not routinely abduct babies, but they snatch minds and spirits.

Causes

Don't delude yourself that only the poor, disenfranchised, and desperate are susceptible, and that your loved ones are exempt and safe from cults. Typical "draftees" to a cult are children who are satisfactory students, with fathers with high-stress occupations, who read newspapers regularly. All youngsters who are searching for meaning in life or spirituality are vulnerable. Many join cults because of frustration with established religion. Some are desperately searching for acceptance. The cultist group becomes their surrogate family; the masculine cult leaders, their father figures. Remember, the cult also serves the specific needs of its followers. Recruits are not usually passive targets overpowered by mind controllers.

Prevention

Once your youngster has joined a cult, it usually is too late for successful action. Prevention is the best, and perhaps only realistic, approach. Never allow your home to be a meeting place for the cult's persistent recruiters. And keep such recruiters out of schools and off its grounds.

Most important of all, broaden the channels of communication with your loved ones. Be open minded, tolerant, and willing to discuss sensitive subjects. You must learn to be an active listener by being totally attentive and not interrupting or imposing your ideas before your youngster has finished transmitting complete thoughts.

Help your youngsters ask appropriate questions and think for themselves. Young people vulnerable to cults often are unable to evaluate and choose among various options. They perceive cults as the only available alternative. As their parents, you should help them develop the art of critical thinking, to discern between productive and nonproductive choices, to make decisions, and to solve problems.

Above all, be a proper role model, and instill in your young people confidence and self-esteem. Should your children seek to detach themselves from a cult and be willing to return home, provide them with love, warmth, and professional counseling.

YOUTH GANGS

A delinquent gang consists of three or more youths who band together to commit crimes. Gang members share common symbols and defend exclusive territory, their "turf." They are extremely dangerous and deadly. The weapons of choice for many of today's gangs are no longer switchblades and baseball bats. Handguns; semiautomatic firearms such as the Uzi, AK–47, and MAC 10; chemical Mace; and machetes rule the day. Particularly in big cities, youth gangs are often just another branch of larger underworld organizations and are involved in the lucrative drug trade. About half of all gang-related crime involves violence. Gangs are comprised of youths representative of all ethnic groups, including whites, Hispanics, Asians, and African-Americans. Most gang members are in their teens, but they may be as young as 7 years, and many are well over 21.

Most cities large and small have a serious gang problem. A 1993 survey commissioned by the U.S. Department of Justice of 115 cities with populations over 150,000 reported 207,285 gang members, 4,349 gangs, and 37,113 gang-related crimes. The number of cities reporting a gang problem, according to the Department of Justice, increased from 72 percent in 1988 to 89 percent in 1993. According to the Attorney General of California, Los Angeles County alone has some 900 gangs with 100,000 members.

As a parent, you should be alert and do everything in your power to prevent your child from joining and participating in gang activity. The Crime Prevention Center of California's Office of the Attorney General warns parents and educators to be on guard for early signs of gang involvement. These signs include drug and alcohol use, low grades, absence from school, a sudden change in friends, staying out late, and displaying lots of money and expensive merchandise that cannot be explained. Additionally, be alert for gang graffiti in your child's bedroom; gang uniforms or colors; special gang hand signals; photographs with gang names, insignia, and symbols; and talk of gang membership.

The best approach is preventative; try to steer your child away from joining a gang before it is too late. Speak to your child about the dangers and consequences of gang involvement; provide close supervision and alternative activities. The primary reasons children join gangs are boredom and lack of a satisfying home life. Contact your school and ask the staff how they can be of assistance or what school programs are available to help your child. Get in touch with community organizations that may be able to provide help and guidance; creating a job bank containing entry-level positions can lead to career developments while offering youths a responsible, lucrative alternative to gang involvement. Seek aid from your religious leaders, who often are knowledgeable about neighborhood programs that strive to prevent gang membership. Form or join a neighborhood watch program, and if you observe gang activity, call 911 or inform your local precinct. Ask to speak to a gang specialist trained in dealing with these matters. Establish a graffiti cleanup program. Organize neighbors and friends to report and remove graffiti in your neighborhood or from local school property. Immediately erasing, cleaning, or painting over graffiti informs the gang that you care about your neighborhood and that gang activity will not be tolerated. Offer alternatives to gang membership by establishing organized activities, including sports, outings, arts and crafts, picnics, barbecues, and trips.

TEEN SUICIDE

Each of us has painful memories of adolescence, and most of us remember incidents that, at the time, we felt we were incapable of surviving. It was a stressful period, but somehow we coped. Too often, however, there are young people who find it impossible to keep going.

Although suicide is generally the nation's sixth major cause of death, it ranks second (after accidents) among adolescents and young adults. More than 2,000 young people, mostly boys between the ages of 15 to 19 (11 adolescents per 1 million people), take their own lives each year. This is an increase of more than 300 percent over the past 30 years. Even more incredible, experts estimate that each year more than 500,000 youths attempt suicide. These figures are alarming, not only for America's parents but also for educators and communities.

Still, many parents, and often educators as well, react unsympathetically to the tribulations of adolescence, but this is precisely the period when teens most need understanding and love.

Physicians treating suicidal teenagers tell us that the preliminary signs of suicide often are vague. Many of these symptoms also signal normal adolescent development. Frequent confusion, moodiness, and depression do not imply that an adolescent is contemplating suicide, although depression alone raises 30-fold a child's risk of committing suicide. It is also important to remember that the availability of a handgun, often kept in the home for protection, substantially increases the likelihood of a successful suicide.

Warning Signs

Warning signs of danger include changes in behavior, actual statements about dying by your teen, and situational factors beyond a youngster's control. Shifts in behavior are usually sudden and may be observed at home or in school. Be alerted especially by a decline in the quality of homework; a general lack of consistency; preoccupation with death; uncharacteristic disregard for appearance; withdrawal from family and peers; marked differences in eating and/or sleeping habits; substantial changes in personality; noticeable boredom; unexplained crying; giving away valued possessions; restlessness, defiance, recklessness, violent behavior, or rebellion; running away from home; and, above all, abuse of drugs and alcohol.

Any reference your teenager makes to dying must be taken seriously. These statements preceded actual suicides: "What would you do if I killed myself?" "Everyone would be better off without me around." "You won't have me to worry about much longer." Of course, prior suicide attempts are a strong indication of yet another try to come at taking one's own life.

Be especially attentive if the foregoing danger signals are accompanied by disappointing experiences, including breakup of a close or intimate relationship, failure to achieve an important goal, serious physical illness, and, above all, the suicide of a peer or loved one.

What to Do

If you observe the danger signals, there are concrete things you should do. First, ask your teenager questions. Don't be afraid to come out and say "I feel as though you have been depressed. Let's talk." Be prepared to drop everything to talk to this person, but, more importantly, be prepared for your teen to say at some point, "I am thinking of suicide." Continue to ask specific questions, and try to assess the real risk. The more thoroughly your child has thought about suicide, the more likely it is that an attempt will be made.

Be attentive and loving, engage in "active listening," where you paraphrase what your child is saying. This technique assures your teen that you are paying attention and are concerned about the problem. It encourages a continuous stream of communication rather than suppressed feelings through parental domination.

Here are some more simple rules: Don't use the word *why* very much; it encourages defensiveness. Try to keep an open mind. Don't make promises you cannot keep, since you can't make everything better. Be honest with yourself, too. Above all, never interrupt or offer advice while your youngster is talking. Children automatically shut down when parents try to offer them advice.

If you sense a strong intention to commit suicide, or even if you are suspicious, remain with your child until you can contact someone else to help you, especially if your attempts at communication are failing. Whatever you do, never handle the situation alone; be sure to enlist the help of someone you trust. You will surely regret not having sought help should anything drastic happen. Call a suicide hotline; you don't have to be the one contemplating suicide to call and get help. You can also contact hospitals, suicide prevention centers, and school suicide intervention programs. For professional help, contact a psychologist, therapist, or psychiatrist who specializes in suicide prevention and treatment. You may even need to turn to close friends, relatives, or other adults whom your teen respects.

COPYCAT OR CLUSTER SUICIDE

More and more cases are reported of young people imitating the suicide of others or simply of a group of people who make a pact to die together. If your teen's friend threatens suicide or actually carries out the threat, your own loved one may therefore be in danger. Although these "copycat" or "cluster" suicides seem to be an expression of the times, there is, unfortunately, no evidence that they will automatically stop over the next few years.

We don't know much about the dynamics of copycat or cluster suicide. What we do know is that youngsters similar to victims in age, sex, and social activities are at a higher risk than others. If your child is exposed in some way to a suicide or a cluster suicide, review the warning signs and suggestions mentioned previously for preventing a lone suicide.

You can also make sure that your youngster's school develops a program to prevent imitation suicides. The key points of this program should include group discussions that provide all peers an opportunity to share openly their feelings, thoughts, fears, and concerns regarding the suicide. Self-esteem and personal confidence should also be addressed. School professionals should be available and accessible to the students, especially those reluctant to talk to a teacher or a group. And if a friend or someone the students know is suicidal, it is imperative that they tell another person.

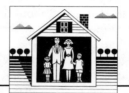

SECURITY FOR OLDER CHILDREN AND TEENAGERS: A CHECKLIST

 1 Teach children security lessons early in life.

2 Protect your children after school until you return from work by designating a secure place for them to stay under adult supervision.

3 Do not permit your children to walk to and from school alone. If children must be home alone, designate a neighbor they can go to in case of an emergency.

4 In the event of an emergency, be sure teachers and supervisors are thoroughly familiar with your children's daily routine, transportation patterns, and personal habits.

5 On Halloween, do not let your children go trick-or-treating alone. Make sure there is a responsible person with the group. Inspect all candy, fruit, or other goodies they bring home.

6 Teach children proper methods for protecting their property, especially bicycles.

7 Teach children to avoid involvement with strangers, to avoid walking or playing in unsupervised areas, to run and yell if threatened, and how to contact police and neighbors in the event of an emergency.

8 Instruct teenagers to let parents know where they are, what they're doing, and with whom.

9 Recognize that teenagers get into trouble, and plan for it with your child.

10 Impress on teenagers the importance of respect for the law.

11 Encourage teenagers to hold jobs.

12 Prevention is the best strategy for protection from cults.

13 Keep cult recruiters out of your house and school.

14 The best protection from cults is open communication and understanding between you and your youngster.

15 Provide your children with support and professional counseling when they decide to leave a cult and return home.

16 Assist your children in the art of critical thinking and choosing properly among competing options.

17 Be alert to signals of gang involvement. Do everything possible to shield your children from participating in gang activities. Seek help from schools, religious leaders, and community organizations in establishing alternatives for young people.

18 Be a positive role model for your youngsters.

19 Monitor all programs and movies that your children watch.

20 Do not permit them to view violent programs with negative role models, including those in cartoons and videos.

21 Don't use television or videogames as a baby-sitter. Get your children involved in hobbies, community groups, or reading.

---

22 Openly explore with your children the characters and actions in programs, and explain any situation that may be unclear to, or misunderstood by, your children.

23 Express your concerns about violent media images to government representatives, TV stations, cable companies, and movie theaters. Enlisting the support of other parents by forming a coalition will give strength to your opinions.

24 Know the warning signals of teen suicide, including sudden changes in behavior and comments regarding suicide.

25 Be aware that many signs of normal adolescent development may resemble symptoms of suicidal behavior.

26 Offer the troubled adolescent support, understanding, and love.

27 If you suspect that a teen has decided to commit suicide, confide in someone you trust. Never try to handle all this on your own. Contact a suicide hotline, a hospital or school intervention program, or a professional, such as a psychologist who counsels suicide individuals.

28 Should your child be exposed to suicide or cluster suicide, be vigilant and provide support, especially if your child shares similar characteristics with the victim.

29 Help establish a suicide intervention program at your child's school. Stress the importance of openly sharing feelings and thoughts about suicide.

30 Impress upon your children the importance of telling an adult if one of their friends is contemplating suicide.

21

DRUG AND ALCOHOL ABUSE AND THE FAMILY

The history of drug abuse is long and checkered. Stone Age people used hallucinogenic mushrooms to alter moods. And like our ancestors, we take drugs that we don't need: painkillers when our only pain is mental, amphetamines to keep us awake when our biological clocks tell us that we should be sleeping, and barbiturates to bring us down from our frenzy of diet pills. We may accelerate the actions of these drugs with a liberal addition of alcohol (the most widely used drug in the world), sometimes with fatal results.

Our children not only abuse the same drugs that we do but also sniff a few of their own: glue, typewriter correction fluid, and some aerosol propellants.

Recent surveys on drug use among teenagers are quite disturbing. Researchers at the University of Michigan also reported a steep rise in marijuana use among high school and junior high school students. As of 1995, 31 percent of 12th graders, 25 percent of 10th graders, and 13 percent of 8th graders reported using marijuana or hashish during the previous 12-month period. The researchers also noted significant increases in the use of LSD and prescription stimulants like Dexedrine and Ritalin, as well as in sniffing glue and paint.

THE LINK BETWEEN DRUGS AND CRIME

Drugs are a major factor in crime, and some authorities believe that drugs are the principal cause of crime. A magazine article on violent crime noted that criminologists estimate that half of all street crime is drug re-lated. Perhaps the most significant of the drug-related street criminals are cocaine users, who finance their addiction through theft, selling drugs, and a host of other crimes, including con-games, forgery, gambling, and pimp-ing. One study found that 243 opiate addicts were responsible for 500,000 crimes during an 11-year period. Two-thirds of this group had from 100 to 365 crime days per year during the time they were taking drugs. Dur-ing periods of abstinence, the crime days decreased to 40.8 each year. An-other recent study of 414 homicides in New York City reported that drugs or alcohol were involved in over 50 percent of these murders.

Drugs alone each year cost the nation an estimated $50 billion in dam-ages and lost productivity, $6 billion in medical costs, $20 billion for drug-related law enforcement, and $50 billion in urban blight—for a grand total of $126 billion. Clearly, the economic and human cost of drugs poses a major challenge for every citizen and every family in our nation.

If you have a teenager with a drug problem, he or she needs help, and so do you. Your family physician, even the child's pediatrician, can provide guidance once it is determined that a problem exists.

RECOGNIZING THE SIGNS OF A DRUG PROBLEM

Because the parent is the most effective person to intervene in a child's drug abuse problem, parents must be aware of the symptoms of drug abuse. First of all, drug use usually produces a variety of noticeable physical changes in a user: sleeplessness, diarrhea, bloodshot eyes, dilated pupils, vomiting, involuntary muscular movements (twitching), runny eyes or nose, inflamed nostrils, and loss of appetite. Other symptoms are lethargy or torpor not unlike intoxication, yellow stains on fingers (caused by the high tar element in marijuana joints), sudden weight loss, craving for sweets, excessive thirst, sweating, shakiness, itching, and, of course, the tell-tale needle tracks, not only on the arms but also on the legs, abdomen, and other parts of the body. The user may be inconsistent in her or his behav-ior—for example, sitting for long periods in a trancelike state and then suddenly becoming hyperactive.

Drug use may also manifest itself in emotional or personality changes. Volatility of temperament, ranging from extreme happiness to blackest de-pression, may signal drug use; so, too, may uncharacteristic anger, radical changes in activity patterns or choice of associates, a sudden deterioration in physical appearance, sloppiness in dress, or inattention to personal hy-giene. School grades may drop, and the drug user may lose interest in things that once held importance, such as school, athletics, and dating. The drug user may seem to be always tired, coming home only to fall asleep. A drug-troubled child may spend considerable time in the house, especially in a locked bathroom. He or she may withdraw from family activities. A previously friendly and outgoing child may suddenly become secretive. A formerly easygoing child may become irritable and overly sensitive. The young abuser may be argumentative and have angry outbursts for no apparent reason.

There may be other evidence of drug use: burned ends of marijuana joints (often referred to as roaches); drug paraphernalia such as a "work kit" with syringes, cotton, needles, and a "cooker" (a metal bottle cap used for converting heroin into a liquid so it can be injected); or small glassine envelopes tucked into a dresser drawer.

A number of stages may be observed in the behavior of those who abuse drugs. In the beginning stage, an abuser is characterized by an ability to take drugs or leave them alone. If the use of drugs becomes more frequent, with periodic or chronic states of insensibility or limited perception, that person is described as a chronic user. Beyond that point, a person who develops a compelling need, as opposed to a desire, to obtain drugs continually, at whatever cost in money or action, is addicted.

FREQUENTLY ABUSED DRUGS

Alcohol

Alcohol is the most widely used of all drugs of abuse. According to the United States Department of Justice, 103 million Americans drink alcohol at least once a month. A 1994 survey by the University of Michigan reported that 50 percent of high school seniors drink alcohol at least once a month, and 39 percent of sophomores had used alcohol during the previous month.

Use of alcohol causes impairment of muscle coordination and of judgment. Prolonged use can cause heart and liver damage. Alcohol contributes to many fatal automobile accidents. In overdose quantities, it may also cause death. Withdrawal may cause anxiety, insomnia, tremors, delirium, and convulsions.

Particularly in combination with other drugs, alcohol is the most deadly of commonly used drugs. According to the United States Department of Justice, medical examiners in 27 of the nation's metropolitan areas reported in 1990 that alcohol in conjunction with another drug was responsible for 40 percent of deaths due to drugs. The National Institute of Drug Abuse reported that 31 percent of hospital emergency episodes in 1990 involved alcohol in the presence of another drug. Alcohol is extremely likely to cause physical dependence, tissue damage, and changes in behavior; the user may also develop tolerances, requiring increasingly larger doses to produce the desired effect.

Alcohol is significantly present in 90 percent of child abuse cases; it plays a role in incest and neglect. Children of alcoholics have compulsions to control their environment and to deny their feelings, and they have low self-esteem, guilt, and a restricted ability to enter into satisfactory relationships. They also tend toward learning disabilities, anxieties, suicidal tendencies, and compulsive achieving.

One issue not much discussed a few years ago concerns children of alcoholic parents. Whether weaknesses concerning alcohol are inherent or acquired, the fact remains that more than half of all alcoholics, some 28 million, have an alcoholic parent; one-third of American families include at least one alcohol abuser. The child of an alcoholic home, in addition to the likelihood of having alcohol-related problems, has the further high risk of becoming alcoholic or marrying someone who becomes alcoholic. It is almost as if alcoholism is a contagious disease.

Problems of the children of alcoholics are quite difficult for others to determine, for these children are usually adept at socially acceptable behavior and tend toward social acceptability. Nevertheless, the number of such children committed to the juvenile justice system—its courts, prisons, and other facilities—is disproportionately larger than that of their counterparts without family histories of alcohol.

Too often, youngsters as well as adults drink excessively at parties or other social functions and then attempt to drive home. The deaths of thousands have resulted from this frivolous behavior. Many accidents could have been avoided by having a designated driver, a friend who had agreed not to indulge on that occasion. Or you could have made a "contract" with your teenagers stipulating that they call you for the drive home should they have decided to drink with their friends.

Cannabis

Cannabis includes marijuana and hashish. In many parts of this country, these particularly popular drugs are the largest cash crop. Cannabis is usually smoked, although sometimes it is swallowed in solid form, often as an ingredient in brownies or cookies.

A sweetish, burnt odor is present when cannabis is used. Some symptoms of abuse are loss of interest in what goes on around a person, lack of motivation, paranoia, mood shifts, infertility, and, sometimes, weight loss. Hazards of using this drug include damage to lungs, heart, and the body's immune system. Although not physically addicting, these drugs can engender a strong psychological dependence. Withdrawal from cannabis may result in insomnia, hyperactivity, and decreased appetite.

Depressants and Stimulants

Drugs that depress the central nervous system are used medically to treat tension and some neuroses, to control pain and severe diarrhea, to minimize the effects of coughs and cold symptoms, and to treat insomnia. Included among the depressants are barbiturates, narcotics, heroin, morphine, codeine, hypnotics, and methaqualone. These drugs are either injected into the veins or swallowed in liquid form or as pills. Drowsiness, confusion, impaired judgment, pupil constriction, lethargy, and needle marks may be valid evidence of the use of depressants.

Heroin use, in particular, has increased dramatically in the 1990s due to lowered cost and the higher concentrations available. About 31,000 heroin-related emergencies were reported by the nation's hospitals in the first half of 1993, up from 21,400 in 1992, a 44 percent increase in a single year.

The lesser hazards of using these drugs include infection, appetite loss, and nausea. More severe hazards are addiction, withdrawal symptoms, and death from overdoses, drug-induced accidents, and/or severe interactions with alcohol. Withdrawal from these drugs may lead to anxiety, insomnia, tremors, delirium, convulsions, and death.

Amphetamines and cocaine are both stimulants, and both are deadly, addictive drugs. Amphetamines are usually taken in pill form, and cocaine is commonly inhaled as a powder. Their availability in liquid form tends to intensify their harmfulness.

Both drugs tend to cause excesses of activity and irritability, and often are accompanied by mood swings—an intense high followed by dysphoria. Even in average doses, they are often fatal, capable of producing loss of appetite, hallucinations, paranoia, convulsions, coma, and brain damage. In addition, there is the distinct possibility of intense psychological dependence. Among withdrawal symptoms are apathy, long periods of sleep, irritability, disorientation, and depression, sometimes leading to suicide.

The Cocaine Generation

Nearly 23 million Americans have used cocaine in their lives. A third of the U.S. adult population reported that they know someone who uses cocaine or crack. According to a University of Michigan survey, 6 percent of high school seniors had used cocaine at least once. So serious is the cocaine problem that Americans consider drugs the principal problem among students.

Cocaine is tricky. It leads you down a primrose path, only to abandon you in the briars and brambles. Initially, it gives you what you believe to be increased confidence and sociability, even control of your environment. You don't realize that your euphoria is mere illusion, at least not until it's too late. But for the rosy early stages, you're on top; you're in total control.

Continued use, though, takes the edge off the feelings of well-being, to be replaced by stress and depression. You also find it takes increasingly greater doses of cocaine to elevate you to the "good" feeling you once enjoyed. You find yourself edgy, confused, and depressed. Your only return to the heights you once reached is more and more cocaine, which produces less and less of the drug's early promise. You find that you require stronger and stronger doses just to maintain mere functional capability; you've lost the ability to get high. You will, by now, have lost your job and your self-respect as well. You've abandoned your friends in your undeviating search for the lost euphoria of coke. In time, hallucinations take hold of you, and finally you mix large numbers of different drugs; then you die.

Crack

What is even more disquieting is the large number of cocaine users who are freebasing, using "crack" or otherwise intensifying the potency of the cocaine they use. A highly concentrated, extremely addictive form of cocaine, crack can easily be produced in the home without sophisticated equipment. Drug dealers sell tiny plastic vials of crack for $5 and $10. Crack is much more dangerous than cocaine because it results in an intense and instant high lasting around 20 minutes called a "rush," which can cause addiction almost immediately. On the other hand, addiction to cocaine, though extremely dangerous, may require months or even years of use before your system is truly addicted (although psychological addiction can begin much sooner). Also, the cheap price of crack ensures greater accessibility to children.

Users claim euphoria, increases in alertness, greater sociability, feelings of increased strength, a decrease in appetite, and a decreased need for sleep. Criminologists are blaming crack for the sharp rise in homicides among teens. According to researchers at Northeastern University, the rate of homicides committed by teenagers aged 14 through 17 increased 172 percent from 1985 to 1994. The expanding crack market since the mid-1980s has fueled a plague in guns and shooting incidents among teenagers. Guns are used more and more to protect the sale of drugs, including crack.

Physicians report that the use of these stronger drugs can induce the most severe of psychological dependencies, which continues and intensifies long after the early exhilaration ceases. As the euphoria abates, it is replaced by aggression and suspicion, even complete psychotic outbursts. Cardiac arrest, sometimes preceded by coma, is the frequent result of cocaine overdoses.

A perplexing question is whether these substances are satisfying natural appetites. Experiments with other primates (monkeys, for example) have produced conflicting evidence. In one experiment, rhesus monkeys refused to smoke tobacco or marijuana. All monkeys, however, will smoke cocaine, preferring it to either sex or food. One monkey, the subject of a cocaine experiment, sat patiently pressing a button almost 13,000 times to receive a single dose of cocaine!

Hallucinogens and Inhalants

Hallucinogenic drugs alter one's perceptions of reality. There is little, if any, medical application for these drugs. There are, however, some experimental uses. Among these drugs are PCP (angel dust), LSD, mescaline, and psilocybin. The latter two occur naturally; mescaline is a type of cactus, and psilocybin, a mushroom native to South America. PCP is often smoked; the others are usually swallowed or injected. The cactus and mushroom configurations are ingested in their natural state.

PCP and LSD are, perhaps, the two most behaviorally damaging drugs. It is little wonder that one of PCP's street names is "killer." In addition to aggressive behavior, users of hallucinogens exhibit slurred speech, blurred vision, confusion, lack of coordination, agitation, hallucinations, illusions, and broad mood swings. These chemicals are particularly hazardous, for they can be stored in the body's tissues and, months after the last use, be released from tissue to profoundly affect behavior. Other hazards are anxiety, depression, breaks from reality, and emotional collapse. Strangely, there is no apparent symptom of withdrawal associated with these drugs.

Inhalants, as their name signifies, are abused by inhaling or sniffing. Among these substances are gasoline, airplane glue, paint thinner, dry-cleaning solution, laughing gas, and amyl nitrate. Abuse of these drugs results in these symptoms: poor motor coordination; impaired vision, memory, and thought processes; abusive, violent behavior; and light-headedness.

The hazards of using these substances include a high risk of sudden death, drastic weight loss, and substantial damage to blood, liver, and bone marrow. Among the causes of death resulting from abuse are anoxia, neuropathy, muscle weakness, and anemia.

Ecstasy and "Roofies"

Ecstasy (the name of a drug) is, perhaps, the heir apparent to the "in drug" mantle. Reports from a trend-setting West Coast university indicate that about one-third of students have experimented with the drug. While research has shown that the drug produces brain damage in animals, there is no clear evidence that it is either toxic or unsafe for human use. The drug has been listed as a Schedule I substance, meaning that it has no known, accepted medical use and that possession is illegal unless government agency approval is obtained, even for researchers.

The substance, a mild amphetamine (often mentholated), first appeared in 1914, intended as an appetite suppressant, but it is possible that it was never used for this purpose. As recently as 1986, it was considered a "small-time" drug by federal authorities. Scant research is available, but there is some evidence that indicates that the drug reduces fear but increases anxiety and defensiveness. This combination could likely produce combativeness and antisocial behavior in users.

Another more recent and, in many ways, more sinister drug is Rohypnol. Commonly known by its slang name "roofies," this drug is 10 to 20 times more powerful than Valium. It has become notorious as the "date-rape drug" because it is tasteless and odorless and can be easily dissolved in a drink without the victim's awareness. Though Rohypnol is neither manufactured nor sold legally in the United States, it is typically available at a cost less than $5 per 1- to 2-milligram tablet. Police began issuing warnings nationwide in 1995 and 1996, as reports of incidents in which roofies had been administered to drugged rape victims became increasingly frequent. And in October 1996, legislation providing for a 20-year sentence for rapists convicted of using Rohypnol was enacted—the first time use of a drug as a weapon was made illegal.

Anabolic Steroids

Anabolic steroids are powerful drugs chemically related to the male sex hormone testosterone, used to rapidly strengthen muscles. For this reason, they are particularly attractive to athletes. Steroids may be taken orally or by injection. They are definitely addictive and may alter the user's mood and cause considerable harm to the reproductive system, cardiovascular system, kidneys, and liver. Other harmful side effects include rashes, gall stones, headaches, and nausea. They can also stunt the growth of children and cause a deepening of the voice during male development. Finally, they increase your risk of cancer and of incurring injuries. Other names for anabolic steroids are juice, hype, or roids.

WHERE TO FIND HELP

The best place for immediate help is a hospital with a staff specifically trained to treat addicts. If your hospital does not have such a treatment facility, it should refer you to one that does.

An effective chemical dependency program is structured to treat the patient's physical and psychological needs by providing expert medical and psychiatric care. A typical program includes a staff of physicians (including psychiatrists), clinical social workers, family therapists, registered nurses, and substance abuse counselors. Drug treatment programs often include components tailored for specific groups such as youths, women, and the elderly. Many programs are divided into five phases, which focus on individual, group, and family therapy. These treatment levels include:

1. Medically supervised evaluation
2. Medically supervised detoxification
3. Rehabilitation
4. Intensive family program
5. Aftercare

Other treatment components include educational and vocational services, urine testing, relapse prevention, and social and community support. The initial four phases of the typical treatment program often last 28 days and emphasize individual and group therapy. Moreover, the patient's family is encouraged to participate in the rehabilitative process. Family members also receive individual and group therapy and attend educational lectures on substance abuse.

An aftercare program is essential because it recognizes the previous and special problems encountered when a recovering addict or alcoholic reenters the community. Therefore, the recovering addict or alcoholic is required, for at least several years, to attend regular "growth group" sessions and to participate in such self-help groups as Narcotics Anonymous and Alcoholics Anonymous. An effective aftercare program also provides counseling and support for family members.

Another possible source of help is a drug rehabilitation center, such as Phoenix House in New York and California, where the drug abuser can be treated as an outpatient or can live on the premises. These centers operate group sessions at which ex-addicts and professional staff members work together to teach people how to live drug-free lives. Through open and honest discussion, the sessions try to determine the root causes of participants' drug involvement and how they must change so that they no longer need drugs as crutches.

Other users may benefit more from one-to-one sessions with a psychotherapist. Here the drug abuser with the help of a trained therapist can perhaps find the road to rehabilitation—possibly more quickly than in group encounters. Above all, studies have concluded that treatment by methadone, other outpatient programs, and therapeutic communities reduce drug consumption and criminal behavior.

PREVENTING DRUG AND ALCOHOL ABUSE

Here are some helpful preventive guidelines for parents:

Curb your own substance use. Children are great imitators. If they see you using drugs, they are likely to follow your example. If you smoke marijuana or drink excessively, you are only asking for trouble. Children may not have the ability to know their limits or to use drugs such as liquor in moderation. Let your children know that alcohol and drugs are unacceptable. Be a positive role model.

Know your children's friends. Perhaps you can view them more objectively than you can your own child. Be sure to meet your children's dates.

Encourage your children to say No to drugs. Teach them how to make responsible decisions and how to resist peer pressure.

Do not keep outdated medications around the house. This is particularly applicable to diet drugs or painkillers. In addition to the obvious opportunity for abuse, there exists the possibility of accidental overdose and even death.

Help your teenager find beneficial activities. The active child—one involved with school clubs, special projects, hobbies, and sports—may not feel a need to use drugs out of frustration and boredom.

Read up on drug abuse. Share current literature about drug abuse with your child, and include materials on related problems such as teen pregnancy, failure in school, crime, and family problems. Correct misconceptions about the incidence of drug use by peers.

Know your child. This is the most important measure you can take. Make time available to talk to your child about problems, worries, dreams, and goals. Teach your child through example that facing problems and coping with them is much better than escaping from them. Escape through the use of drugs is only temporary and creates, in turn, still more problems. If your children know you care, they may decide not to look to drugs as an answer to the questions.

Participate in community prevention efforts. Join and support all communitywide drug prevention activities, including neighborhood watch programs, tenant organizations to combat drugs, and cooperative programs between law enforcement and the community. Also, encourage your school to develop a drug and alcohol curriculum and teacher training on how to manage students with a drug problem.

One observer suggests a unique measure to stem the nation's tide of drug abuse. He notes that there are already on our statute books regulations that permit seizure of automobiles used to transport illegal drugs. How many abusers would have to lose their vehicles before the demand for coke and crack and rock would dry up?

Helping Young People to Just Say No

"Say No to drugs." Young people have all heard this a thousand times, but the National Crime Prevention Council has suggested some effective ways they can use to say No.

❖ Say you have fun things to do rather than take drugs, like go to the movies, jog, watch videos, play sports, and then go out and do them.

❖ Explain that drugs damage your mental and physical health and you want to be at peak performance.

❖ You don't have to explain anything after you say No. If necessary, strengthen your protest by a stronger "No, not ever" or "Get out of here!"

❖ Never attend parties where drugs and alcohol will be available.

❖ Associate only with friends who reject alcohol and drugs.

❖ Learn as much as you can about the harm of drugs and alcohol, and make certain that lines of communication between you and your parents are open on this subject.

If you or a friend needs help and are afraid to go to your parents, call 1-800-COCAINE, a 24-hour hotline, or 1-800-662-HELP (9 a.m. to 3 a.m. EST). Other numbers of local hotlines may be found in your telephone directory, usually under alcohol abuse, drug abuse, crisis services, or under a special listing at the beginning or end of your telephone directory.

Helping A Friend

If your friend is "using," never discuss the problem while he or she appears to be "under the influence." Wait until your friend sobers up. Then, to indicate how much you care, you might say "We have been friends for a long time and I really want to help you. I am very uncomfortable to see you always high and it's painful to watch your deterioration." Be as honest and specific as you can. Don't be surprised if your friend becomes angry and hostile. Also, denying there is a problem is common among users. If you do not succeed on your first approach, wait awhile for what you perceive is the appropriate moment, and try again. Never drink or use drugs with your friend, as this will only worsen the situation and cause harm. Help your friend look up local hotlines and chemical dependency counseling services.

If you are a young person, urge your friend to seek help from your school. You might need counseling as well; do not refrain from seeking professional counseling.

What to Do About Drug Dealers

The first thing you should do of course is to remain drug-free and not sell drugs. If you know someone or are aware of someone dealing drugs, report that person to the police, but do so anonymously for your own protection. If the dealer is a close friend of yours, remind him or her that dealing is a violation of the law. Try to recommend a resource like a school counselor or drug hotline to help if your friend is addicted. Also, you can support laws that are aimed at prohibiting the selling of drugs and drug paraphernalia. Moreover, urge your school system to establish drug-free school zones. Contact appropriate city agencies like the housing and fire departments, and demand that action be taken against a drug den in your neighborhood. These and similar agencies have the authority to issue summonses for violations of building codes. Dealers must be made to realize that drug profits are absolutely not worth the risks involved. If they check out legal jobs, they will be much happier and more truly successful.

If you are a landlord, it is your responsibility to take all necessary legal action to evict persons dealing drugs in your buildings. Contact your local police precinct and the office of your district attorney, and ask for assistance. Also, retain a reputable attorney experienced in landlord-tenant issues.

An "ounce of prevention is worth a pound of cure" is patently applicable in this type of situation. Avoid renting your premises to drug dealers in the first place. Stringent screening procedures are the best way to identify responsible and reputable tenants.

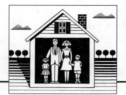

DRUG AND ALCOHOL ABUSE
AND THE FAMILY: A CHECKLIST

1 Be aware of the extent of drug use, especially among young people, and of the links between drugs and crime.

2 Learn to recognize the signs of drug and alcohol abuse.

3 Beware of the physical signs of drug use, which may include watery eyes, dilated pupils, loss of appetite, insomnia, heavy perspiration, and even needle tracks on parts of the body.

4 Watch for sudden changes in personality. A normally happy person may abruptly become hypersensitive and suffer tearful episodes for no apparent reason.

5 If you discover a drug abuser, urge that person to seek professional help. Drug rehabilitation programs are especially useful.

6 Be aware that alcohol is the most widely used of all drugs of abuse and, particularly in combination with other drugs, is the most deadly of commonly used drugs.

7 Set a good example for your children. Remember, if they see you using drugs and alcohol, they are likely to copy your behavior.

8 Make sure that your child is not part of a teenager group that uses drugs for kicks.

9 Do not keep old prescription drugs, particularly diet pills and painkillers, in the medicine cabinet, where they can be found and swallowed by young children.

10 Help your child develop an interest in pastimes such as recreational clubs and team sports. Do not let your child use drugs for "entertainment."

11 Be familiar with the recent literature on drug abuse. Share this with your child.

12 Encourage your child to come to you with problems, even when life is going smoothly. If you keep communication lines open, your child may seek your advice on important matters that otherwise could precipitate the use of drugs.

22

COMPULSIVE GAMBLING AND THE FAMILY

Legalized gambling is increasingly popular. Public acceptance and the desire of governments to generate revenues without raising taxes have stimulated the growth of opportunities to gamble. At present, 48 states sanction some form of gambling such as lotteries, bingo, jai alai, horse racing, and dog racing. According to FBI estimates, gambling is a $300 billion business with an annual growth rate of over 10 percent.

While legitimate gambling may be increasingly acceptable to more and more people, the hazards of losing unacceptable amounts of money and becoming addicted to this habit make it a major threat to family stability and individual safety.

Because in gambling the same person is both the culprit and at least one of the victims, we must ask, "Why do people gamble?" Many people do so for the obvious reason, to win. Moreover, gambling is a social activity. Bingo at the church or the crowd at the track provides a sense of belonging, a feeling of fraternity.

TYPES OF GAMBLERS

Gamblers are not all alike. Experts suggest several categories: casual social, serious social, and compulsive gamblers.

Casual Social Gamblers

Casual social gamblers indulge only occasionally, and do so for entertainment, sociability, and a little excitement. Gambling takes up only a small part of their leisure time.

Serious Social Gamblers

Serious social gamblers, according to experts, bet regularly rather than occasionally, and do so with great concentration and energy. But their gambling is controlled. The money that is allotted for and spent on gambling is well within their means. Their preoccupation is similar to that of the "football junkie" or "tennis nut."

Compulsive Gamblers

Compulsive gambling is described by the National Council on Compulsive Gambling as a progressive behavior disorder in which an individual becomes dependent on gambling to the exclusion of everything else in life. It is a disease with deep psychological and emotional roots. Like alcoholics, compulsive gamblers exhibit an emotional dependence on their activity, suffer loss of control, and fail to function normally in daily life. As with other addictions, tolerance increases and larger and/or more frequent wagers are needed to get the same "high." Emotional and financial suffering afflict not only the compulsive individuals' families but also their employers and the general community. Compulsive gamblers who have depleted their financial resources and credit may turn to crime as a source of income to support their compulsion.

WHO ARE COMPULSIVE GAMBLERS?

Many problem gamblers believe that getting money is the solution to their problems. Compulsive gamblers believe that their troubles (i.e., mortgaging their house, borrowing from a "loan shark," etc.) will be solved with a "big win." Although males have previously comprised about 80 percent of compulsive gamblers, the number of women with gambling problems is on the rise. Women who gamble are predominantly employed in support positions, such as secretaries or clerks. Women are also more likely to siphon family funds for gambling but are less likely to commit serious criminal acts to support their habit.

Most women start gambling as adults, whereas men usually begin in their teens. Over half the women who suffer from compulsive gambling do so as a means of escape from personal problems or to combat loneliness or boredom. Gambling may even provide an escape from an abusive home. In addition, there is a greater stigma against female gamblers than males. As a result, they are less likely to seek help for the problem.

Problem gambling has also been associated with other addictions, such as drug and/or alcohol abuse. A study at South Oaks Hospital in Amityville, New York, found that about one-fifth of alcohol and drug addicts were also problem gamblers. Some experts suggest that this is due to an addictive personality.

BEHAVIORAL AND EMOTIONAL EFFECTS OF PROBLEM GAMBLING

The Valley Forge Medical Center and Hospital has specified nine behavioral and emotional effects that may occur in a progressing gambling problem. These are:

1. Getting a tremendous thrill from gambling and dreaming about winning big, the gambler makes larger and more frequent bets. The individual may even experience a winning streak or a "big win."
2. The gambler loses bets, starts borrowing money, and becomes irritable and withdrawn. Gambling begins to take precedence over work and family.
3. Desperation sets in, and there is no longer caution in gambling. The gambler blames others for all losses. This is accompanied by alienation from family members and further cheating, stealing, or lying in order to continue gambling.
4. The gambler starts to feel guilty and deeply depressed, and may suffer a nervous breakdown and start to abuse alcohol and/or drugs.
5. The "critical point" is when the individual's world is destroyed. The gambler may even attempt suicide or ask for help to prevent it.
6. At this point, when compulsive gamblers admit having a problem and begin to reassess their lives, they may seek treatment.
7. They become hopeful once again and are more open to others. They begin to work on realistic goals.
8. The gambler starts to rebuild his or her life and relationships with loved ones.
9. The individual learns to struggle with the problem one day at a time through Gamblers Anonymous or another treatment program.

RECOGNIZING AN INDIVIDUAL WITH A GAMBLING PROBLEM

Recognizing compulsive gamblers in the early phase of their problem is not so easy. The obvious behavioral changes have not yet occurred. Yet a number of indicators, in combination with one another, suggest a gambling problem:

❖   *The amount of time spent gambling.* Keep alert for any increase in the amount of time or energy spent gambling, especially if you notice a surge in a person's activities away from home, in other cities, for example.

❖   *Growing size of bets.* You should recognize any sharp increase in the amount of bets. If $5 to $20 bets increase to $50 or $100, you can be sure that compulsiveness is imminent.

❖   *An intensity of emphasis on gambling.* The compulsive gambler finds it exciting to talk and boast endlessly about that activity, and searches out special occasions for gambling, like sporting events, parties, and junkets.

❖   *Loss of interest in other activities.* Gambling becomes the most important event in the gambler's life. You should be alert to a gambling spouse whose interest in you and the children begins to wane.

❖   *Suspicious absences from home and work.* Strong indicators of compulsive gambling are absences from work and home, without explanation or with only suspicious explanations.

❖   *Shifts in personality structure.* The stress associated with winning and losing often produces belligerent behavior, impatience, and irritability.

❖   *Siphoning off family funds.* When the compulsive gambler begins cashing in insurance policies, redeeming securities or savings bonds, and draining the family savings account, you can be sure that gambling has reached the addictive stage.

GETTING HELP

When compulsive gamblers finally accept help, there are basically two sources: Gamblers Anonymous and professional counseling.

Gamblers Anonymous (GA) is the only national voluntary organization for compulsive gamblers. Founded in 1957, it is structured along the lines of Alcoholics Anonymous. There are over 700 branches of GA in the United States, as well as 20 international ones. Like Alcoholics Anonymous, GA has a 12-step program beginning with the admission that you have a problem. GA members consider anonymity, confidentiality, and mutual support of the utmost importance.

Gam-Ateen is the treatment program for teenage problem gamblers. Gam-Anon is the GA counterpart for family members of the compulsive gambler. These group meetings provide support and teach the family members ways to cope with the gambling problem of their loved ones. Look in your telephone directory for the local chapter of Gamblers Anonymous, or contact their national office at:

Gamblers Anonymous
National Service Office
P.O. Box 17173
Los Angeles, CA 90017
(213) 386-8789

On the whole, treatment centers restricted to compulsive gamblers are in short supply. One such program is at the Valley Forge Medical Center and Hospital in Norristown, Pennsylvania. You can call them for additional information and a confidential consultation at (215) G-A-M-B-L-E-R. The next best treatment alternative is traditional psychotherapy, either with a professional in private practice or at a psychiatric clinic or community health center. For referrals to local sources of assistance, contact:

The National Council on Problem Gambling, Inc.
P.O. Box 9419
Washington, DC 20016
(800) 522-4700

Do not delay; compulsive gamblers are unlikely to overcome this problem by themselves.

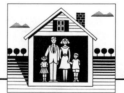

COMPULSIVE GAMBLING
AND THE FAMILY: A CHECKLIST

1 Know the behavioral signs of problem gambling. These include increased time spent gambling, increases in size of bets, and a drop-off in other activities.

2 Watch for sudden changes in personality.

3 Be especially careful about gambling if you abuse drugs or alcohol or suffer from any other addiction.

4 If you think you yourself are at risk of getting "hooked" on gambling, you should avoid gambling with money you cannot afford to spend.

5 Avoid borrowing money or using credit to finance your gambling.

6 Allocate a limited amount for gambling. Avoid using money that has been set aside for other purposes.

7 Do not gamble to get money with which to pay debts or to otherwise solve financial problems.

8 Do not gamble illegally, as with a bookmaker.

9 Do not allow gambling to involve you in illegal activities.

10 Avoid using gambling as an escape from problems or personal troubles.

11 If you or a loved one has a gambling problem, call Gamblers Anonymous, or learn where to find help in your community. Do not try to fight the battle alone.

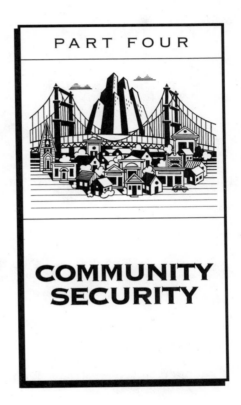

PART FOUR

COMMUNITY SECURITY

23

NEIGHBORHOOD CRIME PREVENTION

A citizen patrol unit was driving along Crenshaw Drive between Fourth and Fifth Avenues when they spotted a man breaking into a blue 1989 sports car. They immediately called 911 and watched as the man attempted to penetrate the steering column of the car with a screwdriver. Then the police arrived, and the would-be car thief was arrested. "Arrests like that make me feel great because I feel like I'm contributing to the neighborhood," said R. Estes, one of the members of the citizen patrol. "Bad guys will think twice before coming into our neighborhood."

The best way to avoid becoming a victim of crime is to prevent it in the first place. Recent statistics show that 1 in 12 households in this country is victimized by burglary. With the rise in single-person households, two-wage-earner families, and the smaller number of children per marriage, many households are completely empty 5 days a week. It is now more important than ever for neighbors to join together to keep crime out of the neighborhood.

CITIZEN CRIME PREVENTION

The crime issue provides us all with an opportunity to become personally involved. Citizen crime prevention exemplifies the main philosophy of this book: to deal with crime in a proactive rather than reactive manner.

Citizen crime prevention programs may be divided into programs involving cooperative citizens efforts; steps individual citizens can take to protect themselves, their families, and their homes; and environmental design.

COLLECTIVE CRIME PREVENTION INITIATIVES

A very productive way of protecting yourself from crime is through collective and cooperative citizen efforts. Approximately 5 million Americans in about 2,500 communities belong to some sort of crime-stopping organization such as a Neighborhood or Block Watch, and one out of every five people polled in a recent survey said they participated in some kind of crime prevention program. Some programs strengthen the crime prevention posture of your neighborhood, while others increase the efficiency of criminal justice agencies charged with combating crime. These programs are not difficult to develop, and they have been found to reduce the chances of victimization. At the very least, the programs will increase the cohesiveness, unity, and solidarity of your neighborhood; these characteristics alone will have an impact on crime.

Block Clubs

Some clubs consist of the residents of one block. Among the activities of these groups are systematic and organized efforts to educate neighbors and make them aware of crime and public safety. Many block programs also conduct street surveillance. Block club participants, including children, are encouraged to report crimes and suspicious-looking people to the police.

Neighborhood Watch

Neighborhood Watch programs are similar to the block club but cover a broader area. Citizens are trained to report crime and suspicious events or people in the neighborhood. Special telephone numbers to police headquarters often are provided in case of an emergency. Neighborhood Watch programs may provide extended services beyond their traditional functions of observation, crime reporting, and crime deterrence. Many offer short- and long-term victim assistance, including emotional support after the crime, such as listening to the victim and giving support and direction on how to get through the complexities of the criminal justice system.

Interviews with criminals reveal that the Neighborhood Watch program is a very effective deterrent against robbery. Most burglars claim that they would leave a neighborhood if they were observed or challenged by a resident. These programs have demonstrated that improving crime reporting reduces crime—and the fear of crime. Contact your police or sheriff's department for information on the national Neighborhood Watch program.

Citizen Patrols

The fear of crime has motivated citizens to organize crime patrols. In some areas, residents carry out the patrol activities, and in others they hire professionally trained security officers. Some patrols concentrate on specific buildings or housing areas, while others cover entire neighborhoods. The patrols are usually equipped with citizens band radios. Thousands of such groups, comprising everyone from young adults to senior citizens, have been formed throughout the country.

The Beverly-Fairfax Community Patrol based in West Hollywood is a visible citizen patrol. The patrol begins during early evening and ends around midnight. Two community volunteers drive their own cars with signs indicating they are on patrol. Each team is given a portable two-way radio, a powerful spotlight, and a bright-yellow jacket that indicates they are community volunteers.

Many neighborhood patrols have followed the lead of the police and have taken up bicycle patrols, which offer more visibility and mobility than foot patrols, and which offer more citizen interaction than motor vehicle patrols. Bicycles can also get into areas automobiles can't, such as alleyways and parks.

Unlike building patrols, which may prevent unwanted visitors from entering buildings, neighborhood patrols cannot deny people access to their streets. Instead, they concentrate on uncovering suspicious and criminal behavior, which they report to the police. Some patrols also perform social service functions, such as escorting senior citizens and providing job opportunities for teenagers. Others monitor police activities. These patrols are often organized when police-community relations need improvement.

Symbolic marches can be held by neighborhood residents to show that they won't allow criminal behavior to take over the area. In an area of Los Angeles where drug dealers and prostitutes had recently appeared in alarming numbers, local citizens marched in protest, holding signs and chanting "We want safe streets!" as passing drivers honked their horns in support.

How effective can individual initiatives such as these be? A resident of a large southern city who works nights is involved in protecting himself from crime. First of all, he and his wife formed a Neighborhood Watch unit. He thus became acquainted with many of his neighbors.

All of his efforts on behalf of his family and his neighbors paid off. He was working in his yard when he saw a man breaking into a neighbor's house. He called the police. He had made advance preparations for such an occasion. He had entered the police emergency telephone number on his automatic-dialing equipment. Keeping watch on the window through which the intruder gained entry into his neighbor's home, he reported the break-in. The police arrived a minute later, according to the good neighbor's report. Not only was he able to assure the police that the intruder was still inside the structure, he was also able to advise them that there were several firearms in the house, a fact he had learned when organizing the Neighborhood Watch organization.

This action may have prevented a tragic attack on an unwary police officer. Rather than barging into the crime scene, the police radioed for a tactical (SWAT) squad. Because the doors of the house were protected by double-cylinder deadbolt locks (which can be opened only by a key), the intruder was unable to escape.

This incident is a "small" crime, but one that was almost certainly repeated many times on that day. It was also a very large crime, because it proved, beyond doubt, that we don't have to be held hostage to the thieves and other criminals who prey on us. In your hands lies the answer to protecting yourself from crime. It is you!

Crime-Reporting Programs

In selecting crime-reporting programs for your community to participate in, you may want to consider some of the following alternatives:

❖ *The Whistle-Stop program.* Whistle-carrying citizens sound off when they are victimized or when they see a crime in progress. The whistles serve as a community signal system. Neighbors who hear the sound also blow their whistles to disrupt crime and alert the police.

❖ *Radio watch projects.* Radio-equipped autos patrol neighborhood streets, looking for criminal activity or suspicious people. When they spot something amiss, they report it, either to a dispatcher who then notifies the police or directly to the police on special emergency frequencies.

❖ *Special telephone or secret-witness programs.* These projects provide special telephone lines so that people may report suspicious behavior or can report criminal activity without revealing their identity. Rewards are frequently offered to citizens for their assistance. "Crimestoppers" is a successful example of this type of program.

❖ *Drug watch.* This recent but excellent program involves the community in combating drug dealing. One specific program in New York City known as Westside Crime Prevention provides its members with drug-watch training sessions. Participants are shown slides of drug arrests, drug-selling locations, and visible signs of drug transactions. A retired police lieutenant with experience in narcotics enforcement teaches how to accurately report dealing to the police. Members are taught that it is not enough for the police to hear that someone is selling drugs in their neighborhood. Participants of Westside Crime Prevention learn that descriptions to the police must be specific enough to identify the perpetrator and to provide probable cause.

Community-Based Adolescent Diversion Projects

In several university communities, the schools have joined forces with the local criminal justice system to help juveniles in trouble. These youths are referred to the project, rather than the prosecutor's office or juvenile court, and are assigned to student volunteers who develop special programs for them. The students are trained and supervised by experienced psychologists, and they receive credit for their efforts. Project New Pride began in 1973 in Denver and today stands out as one of the most successful programs for redirecting "hard-core" youths back into the mainstream of their communities.

Other Community Programs

The following community programs may give you further ideas:

❖ *Anticrime campaigns.* These involve special citizen groups organized to combat crime and improve criminal justice agencies such as police, courts, and corrections. The Kansas City AD HOC Group Against Crime, (Detroit) Michigan's "Reach" and the Philadelphia Crime Commission are examples of organizations that have conducted successful anticrime campaigns.

❖ *Police-community relations programs.* Thousands of programs in which police officers and citizens work together have sprung up throughout the nation. Their objectives are to improve formal and informal communication between local police and neighborhood residents, to prevent crime, and to combat juvenile delinquency. A successful illustration of this type of program is the 3,000-member Association of Chicago Beat Representatives. These volunteers periodically receive community crime information from the local police commander at special meetings. Acting on this information, they have assisted the police in solving homicides and robberies. Also, these representatives have helped the police rid neighborhoods of youth gangs.

❖ *Community policing.* This style of policing affords greater opportunities for citizen participation than traditional policing. Private citizens work together with individual police officers to develop creative ways to combat "quality of life offenses," including public drunkenness, prostitution, and low-level drug dealing, and such neighborhood deterioration problems as uncollected trash, run-down housing, and absence of drug treatment facilities, all of which set the stage for social decay and criminal behavior. Citizens are also empowered to take a proactive role in solving neighborhood crime problems. For example, citizens might serve as volunteers to staff local police stations, offer information on local crimes, help identify neighborhood toughs and crack houses, or supervise sports activities for community youth.

Police departments in Madison, Wisconsin; Newport News, Virginia; Edmonton, Alberta, Canada; and Los Angeles, California, have introduced successful community policing programs in recent years. For more information on programs that could work as a blueprint for your local community programs, contact the following sources:

The Neighborhood Resource Team, Dade County, Florida
Contact: Detective Ronald Tookes
Metro-Dade Police Department
10155 Circle Plaza West
Miami, FL 33151
(305) 254-5834
(305) 254-5837 (fax)

The Neighborhood Network Center, Lansing, Michigan
Contact: Officer Don Christy
Neighborhood Network Center
735 East Michigan Avenue
Lansing, MI 48912
(517) 483-4600

PACE, Norfolk, Virginia
Contact: Corp. Jesse Moore, Chairperson, PACE Support Group
302 City Hall Building
Norfolk, VA 23502
(757) 664-4626
(757) 664-7001 (fax)

❖ *Auxiliary or reserve police.* Many police departments—including the nation's largest, the New York City police, because of fiscal restraints and limited personnel—have helped organize auxiliary-police organizations. Civilian volunteers are trained in police methods and procedures. They wear uniforms similar to those of police officers, and they often patrol on foot and in vehicles supplied by the police department. Their main function is crime prevention and deterrence. They report crimes to the police, but they will come to a person's aid if necessary. Auxiliary police officers are usually discouraged from making actual arrests. Instead, they are urged to summon police officers to do this. Auxiliary police officers often assist regular police officers in crowd and traffic control, at demonstrations, or at an accident scene.

PRIVATE-SECTOR SECURITY

Private security elements play an increasingly important role in the battle against crime. Lacking most of the police powers of their public-sector counterparts, the private industry has long emphasized the prevention of crime. Private security is not concerned with arrests, only with preventing incidents.

These services are increasingly used because they are effective. Business is using private-sector security more than ever, often in capacities once performed by the public police, such as in employee or customer protection or in escort service to parking areas. In this way, private security does not supplant the public police; it supplements them. The private sector of the criminal justice complex is characterized by an ever-increasing number of private security personnel. Private security people are now more numerous than state and local police by a factor of 3 to 1.

As public forces suffer from insufficient funds and private forces increase enormously, a loose, undefined, and totally unofficial partnership—or at least a division of labor—seems to be emerging. For example, with the restriction of beat cops or prowl cars, wealthy individuals and neighborhood groups are now engaging private security officers to perform the patrols that were cut back in the public sector. No formal agreements forge this public/private relationship. The police were forced to cut back services, and the private firms were able to provide these services to businesses and groups of individuals with common property interests. Private security in various parts of the country is also expanding its role in public-building protection, residential-neighborhood patrol, traffic control, parking enforcement, crowd control, and court security.

However, the major problem with private security forces is that an ill-trained private security force can be more dangerous than no private security force at all. Abusive or unwarranted behavior towards citizens by a private security officer can lead to lawsuits or violent confrontation. Hire security officers from a reputable company that ensures stringent standards of recruitment, screening, and training. On the whole, private-sector security is a good idea because it can complement traditional venues of security. But remember: It is unwise to believe that writing a check is going to make someone safe. Personal safety starts with personal responsibility.

INDIVIDUAL CRIME PREVENTION EFFORTS

Individual efforts have been successful in providing protection from crime. Programs similar to those that follow may be useful in your neighborhood:

❖ *Residential security surveys.* A residential security inspection offers a practical and simple solution to security evaluation. It usually consists of a thorough examination of your residence to identify its security deficiencies. The survey determines the protection required and shows how to minimize opportunities for criminals. Studies have shown that such surveys reduce your chances of victimization.

❖ *Property-marking programs.* Citizens borrow marking equipment, often from the police department or a civic organization, and engrave identification numbers on portable property. The numbers are then recorded with the police. Program participants post decals on their doors or windows indicating that their property has been marked. Marked property is less appealing to a thief, and in the event of a theft, your personal property may be identified and returned to you. This crime prevention effort became popular over the last few years and has been shown to reduce burglary rates. (See Chapter 2.)

Individual crime prevention efforts may be as simple as replacing a burned-out lightbulb for an elderly neighbor, thus increasing his or her nighttime security. Such efforts include accompanying a neighbor going shopping. In so doing, you add to that person's well-being, as well as your own, through doubling your protective capabilities.

Take your elderly neighbor to the bank to deposit a Social Security check, and, while you are there, point out the advantage of electronic mail deposits to eliminate the possibility of mailed checks being diverted to criminals.

A nosy neighbor can be a neighborhood treasure who will tell you when your floodlight is out, remind you that you have allowed the vegetation to grow too high around your trashcan area, or advise you that you failed to lock your garage. When you reciprocate and advise your neighbors of security shortcomings at *their* homes, you have the beginnings of a crime-fighting neighborhood organization.

Still another valuable service, which even senior citizens can provide, is to serve as "block parents" who can offer guidance or shelter for neighborhood children who may need assistance. On a more formal basis, Mc-Gruff Houses performs these and other services and has the additional advantage of being part of a nationally advertised endeavor to provide for neighborhood children. This is a very important consideration, because in today's families, both parents are often working.

CRIME PREVENTION THROUGH ENVIRONMENTAL DESIGN

Because the physical environment directly affects criminal activities, changes in the structure and design of the environment may reduce opportunities for crime. Thoughtful physical design of buildings and landscapes can make your environment safer and even motivate you to engage in additional crime prevention behavior. Increased surveillance may be accomplished by eliminating places of concealment, such as dense shrubbery, overgrown hedges, unpruned trees, garbage accumulations, and dark, isolated parking lots, alleys, hallways, elevators, lobbies, and stairwells. Increased lighting in streets, parks, and sidewalks also helps. With greater visibility, you and your neighbors can look out for each other and perhaps offer assistance if needed. (See Chapters 7 and 8.)

Environmental design can make it easier to distinguish between people who belong in an area and those who don't. Common lawn areas can be divided into private yards or patios, using small picket fences, well-trimmed shrubbery, or concrete curbing. In effect, these measures extend the social control of residents from their houses and apartments into nearby common areas. This approach can be further enhanced by limiting the number of public access points to the area and by providing the remaining entrances with adequate lighting, visibility, and security.

The environmental design of streets also may be modified to reduce crime. Traffic can be rerouted so that the residential character of neighborhoods is preserved. Certain avenues can be narrowed and selected streets turned into cul-de-sacs to avoid through traffic.

Improving the appearance and attractiveness of your house, property, and areas shared with your neighbors will promote a sense of responsibility among all of you. Decorative painting, lighting, installation of benches at strategic spots, and careful landscaping will motivate neighbors to care for each other's welfare and safety. These steps also will tend to intensify the use of streets, parks, and surrounding land structures by local residents. Criminals are less likely to commit crimes in attractive, well-populated neighborhoods than in run-down, deserted areas.

Many experts recently have examined personal security from the perspective of the perpetrator. Criminals form mental images of potential targets often based on nonverbal cues given off by the target. These messages convey meanings about opportunities, risk, and ease of committing crime. Social psychologists suggest that burglars weigh five sets of questions before committing a crime:

1. Am I detectable? For example, where are the doors and windows positioned, and what is the distance from the street to the house?
2. Are any meaningful barriers present? Does the structure have a gate, strong locks, or an intrusion alarm?
3. Are there any signs or symbolic barriers like Neighborhood Watch or private patrols that define territoriality and vigilance?
4. Are residents active in the streets and yards? Are lights on in the homes? Are newspapers still lying in the driveway?
5. Is there a positive social climate in the area? Are people suspicious of me, staring at and questioning me, or can I go about my nefarious business without interference?

These issues provide deep insights into the criminal mind that can be used for environmental design that offers maximum security.

Remember, you should know your neighbors. You should assist your neighbors in keeping an eye on their property, and vice versa. If you've set up a neighborhood watch, every member should have a map of the area, with each neighbor's name, address, phone number, and the kind of vehicles they own. The idea isn't to "butt in" on anybody's privacy but to keep an eye out for anything out of the ordinary. However, keep the map in a very safe place; in the hands of a burglar, it could be very valuable.

Finally, if you start, or get involved with, a Neighborhood Watch program, good for you! Now stick with it. The biggest problem with these programs is that members have a tendency after an initial rush of activity to let the organization stagnate, to stop participating. A nonoperating program will assist only those whose activities it was designed to curtail.

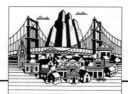

NEIGHBORHOOD CRIME PREVENTION: A CHECKLIST

1 Join a cooperative crime prevention program in your neighborhood. Programs include block clubs, neighborhood watches, citizen patrols, crime-reporting programs, police-community relations programs, and other anticrime campaigns.

2 Organize a citizen crime prevention program if none is available in your neighborhood.

3 Participate in all community programs tailored for individual crime prevention, including residential security surveys and property-marking programs.

4 Even simple crime prevention acts are useful, such as replacing a burned-out light bulb for an elderly neighbor, accompanying your neighbor on a shopping excursion, or driving your neighbor to the bank to deposit a check.

5 Set up after-school activities for the youth of the neighborhood.

6 Consider if your neighborhood needs a drug-watch or gang-control program.

7 Design your residence and its surrounding area to increase visibility from the street and to reduce the opportunities for crime.

8 Reduce places of concealment for criminals by cutting and trimming overgrown bushes, trees, and shrubbery.

9 Increase lighting in parking lots, alleys, corridors, lobbies, elevators, and stairwells.

10 Divide common lawns and areas into private yards and patios.

11 Limit the number of public entrances to your apartment building or condominium.

12 Route heavy traffic away from your streets so that the residential character of your neighborhood is preserved.

13 Provide adequate maintenance for your property, and continuously upgrade its appearance.

14 Examine the possibility of private-sector security services for your neighborhood. But remember, writing a check won't solve all your safety problems. Personal safety starts with personal responsibility.

24

SCHOOL AND CAMPUS SECURITY

A 1993 survey by the Metropolitan Life Insurance Company found that 1 in 4 students and 1 in 10 teachers had been victims of school violence. Moreover, 13 percent of students admitted bringing a weapon to school. A 1993 Harris poll reported that 60 percent of high school children reported that guns were easily accessible, and 35 percent feared being shot. According to a recent National Crime Victimization Survey, 15 percent of the nation's students reported gang activity in their schools, and 16 percent said that a student had threatened or attacked a teacher at their school. On a local level, for the 1995-1996 school year, New York City junior and senior high schools reported over 22,000 serious crimes including assaults, sex offenses, and illegal-weapons charges. Obviously, this problem is grave.

Since knowledge is often power, it is up to parents to teach their children early on how to defend themselves. Unfortunately, many parents believe this means allowing their children to carry weapons. This strategy serves only to escalate tension, fears, and violent attacks. Instead, school children should be taught to follow certain safety rules and to practice caution.

SECURITY FOR STUDENTS

By the time children are old enough to attend school, they spend more time away from the security of the home, and thus need increased protection. They should already have been educated in the basics of personal safety. Still, until you are sure they can travel alone and know their way, drive or walk with them to and from school.

If they travel on their own, do not allow them to take dangerous short-cuts; they should not not walk past construction sites, empty stores, or deserted buildings, and should avoid walking near or through parks. Check immediately on any delay in their trip to and from school. Forbid them to hitchhike or to accept rides from anyone other than those you have designated beforehand. They must learn to inform you and their teachers or principals of any strangers who approach them.

For the older child, additional precautions are necessary. Remind your children not to take large sums of money to school and to keep as few valuables with them as possible. If they take the subway to school, instruct them to wait near the token booth until the train comes. Encourage them to place all personal possessions in locked school lockers and never to give out the lock's combination. Incidents of crime or situations involving drugs or alcohol in or around the school must be reported to the school's main office, or at least to you, the parent. Then it is up to you to alert the school.

No matter what their ages, your children need to be warned of the dangers involved in walking alone in deserted hallways, corridors, or stairwells. Not only strangers and peers but even some school personnel might be a threat. Older children may benefit from learning jujitsu, karate, or another form of self-defense, especially if they express an interest in these martial arts. Martial arts encourage self-confidence and discipline and may assist your child if she or he is confronted by a threatening person.

These precautions do not imply that your children need be completely isolated during their school years or mistrustful of everyone they meet. The key is not to be constantly suspicious but always cautious.

Encourage your children to tell you everything, and keep open the lines of communication. They and their friends may even be contributors to unsafe conditions in school, not the victims. With communication, love, and understanding between you and your child, plus the help of the school, other parents, and professionals, you can work through problem situations. Above all, if your children or their friends are suffering from drug or alcohol abuse or any emotional problems, seek advice and support from their teachers or school counselors.

Know your children's playmates, friends, teachers, and school officials, and communicate with them. By knowing your children's peers, you are better able to exclude bullies and thugs. Within the school as a whole, parental support for security and discipline is vital to proper protection of students and teachers. Demand proper security measures in the schools, especially in high-crime areas. If weapons and violence are threats to your child's safety, insist that the school install metal detectors, X-ray bag scanners, and ID-card-controlled access systems. These technologies have been found successful in reducing the number of illegal weapons brought to schools by students as well as intruders. Also, insist that your school have an adequate staff of well-trained school safety officers. Suggest self-defense instruction. Become involved in the school board, even if only by voicing your dissatisfaction and insisting upon safe conditions in the schools.

The learning environment is also jeopardized by violence and vandalism against the school. A number of programs have been designed to reduce or minimize this likelihood. One includes a Neighborhood Watch that enlists neighbors near the school to help in watching the school and reporting suspicious incidents to authorities. Other programs focus on student involvement in deterring vandalism and repairing its consequences. You must stress the undesirable effects of destructive behavior and encourage your children to report vandals to school authorities or to you. Promote the idea that it is their school, and encourage them to work with teachers and school personnel to improve awareness, protection, and prevention.

The School Administrators Association of New York State offers the following advice to reduce school violence. Teach children at an early age how to resolve arguments without fighting, how to develop friendships, and how to manage anger, jealousy, fear, sadness, and loss. Children must be taught how to communicate, because children who can express their feelings are less likely to act out violence. Teach your child how to listen to others, especially other kids, and to try to understand her or his feelings. You should teach your child never to interfere in a fight, not to call other people names, to be honest, and to make a sincere attempt to solve problems in a well thought-out and reasonable manner. Conflict resolution, problem solving, peer mediation, and designating peacemakers are important techniques for reducing conflict and violence.

SPECIAL CONSIDERATIONS FOR TEACHERS

Communication is a basic necessity for effective teacher-pupil relationships, but in some cases it may not be enough. Because of increased levels of drug and alcohol abuse in schools, teachers are confronted with increasing violence and abuse. To protect themselves and at the same time fulfill their professional obligations, teachers need to develop appropriate strategies worked out in detailed tactics.

Establish good communication with your students, and involve them in setting up classroom rules, but be sure they understand that you are still in control. When trying to control students, never use sarcasm, shouting, or embarrassment, and do not threaten punishments unless you are willing to carry them out. Know the problem students, and consult with other school personnel to determine how to handle them.

Immediately report any threats by students to administrators and the police. Never walk in secluded areas alone or stay late at school without others present.

Most of all, try to be a friend to your students, support their successes, and guide them through their failures. Most students still look up to their teachers; your advice and friendship may be just what they need.

COLLEGES AND UNIVERSITIES

In a nationally publicized incident, a young student at a Pennsylvania university was raped, tortured, and murdered during a robbery of her dormitory room. The murderer was a student and employee of the college. In another incident, a student with a sawed-off shotgun murdered two other students on a Michigan campus.

Although many young adults between 18 and 22 feel that they are immune to crime, stories and statistics such as those above prove otherwise. The perpetrators of crimes on college campuses are usually outsiders who engage in theft and sexual assault, or students who commit mainly sexual assaults. (See Chapters 29 and 30 on protecting yourself from rape, and Chapter 31 dealing with sexual harassment and stalking.) Campuses are also plagued by hate crimes—threats or acts of violence against individuals, groups, or property which are motivated by race, color, religion, national origin, age, disability, or sexual orientation. (See Chapter 33 for a more detailed discussion of hate crimes.) Be sure to report to campus authorities any signs or incidents of sexual assault and any information you may have about perpetrators of a hate crime.

The Federal Student Right to Know and Campus Security Act ordered colleges and universities to collect and publish statistics on campus crime each year beginning September 1, 1992. One purpose of this bill is to inform prospective students and parents about campus safety issues so that decisions regarding choice of college can be based on facts.

A 1994 FBI survey of 831 colleges and universities (each with an enrollment of at least 5,000 students) reported about 5,500 serious violent offenses, including 19 homicides, 1,001 forcible sex offenses, 1,375 robberies, and 3,049 aggravated assaults. In addition, there were 19,172 reported burglaries and 6,624 reported auto thefts.

Choosing a College

Most parents and teenagers select a college based on its tuition, size, location, and type of student body, as well as its reputation for teaching, research, and social activities. Probably the last thing in your mind and the mind of your teenagers is the incidence of crime on campus. However, this is an increasingly important consideration.

When considering a college, always ask about its safety record and security features. Consult the FBI's *Crime in the United States: Uniform Crime Reports,* available in all major libraries, which each year has expanded coverage on crime on the nation's campuses. Your final academic selection should also include information about crime prevention orientation, a mechanism for immediately informing students about serious crimes, a student newspaper that provides information on campus crime, and strictly enforced policies on drug abuse, alcohol consumption, sexual harassment, and sexual assault.

Compare the per capita expense that the college or university spends in their entire law enforcement or security program with other schools. Research the amount of incidents that occurred in the preceding three years. Find out if the school president is serious about safety and security on campus.

Be certain your college or university has enough campus law enforcement officers. *Crime in the United States* also provides data on the number of officers and civilian law enforcement employees who work at selected campuses, or request this information from your college representative, admissions officer, or counselor. Many factors determine the number of security officers, of course, including campus size, number of students, location near or in a major urban center, and the incidence of campus crime.

No-Hassle Security

The college campus is something like a small city. Student dorms are, in fact, apartment buildings, and the security measures the student takes in a dorm must be no less serious than those for an apartment. There are also special considerations for dorm students, who are in much closer contact with others, i.e., their dormmates. Many more people are likely to be in and out of one's room than in a typical apartment situation.

As a college student, you should protect your residence by following a few simple "no-hassle" security rules. First, note the conditions of the door and window locks, as well as the lighting both outside and inside your room, and demand improvements if necessary. Become familiar with your roommates and neighbors, and encourage their efforts at crime prevention. Prepare for dangerous encounters by discussing what you would do if you were threatened or attacked. If you can't agree with them, request a room change. Always look out for each other's safety, and report any crime to the campus police. Always lock your doors and windows, even if you plan to be gone only a short time. Don't keep valuables or large sums of money in your dorm room.

Keep a complete and up-to-date inventory of your valuables. Determine whether the campus security office has an organized tagging or labeling system for stereos, TVs, computers, and the like to deter thieves and aid in recovering stolen items. Always lock your bike or vehicle securely, and be cautious in parking areas. Park only in well-lighted areas that are well traveled.

In addition, follow these rules: Maintain a record of anyone with a key to your room, and be sure to request a change of lock if a key falls into the wrong hands or even if it is lost. Do not allow your room to be left unlocked, and do not leave visitors alone in your room when you are away. Never let a stranger into the room, especially if you are alone.

Exercise caution when giving out your phone number. Beware of telephone solicitation calls or wrong numbers, and never divulge your name, address, or any other personal information to such a caller. Hang up immediately if you receive an obscene phone call. If the caller persists, discourage additional calls by removing the receiver from the hook for a brief period. Near the phone, keep a list of emergency numbers, including campus security. Always provide an updated list of emergency and next-of-kin information to the college's registration office. Do not give your student ID number or Social Security number to anyone other than college faculty, administration, or staff. Never leave lying around any papers that have your ID number on them, especially in registration areas.

Secure your personal belongings in class, the restroom, library, cafeteria, and computer facilities. Never leave your pocketbook, books, or backpack out of your sight. Many students have experienced thefts while leaving pocketbooks or backpacks hanging from a chair for only a few minutes.

Never travel alone after dark. Avoid deserted and isolated areas such as empty classrooms, stairwells, elevators, library stacks, and laboratories. Also, stay away from department offices after hours, when no one else is around. If you must go to the office to copy or type something, use a buddy system, or at least inform your friends where you are, and maintain contact. Be careful, and follow safety rules when walking alone off campus. Be especially alert if the surrounding area is a high-crime neighborhood. Check with the security office for an escort or shuttle service across campus at night, or form your own. Do not use unlighted or unfamiliar shortcuts, and never hitchhike. Avoid exercising or jogging outside at night or early in the morning, unless with a group.

Finally, ask your security office for further crime prevention tips, and be aware of security problems on campus. If the security office is unresponsive to your complaints or concerns, bring this to the attention of college administrators and the student government. Above all, make an effort to determine the level of crime at the college of your choice before you make your final decision.

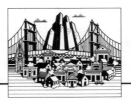

SCHOOL AND CAMPUS SECURITY:
A CHECKLIST

1 If you are a parent, teach your children from an early age about crime and how to protect and defend themselves.

2 Don't allow your children to carry weapons or firearms.

3 Accompany children to and from school until they know their way, and set strict rules regarding routes and contact with strangers.

4 Remind your children not to carry extra money or valuables to school.

5 Teach your children to secure their personal belongings in school lockers and not to give out combinations.

6 Warn your youngsters about dark corridors and deserted staircases in schools.

7 Encourage your children to learn martial arts, especially if they express an interest.

8 Open the lines of communication with your children, their peers, friends, teachers, and school officials.

9 Be aware of bullies and troubled youths, and do not tolerate their presence.

10 Urge that those who have drug- or alcohol-related problems be required to seek counseling.

11 Forbid your children to engage in vandalism, and encourage them to protect their school.

12 If you are a teacher, establish effective communication with students, and invite their input, but be sure they remember that you are the authority.

13 Never ridicule, chastise, or harass students, especially in front of others.

14 Be aware of problematic students, and prepare ways to handle them.

15 Report any threats to the proper authorities, and increase your self-protection.

16 In selecting a college and dormitory, be aware of high-crime rates and security effectiveness.

17 If you are a dormitory resident, examine door and window locks for their dependability, and insist on adequate lighting in your room and around your

room. Always lock your door, even if you expect to return in a few moments.

18 Keep a record of valuables, and participate in equipment-labeling programs. Never keep valuables or large sums of money in your dorm residence. Secure all personal belongings at all times.

19 Don't allow guests to remain alone in your room, and never let a stranger into your room.

20 Keep a record of everyone with a key to your room. Should the key be lost or stolen, change the lock.

21 Restrict the distribution of your phone number. Keep emergency numbers posted by the phone. Hang up immediately on obscene phone callers; report all incidents to the campus police.

22 Provide the registration office with updated emergency-contact information.

23 Be cautious in displaying your student ID number.

24 Never travel alone, take shortcuts, or hitchhike, especially at night. Stay away also from deserted or isolated locations on campus, such as empty classrooms, stairwells, library stacks, and laboratories.

25 Be especially alert in the neighborhood surrounding the campus.

26 Lock up any vehicle properly, and be cautious in parking areas.

27 Protect yourself against sexual assault, including date rape. Report all incidents to campus authorities.

28 Voice your concerns and problems to parents and to any school association. Be sure to give them any information you may have about perpetrators of hate crimes on campus.

25

SECURITY IN HOSPITALS AND NURSING HOMES

A 72-year-old man, waiting in City General Hospital for routine surgery to repair a hernia, decided to take a short walk around his hospital floor. When he returned to his room, all his personal valuables had disappeared, including his wallet, credit cards, watch, gold ring, keys, and even dentures. He immediately reported the theft to the nurse, who summoned hospital security.

As hospitals and nursing homes become more crowded, the need for security and safety is increasing. You can, therefore, understand how important it is to be aware of your personal safety and property while in one of these facilities. Patients, staff, family, and other visitors need to exercise special care to protect themselves and their loved ones. A hospital, nursing home, or convalescent center should have a security department or plan. Report anything unusual to the security department; they are there to help you.

IN THE HOSPITAL

Hospitals present unique security problems because, unlike many offices, they operate 24 hours a day to admit the sick and injured. They also admit family members and other visitors at all hours. All day and night, large numbers of staff members—including physicians, nurses, health aides, pharmacists, cashiers, clerks, and repair and maintenance people—enter and leave through the many often-unlocked entrances and doors. The patients, on the other hand, are unable to provide minimum defense against crime, because they are often too ill to walk, move, or talk.

Not only patients but hospital personnel also are at risk. While probably not aware of the precise statistics, criminals must have a good idea that over 70 percent of hospital employees are women and that during late-night hours more than 95 percent of the workforce is female. Where the lure of patients' property is enhanced by the prospects for rape and perhaps stealing drugs, hospitals can be seen as very attractive targets for criminals.

In such circumstances, staff, patients, family, and even visitors must take special precautions. Research conducted by the International Association for Hospital Security and Safety (IAHS) found that theft was the most common crime occurring at hospitals. Thefts for each hospital bed per year are estimated at between $1,200 and $2,300 on average. Even more startling, $5.5 billion is lost each year due to crime in health-care institutions. Patients should not have to be robbed while recovering from serious illnesses. The patients themselves need to contribute to their own protection, however. Many simple and specific actions can reduce the hazards of crime in hospitals.

Determine, in consultation with your doctor, if a hospital stay is absolutely necessary. A second opinion on this decision is a good idea. Many minor procedures can be performed in a doctor's office or as an outpatient at a hospital.

If a hospital stay is necessary, check unneeded valuables in the hospital vault or, better yet, leave them at home. Some hospitals require waivers absolving them of responsibility for valuables not secured in their vaults. Patients who are too ill at the time of admission to secure their personal belongings can request that a nurse provide a safe-deposit envelope to store valuables. The envelope should be sealed in the patient's presence, signed on the outside, and signed as well by the hospital representative. Then someone specifically named can be held accountable if the patient's property is lost, stolen, or damaged. The receipt should be stored safely in a table drawer until it can be given to a family member for safekeeping.

Other rules for protection against hospital crime are simple and obvious. Do not wear expensive jewelry. Keep only small change and a few small bills in a drawer next to your bed, and don't leave clothing or drugs lying around. In addition to your wallet, check your credit cards, keys, rings, watches, and other valuables. In many cases, pocketbooks or purses with housekeys have been stolen by thieves who were able to determine the patient's address. Then the thief had all the time in the world to ransack the patient's home, knowing full well that the victim was lying helpless in the hospital.

Do not place dentures, hearing aids, eyeglasses, radios, or similar objects in the safe-deposit box, because they are likely to be damaged during handling and storage. Many hospitals require patients to remove their dentures, because precious metal in them attracts thieves. Remember, if there is a theft, notify hospital security at once.

Be aware of your rights as a patient, and make sure these are enforced. A list of these rights may be obtained from your doctor or hospital, local area agency on aging, or from your library. Knowing these rights is essential, as they include numerous protective measures, such as your right to a living will, your right to approve or refuse treatment (and to be advised if such treatment has any complications or is in the experimental stage), your right to privacy and confidentiality, and your right to question any and all expenses incurred during your hospital stay. Many hospital and health care facilities provide security brochures. When you are admitted ask for a copy of the facility's security rules or brochure. Make use of the security suggestions and services that are offered.

It is of the utmost necessity to check your hospital bill. Question anything you find suspicious or in error.

Emergency Room

The emergency room is a particularly risky area, because that is where victims of drug overdoses, shootings, stabbings, and other crime-related injuries are treated. Intoxicated individuals, people high on drugs, criminals, and disoriented people filled with rage, resentment, and violence arrive regularly at emergency rooms. Many of them have been brought there against their will by friends or family members, who may also be under the influence. Some patients or visitors may still be carrying concealed weapons, including guns, knives, brass knuckles, or blunt instruments. These angry and hostile individuals often provoke verbal attacks, physical attacks, and other forms of disruptive behavior. They may destroy property.

Often, the long waiting periods before treatment irritate emergency room patients, making them tense, nervous, and anxious. Other patients should be alert to overwrought individuals and under no circumstances attempt to calm them down or provide assistance to resolve a dispute. They should stay calm and not mix in. It is the job of hospital personnel, especially the security department, to handle these highly volatile and sensitive situations. Hospital personnel are trained for these difficult and dangerous tasks. If someone nearby is disruptive or abusive, a patient can change seats immediately, as far as possible from the area of disturbance. The new seat should be near the nursing station, or at least within sight of the emergency room security officer or other hospital personnel.

Be particularly careful if no security officer is on duty, as on the late-night shift or at small hospitals. Do not wander around hospital corridors or hallways while waiting for treatment, especially at night, when many areas are deserted. Also, people accompanying you should be instructed regarding this potential danger. Although emergency rooms and adjacent areas are critical for delivering essential medical care rapidly, they can also be dangerous places.

Maternity Ward

The safest place in a hospital ought to be the maternity ward, where mothers can peacefully recover from the travails of childbirth and rest assured that their newborns are safe and sound. Unfortunately, maternity wards have become the most dangerous areas in the hospital because of infant kidnappings.

Dressed as hospital personnel and as nurses and physicians, kidnappers may gain entry to the newborn section or nursery and abduct infants. Hospitals have increased security to prevent such incidents. In addition to increasing patrols, hospitals are now requiring identification badges for visitors.

Once an abduction occurs, it is obviously too late to take precautions. Serious thought must be given in advance to every aspect of security for the child and its mother. Find out about your obstetrician's hospital affiliations before choosing a hospital. Then check the security procedures for the maternity ward and newborn nursery at that hospital. Most important, be assured that there is adequate control over access to these areas. Make certain that the entire maternity ward is a restricted area. At the very minimum, the newborn section should be locked at all times, with carefully monitored visiting privileges.

Choosing a maternity facility can be a lengthy process. Special consideration should be given to security in the maternity ward. Some institutions provide sophisticated monitoring of patient rooms and nurseries as well as systems to prevent and detect possible abductions. Other methods, such as identification cards and card key systems, which have proved useful for access control, can be tested by a single visit to the maternity ward. Are you challenged when you walk past the entry point into the ward? Do all hospital personnel who care for the babies wear uniforms of the same type and color, bearing special employee identification badges? If not, anyone could don hospital garb, mix with the staff, and walk off with your newborn.

Stroll through the corridors, and get a sense of the level of safety and security. If you feel uneasy or dissatisfied, there probably is something wrong. Discuss your impressions with a hospital representative. If you are unhappy with the response, choose another hospital. Most hospitals use infants' footprints, a relatively simple procedure, to aid in identification. This not only provides some help with administrative problems but may also prove useful in kidnappings.

Parking Areas

Parking lots at hospitals may be even more isolated and deserted than those at shopping centers or malls. Often they sprawl over large areas and are accessible to anyone 24 hours a day. After the stress and tension of visiting a sick loved one, the last thing you want is to return to your car and find that it has been vandalized or has disappeared. Even worse, on the way to your car you may be robbed and/or raped. Most hospital security departments are willing to provide you with an escort to your car. If you feel at all uncomfortable going to your vehicle alone, do not hesitate to take advantage of this service. Many of the security procedures discussed for parking while shopping should definitely be followed for hospital parking (see Chapter 14).

Precautions for Hospital Staff

If you work for a hospital, particularly as a physician, nurse, or aide, your schedule usually varies over 24 hours, and you frequently come and go at odd hours or during off-periods. Be especially careful to follow the procedures outlined for safe access to your auto. Remember, every addict craving a fix knows that hospitals store large quantities of drugs. These desperate individuals may force you to obtain some for them. If your hospital separates employee from visitor parking, take advantage of this safeguard. Allow security to protect you by spotting loiterers who can be easily identified between shift changes.

Always be aware of your responsibility to protect each patient's property. Be alert in recognizing suspicious people in patient-care areas, particularly the maternity ward, and, even more, the newborn nursery. A stranger should be asked, politely but firmly, what business he or she has in the area. But a kidnapping may be perpetrated by a person upset by such a question. If you are suspicious or intimidated, act as if nothing is wrong, and call for assistance. The security staff is trained to handle these situations. Let them do so.

Be especially alert and cautious in instances where police officers bring a prisoner to be treated at the hospital. These situations require increased security. Needless to say, during these incidents hospital staff, as well as patients, are at risk of serious and even fatal injury.

Some hospitals have provided training in security procedures for all employees using films and police instruction. Topics covered include managing intruders, recognizing the beginning stages of altercation, and intervening without escalating the altercation. Finally, be alert as you walk around the maze of deserted hallways typical of most hospitals.

IN A NURSING HOME

Five percent of the elderly population, or over 1.5 million people, currently reside in the nation's more than 25,000 nursing homes. However, the number of institutionalized elderly is expected to reach nearly 3.5 million by the year 2030. As the elderly population becomes larger, the number of nursing homes will increase, and they will differ according to cost, level of medical care, convenience of location, visiting rights, accreditation or licensing, quality of food, privacy, adequate lighting, proper staffing, numbers of personnel, and atmosphere. Other criteria in your final choice are security and safety. Highly publicized scandals and investigations into criminal misconduct by nursing home owners over the last 15 years have highlighted the terrible dangers and conditions found in some nursing homes. Several even had connections to organized crime.

When you are searching for a source of elder care, investigate alternatives to resident nursing homes. Part-time domestic help, a nurse, or aide may be a better option. This allows an elderly person to remain at home with a higher level of independence and in familiar surroundings. A study conducted by the Office of the Inspector General reported that nearly 95 percent of respondents agreed that abuse in nursing homes is a problem. In addition, they found that the problem is progressively worsening.

Staff Problems

Because abuse by nursing home staff is not uncommon, you must exercise extreme caution in your selection. Be sure the nursing homes you are considering are certified, and that the staff is thoroughly screened.

Horrible experiences can be avoided by visiting nursing homes with members of your family before making your final selection. Ask your doctor, local health department, or area agency on aging for references to several nursing homes. The more homes you visit, the easier you will find spotting a quality home. Spend several hours at each, preferably during an event or activity. During your visit, ask questions of the staff and residents. Request to see the home's latest state survey results that report any problems the facility has had, and compare these, as well as different ones, with past reports at the same nursing home. State surveys are done at every licensed nursing home. Do not admit yourself or a loved one to a home that does not allow you to see this report. The administrators may be hiding the report for a good reason.

Find out whether the staff is caring, compassionate, understanding, and energetic. Observe how attentive (or inattentive) they are to residents' needs. For example, see if they ignore residents that approach them, or how quickly they respond to call bells. Make sure the staff also respects and adheres to basic patient rights, such as confidentiality and privacy and safety from exploitation. Determine what residents think about the nursing home. If they are unhappy, you are sure to be displeased as well. Make sure residents look clean and healthy, and that if any elderly are restrained, it is for safety purposes only. Another key aspect to look for is resident awareness. A lot of nursing home residents who appear "drugged" is a bad sign. Avoid nursing homes that have had a record of abuse.

Some staff working conditions that are likely to decrease incidences of abuse include the following:

❖ High staff-to-resident ratios
❖ Highly skilled and trained staff
❖ Low staff turnover rates
❖ Sufficient staff supervision
❖ Well-paid staff
❖ Low-stress working conditions
❖ Minimal number of critically ill patients
❖ Staff empathy and understanding of the elderly and their needs

Although any member of a nursing home's staff can abuse residents, research results from the Office of the Inspector General indicate that respondents felt that aides and orderlies, those most responsible for daily care, contribute more than others to all aspects of abuse, with the exception of medical neglect. The report also found verbal and emotional abuse and physical, verbal, and emotional neglect, to be among the most common forms of abuse according to nursing home residents. Be sure to review the procedures in this book for preventing elderly abuse. (See Chapter 18.)

Another matter of concern is the cost of a nursing home. There have been many recent cases of exploitation by nursing home owners who pay themselves salaries in excess of $1 million annually, while robbing the elderly (and Medicaid). One study in 1992 revealed that about 4 of 10 profit-earning nursing homes in New York City generated profits of over $1 million. These extraordinarily high profits and salaries continue despite the fact that state guidelines recommend that the salary limit be set at $119,800, even at a large nursing home.

Nothing undermines the morale of a resident more than an unsafe nursing home. While theft is the most common crime in many nursing homes, there have also been many cases of physical and sexual assaults, robberies, and even homicides. Be sure, therefore, that the nursing home administration is truly concerned about the security of your family member, and that its plan of action ensures a safe environment. Review the guidelines offered in the previous sections concerning hospitals, which apply equally to nursing homes.

Since theft is the most common crime in nursing homes, both patient and family should sit down with the administrators and determine which valuables (if any) should be brought along. These should be put in a safe-deposit box maintained by the nursing home or placed in a locked property-storage container mounted on a wall, cabinet, door, or similar convenient location. An alternative—less convenient but safer—is to have the nursing administrator or the patient's family make arrangements to store valuables at a local bank. If the person is mobile, this arrangement also requires an occasional trip to town and affords a chance to see people not associated with the nursing home. A change of scenery is a great morale booster.

If your nursing home has a property identification program ("Operation ID") by which valuable personal property can be engraved with a unique identification number, it should be used. Then a special decal can be displayed to indicate that expensive belongings have a serial number and that the thief will have difficulty disposing of them. A complete inventory should be made of all personal property. This inventory should be updated frequently as it will be useful in identifying property and in recovering lost or stolen items.

Hallway Watch

At some nursing homes, residents on the same floor have gotten together and organized a hallway or floor watch. They meet periodically to discuss security and arrange to watch out for each others' safety the same way groups of neighbors do in the Neighborhood Watch program. (See Chapter 23.) It is highly recommended that such a watch be organized at every home. The hallway or floor watch is useful for preventing crime by both outsiders and employees. Members of the hallway watch should always be alert for strangers, suspicious persons, and people having no legitimate business in the nursing home. Missing property should be reported to the nursing staff as soon as possible. A thief who finds it easy to steal will try again at the same spot or nearby.

For more information on how to select a safe and secure nursing home suitable for your needs, check your local agency on aging or write to:

American Association of Retired Persons
Health and Long Term Care
601 E Street, NW
Washington, DC 20036
(202) 434-2230

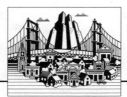

SECURITY IN HOSPITALS AND NURSING HOMES: A CHECKLIST

1 Determine if a stay at a hospital or nursing home is necessary. Look into the possibility of outpatient procedures or home care for the elderly.

2 Before entering a hospital or nursing home, become familiar with patient's rights. Make certain these are enforced during your stay.

3 Check the level of security at the hospital or nursing home of your choice. Stay informed of security procedures and services.

4 Deposit your valuables in the vault provided by the hospital or nursing home, or, better yet, leave them at home or with trusted relatives.

5 Check all medical and hospital bills for overcharges and report faulty bills.

6 Do not place dentures, hearing aids, eyeglasses, radios, or similar objects in the safe-deposit box, because they are often damaged due to faulty storage facilities.

7 Notify the security office at your hospital or nursing home if you are aware of a theft.

8 Never meddle in an altercation in the hospital, especially in the emergency room. Notify hospital staff.

9 To safeguard against infant abduction, maternity wards should be restricted areas. The newborn section should be locked at all times and carefully monitored.

10 Never wander aimlessly around hospital corridors or hallways.

11 If you work at a hospital or nursing home, be alert for suspicious individuals. Find out the purpose of their presence, and if you are not satisfied, notify security.

12 To protect yourself when parking at the hospital or nursing home, park your car within view or earshot of parking attendants or pedestrians and in an adequately lighted place. Be alert for suspicious persons. Always lock your car.

13 Investigate a nursing home fully before you or a loved one stays there. Spend at least a few hours there observing the staff and residents.

14 Be certain that the nursing home you are considering is certified and that all employees are thoroughly screened.

15 Pay attention to how the staff treats residents. Make sure their working conditions do not make them more potentially abusive.

16 Avoid nursing homes with a history of scandals, corruption, or ties to organized crime.

17 Make sure all residents appear clean and healthy, and that any restraints used are only for the resident's safety.

18 Look for resident awareness. If too many nursing home residents appear "drugged," they may well be so unnecessarily.

19 For their own self-protection, residents should report all incidents of abuse to their families and the nursing home administrator.

20 To protect themselves and their valuables, residents should take advantage of all programs offered by the nursing home, including Operation ID and a hallway watch.

26

ELDERLY VICTIMS
OF CRIME

The number of elderly citizens in this country is increasing rapidly. By the end of the century, the number will reach just under 35 million. The fastest growing group is those aged 75 and older, because of increasing life expectancy. The age group of 85 and older is expected to increase by 60 percent over the next decade. Because of these population changes, there will be more targets for crime among the elderly.

CRIME AND THE ELDERLY

Although the elderly have the lowest crime victimization rates of any age group, they are particularly vulnerable physically, psychologically, and financially. The elderly are more likely than younger age groups to be robbed by a stranger and to be confronted by an armed assailant. Elderly victims are targeted often because they are less able to flee from danger than are younger victims, and less likely to try to protect themselves. Most elderly citizens who do use protective measures utilize nonphysical means of self-defense, such as arguing, screaming, running away, and even reasoning with the perpetrator.

The elderly person's worst enemy, as far as crime is concerned, is often him- or herself. Three-quarters of the burglaries victimizing older people involve unlocked doors or windows. And strange as it may seem, half of these burglaries are never reported to anyone. The risk of burglary and other crimes increases when an individual lives alone, because of lack of activity around the residence. The burglar is not the senior citizen's only threat, though. Purse snatching and pickpocketing are the most frequent crimes against the aged. The typical purse theft involves grabbing a purse with one hand, shoving the victim with the other, and running away. Broken bones commonly result from this type of crime—often more serious than the loss of the contents of the purse.

Payday for the robber, mugger, purse snatcher, or burglar often coincides with delivery day for government checks. It is so easy to avoid losing money to thugs by using direct deposit, in which funds are transferred directly to the bank for deposit. Many communities have at least one bank that provides free checking accounts to seniors. Yet many older citizens continue to make the regular "payday" trip to cash a check and all too often provide a payday for someone else. If your Social Security check is more than three mailing days late, call the Social Security Administration at (800) 772-1213. In emergencies, a replacement check can take as little time as a week. A post office box provides additional security for checks and mailings.

Three of the leading crimes committed against the elderly could be drastically reduced by three simple steps:

1. Lock doors and windows.
2. Don't carry more money than you can afford to lose.
3. Don't carry a purse.

Instead of a purse, use pockets in slacks, jackets, or coats. If necessary, sew pockets in your clothing. Although you don't have a purse, you may still be stopped on the street and robbed at gunpoint, but you're less likely to get the broken leg that could result from being knocked to the ground.

What Senior Citizens Should Do

Senior citizens should establish daily telephone contact with their children and/or friends, encourage frequent visits, and check with neighbors on a regular basis. If no one is available for daily contact, join a neighborhood program that provides this service. The U.S. Postal Service, for example, has mail carriers report when elderly residents have not picked up the previous day's mail. Many utility companies sponsor similar programs. It is a good idea for an elderly person to join others for mutual self-protection such as in a citizen crime prevention group, a property identification program, or similar activity.

Help aged people you care about improve their residential security, and give them a few useful tips without frightening them. Many elderly are so frightened by media stories that they are afraid to leave their homes. A crime prevention specialist from your local police precinct can give your residence or a loved one's residence a home security survey. If you are moving to a senior complex or nursing home, ask someone to go with you to check security standards and to make sure it is not a rip-off. (For additional information on nursing home security, see Chapter 25.)

If you're returning home, have your key ready, and don't linger at the door. Whenever possible, have someone walk you home, especially at night. If you observe suspicious-looking people around your entrance, don't go in. Go to a nearby store or to the house of a neighbor, friend, or relative, and call the police. If you live in a building and someone is standing near your apartment door, ring a neighbor's bell and pretend to be a visitor. Establish a light-up/lock-up routine on retiring for the night. Be sure to close drapes and pull down shades at that time too.

When you need to go shopping or on other excursions that take you out of your home, follow the guidelines described in Chapters 12 to 14. Try to bring a friend or relative with you when shopping or running errands. There is safety in numbers.

Criminals are on the lookout for predictable schedules, so it is best to vary your routes and routines. This is particularly important when making a trip to the bank, especially at the beginning and end of the month when checks are often received.

If driving, park as close as possible to your destination. If you have a health problem or disability, ask your doctor about your eligibility for a "handicapped sticker" for your car. This sticker will allow you to park near entrances.

Check references of anyone who wants money from you for any reason. Seek trusted advice before signing any contract or making any major expenditures—especially insurance purchases. Mail offers that seem too good to be true are probably just that. Before undertaking any medical treatment suggested by someone who approaches you, check it with your own physician or community health clinic. Get a receipt for any significant expenditure you make.

Federal crime insurance is currently available in most states. For a premium of only a few dollars per week, a victim of crime can be reimbursed for damages and stolen property. However, to qualify, the applicant must have window locks and deadbolt locks on doors.

What Senior Citizens Should Avoid

Don't let strangers stop you for conversation, and avoid parked cars with running motors. Don't be conspicuous wherever you may be; dress simply and avoid displays of cash or valuable jewelry. Avoid large groups of adolescents. Avoid isolated, sparsely traveled streets or roads. Don't carry a purse if at all possible, and, if you must, never let it out of your sight. Never keep your keys in your purse or in the same pocket as your wallet. If your purse or wallet is stolen, the criminal will also have your address (from identifying cards). If your keys are stolen also, your locks must be changed immediately.

Don't be a hero—surrender valuables if you're robbed. When you are home, follow the security guidelines as outlined in Chapters 1 to 4.

The elderly are particularly vulnerable to con-artists and con-games, and the risk of becoming a victim of fraud increases as a person gets older. Be particularly cautious when purchasing items over the telephone. Legitimate phone order operations have detailed warranty and return policies and will gladly answer any questions you may have. If they are evasive or use high pressure tactics, go elsewhere with your business. (Read Chapter 27 for tips on protective measures against con-artists and con-games.)

Under no circumstances should you take any of these risky actions:

❖ Don't give "good-faith money" for any investment that hasn't been thoroughly checked by someone you have known and trusted for many years.

❖ Never disclose personal information, bank account numbers, or credit card numbers to a telephone caller, even if the caller claims that he or she is a bank official or that you have won a prize. Also be wary of mailings that offer prizes, especially when they request money.

❖ Do not withdraw any of your banks funds as a part of an alleged investigation of bank procedures.

❖ Don't pay in advance for any significant purchase, unless you are buying from a reputable merchant with whom you have traded for years.

❖ Don't sign any contract whatsoever without first checking with your children, a trusted friend, your attorney, or the Better Business Bureau. To be even more protective of your assets, place a call to the police department's fraud or bunco squad. Other sources of assistance include your local consumer affairs office, the district attorney's office, and your attorney general. Just make certain that the correct date appears on anything you sign. Even if you don't fall for a scam, report it. You could prevent someone else from falling into a trap.

Though you may have done everything suggested in this chapter, it is possible that something has been overlooked. Perhaps you made a mistake and entered the wrong date on the order form, or maybe the salesperson took your copy of the contract, and you were left holding the bag. Call the police anyway, or the district attorney or the local consumer protection office. More than likely, a crook who victimizes you will also have victimized others, and your identification could be the piece of evidence that would bring an end to this particular fraud.

WHERE TO FIND HELP

First of all, in finding help, don't be afraid of "being a burden" to your children. You were there when they needed you!

Know emergency phone numbers: In most communities, help is available by dialing 911 or the operator (0). Keep a list of emergency telephone numbers next to your telephone, including those of friends or relatives nearby who can help when needed. Help is always available at a police station, a fire station, and sometimes even at a business that you patronize.

One word of advice: If you need help, ask for it. Don't wait for someone to come to your aid. If you wait, you may attract the wrong person— a scavenger after easy prey. Local sources of help are usually best, because they are nearby and are more familiar with the special needs and aspects of your community. Make a list of telephone numbers and addresses of local resources for easy reference. Keep this separate from your emergency list. If you are the victim of a crime, report it!

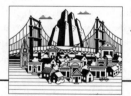

ELDERLY VICTIMS OF CRIME: A CHECKLIST

1 Establish daily telephone contacts with relatives, arrange frequent visits, and check with neighbors on a regular basis.

2 Be on guard at all times for criminals who will take advantage of your weaknesses.

3 You can eliminate many crimes against the elderly if you lock doors and windows, limit the amount of money or valuables you carry, and keep the carrying of handbags at an absolute minimum.

4 Make arrangements for direct deposit of all government checks in your bank account.

5 For your own self-protection, you should do the following:

    a. Call your police precinct for a home security survey.
    b. Establish a light-up, lock-out nighttime routine.
    c. Have your key ready for use when coming home. Go for help if a suspicious-looking person is loitering around your entrance.

    d. Keep shopping money separate from lunch or transportation funds.

    e. Ask your doctor if you're eligible for a "handicapped sticker" for your car.

    f. Check references and seek advice from those competent and trusted before making any significant expenditure—especially on medical insurance or home repair—and get a receipt. Use credit cards or checks for payment, never cash.

6 Avoid the following risks:

    a. Unsolicited conversations with strangers

    b. Conspicuous dress or actions

    c. Congregations of adolescents

    d. Isolated, sparsely traveled streets

    e. Carrying valuables

    f. Letting unknown visitors into your home

    g. Doing business with a stranger whose reputation is unknown

7 The telephone can be an invasion into the security of your home. Be very cautious in using the telephone.

8 Never disclose personal information, bank account numbers, or credit card numbers to a telephone caller, even if the caller claims to be a bank official. Also be wary of mailings that offer prizes, especially when they request money.

9 Do not withdraw any of your banks funds as a part of an alleged investigation.

10 Learn where to find help in your community. Seek help; don't wait for help to find you. Your ostensible helper may actually be looking for your valuables.

11 Above all, if you are the victim of a crime, report it.

27

$\approx$

CONSUMER FRAUD, CON-ARTISTS, AND CON-GAMES

The doorbell rang at the suburban Long Island home of Ms. Margaret Wilson. She opened the door to find a man claiming to be an oil company repairman. She showed him to the basement, where he completely dismantled her heating burner. He then demanded cash in advance for the repairs he said the burner needed. Ms. Wilson later found out that the man had no connection to the oil company, and the "repairs" he made were completely unnecessary. To add insult to injury, she realized that while in the house, he helped himself to a few of her personal items.

Con-artists, con-games, and "scams" may seem antiquated to the reader, swindles one finds only in a Damon Runyon novel or in movies such as *The Sting.* We all like to think we're too smart to "fall for the bait." However, all too often we fail to realize that we're being baited in the first place. According to one study, each year in the United States, millions of people are so victimized, resulting in losses of more than $100 billion.

CONSUMER FRAUD

Most businesses are honest. However, there are always those that will try to cheat you if they think they can get away with it. It is usually safer to do business with a firm that has been recommended by your relatives or trusted friends. Before contracting for a service or making a major purchase, check the reputation of the company by calling a consumer service bureau, such as the Better Business Bureau. The local office of the Federal Trade Commission may give you information on similar types of businesses, if not the actual firm you are checking.

Unscrupulous Contractors

Remember, even though a business may be licensed, there is no guarantee that its personnel are honest or that it provides quality work. Before you authorize any work from a contractor, get a *written estimate*. Later, ask the contractor to itemize each item of cost before you approve the estimate. If you need clarification, do not be ashamed to ask questions or to get a second or third estimate.

Advertising Swindles

Advertising by its very nature is meant to persuade the consumer to buy the product or use the service that's being advertised. Even legitimate businesses may employ questionable practices, from "fine print" to misleading statements in an attempt to create interest in their wares. Unfortunately, fraudulent promoters have practically made an art form out of bending (and breaking) the already confusing laws concerning truth-in-advertising to hawk their own illegal or worthless products or services.

Every advertisement you encounter (and you are probably exposed to a countless number each day) should be taken with a grain of salt; however, fraud and inaccuracy are most often associated with ads involving medical aids, wonder cures, sure-fire investments, work-at-home opportunities, travel opportunities, credit repair, and weight loss or fitness programs.

Offers that appear to be too good to be true—such as "overnight weight loss" or "earn thousands a week" or "bad credit history erased"—are almost always worthless and expensive scams. Any ad that directs you to call a 1-900 number for information (which can result in charges to your phone bill of anywhere from $3 to $50 a call) is most certainly not legitimate; unfortunately, even some 1-800 numbers now charge for the call. A business that offers an honorable product or service should not charge you just to get you to know more information about it.

Remember, con-games (including false advertising) are not always officially illegal; you may be charged exorbitant (but legal) fees or prices for unnecessary services or worthless items. You do not need to call a 1-900 number to get a report of your credit history; this may be obtained free of charge or, for a nominal fee, from the credit bureau in charge of your records. However, you are entitled to a free credit report if you were turned down for credit. Also, reputable modeling/acting agencies or agencies that are trying to find you employment don't charge cash fees to list your name in directories; they usually work on commission. Remember, if an ad has fine print or lists several conditions, you *must* carefully read all the lines before making a decision. Never buy on impulse because of the selling power of an ad. Something that's truly good today will still be good tomorrow, after you've had time to think about it. The only person you hurt by ignoring these warnings is yourself.

Retail Swindles

Beware of consumer rip-offs when shopping in retail establishments. Signs such as "Lost Our Lease" or "Everything Must Go" may be used to lure shoppers into the store. When paying by check, make the draft payable only to the company, not to an individual employee of the store.

Always have a secondhand car checked by a mechanic before you buy. Used-car dealers are skillful at hiding the defects of their wares. At a supermarket, even if it uses a scanner to record your purchases, watch as the checkout clerk rings up each item. Price mistakes are often made unintentionally, but also deliberately.

When making a major purchase, such as an air conditioner or microwave oven, shop around and compare warranties. Some warranties offer full service, while others provide minimal coverage on certain parts of the product. Ascertain who guarantees performance under the warranty and the ability and resources of the guarantor to meet the contractual obligations. Save all receipts, and note the installation date. It is possible that you will wish to file a complaint against a company, and this information is essential. Describe to the person who has the authority to resolve your problem what is wrong with the merchandise and what you want done about it.

If you aren't satisfied, you may want to take the matter to court. Small-claims court sessions are held at night in many jurisdictions, and often you will not need to hire a lawyer. Payment of a small filing fee will usually ensure that your case will be heard in a month.

Mail and Telephone Fraud

Two associated areas of widespread fraud are mail fraud and telephone fraud. Frauds involving these venues are often categorized as legitimate business transactions—and as a matter of fact, some technically are. The fraudulent elements in these types of swindles are often overpricing or inappropriateness. Some transactions involve actual lies, and their promoters rely on inertia on the part of their victims. Promoters figure that instead of contacting the proper authorities or going to court, their victims will just chalk up their mistakes to experience. Remember, anyone with a phone or a mailbox is a potential mark. The question is: Once approached, will you take the proper steps to avoid being a victim?

Fraudulent activity involving mail or phone lines includes insurance offers (especially health insurance); debt consolidation; magazine subscriptions; land, property, and condominium offers; securities and oil leases; franchise deals; work-at-home plans; publish-your-own-book arrangements; home improvements; medicine and miracle cures; weight loss or fitness programs; sweepstakes opportunities; travel opportunities; and discount purchasing clubs.

Be wary of mail order or phone swindles for work-at-home schemes that require cash deposits or payments, or that require you to call a 1-900 toll charge number to receive information. If you are looking for work, there are many ways to go about it free of charge (classified ads) or by payment of a standard commission (to a legitimate temporary agency). One of the fastest-growing frauds is a telephone call or a postcard that promises an exotic vacation, an exorbitant gift, or a cash-money windfall in exchange for a processing fee, or for your purchase of an item the caller or postcard is hawking. Remember, it is the *law* that no purchase is required where a sweepstakes is concerned. For a good clue to the legitimacy of a "prize" offer, check the postage on the letter; if it's bulk rate, you haven't won anything of value—in fact, thousands of other people have received the same notice as you. As for the phone, remember you have no obligation to stay on the line; it is your right to hang up at any time.

Obviously, one reason why mail order and phone scams have become so popular is that legitimate purchasing through the phone and mail has become widespread. Remember, all legitimate mail and phone order operations have clearly detailed return and warranty policies and will gladly answer any questions you have; they seek your *repeat* business. If they are unclear or evasive about their policies, or use high-pressure tactics to get you to commit, go elsewhere with your business.

Remember, never give out your credit card number, your Social Security number, your telephone calling card number, or any personal information for that matter, without fully understanding to whom and why you are giving this information. The only information that you would possibly have to give is your credit card number, and that should only be on a call you initiated with a business of confirmed legitimacy. *Never* send cash in the mail.

Be on the lookout for a phony IRS agent calling, saying he needs an immediate cash payment to settle a problem, or your Social Security or credit card number so that he can set up an "audit." Ask for an ID and a number you can call back. You can call the IRS hotline, (800) 366-4484, for verification.

Finally, beware of organizations offering to find you a low-interest credit card or to repair your credit history. The Consumer Credit Counseling Service, (800) 388-4484, is a legitimate organization that can help a person get out of debt.

CON-ARTISTS AND CON-GAMES

The con-artist is sometimes glorified in movies and literature. In the real world, these swindlers are despicable criminals, preying on the uninformed and elderly, often taking their life savings and leaving them to blame themselves for a life of privation and despair.

Stranger at Your Door

This book repeatedly cautions you not to admit anyone into your home unless you know who he or she is and why he wants admittance. One of the many good reasons for this advice is that such people may be con-artists. Here are a few ways in which they operate.

One of the simplest cons is initiated by a person who knocks on your door and asks for a glass of water. As he or she is ushered into the kitchen, an accomplice sneaks in and steals money, jewelry, credit cards, or other valuables.

Another favorite scam involves the con-artist masquerading as a repairman, often for a utility or electric company, or perhaps a cable TV company. It is highly unlikely that any of these people would show up at your door without giving you prior notification. In any case, always demand to see proper ID and documentation, and don't be afraid to refuse entrance until you contact the worker's employer and verify his legitimacy.

Another particularly vile con involves the "funeral chaser," who reads the obituary notice and shows up at the home of the deceased with highly overpriced merchandise that the deceased ostensibly ordered. Of course, it isn't true, but the salesperson can be most persuasive, often threatening to tie up life insurance proceeds and employing other such tactics.

On another occasion, a caller claiming to be a bank examiner requests your help in trapping a dishonest bank employee. You are asked to withdraw funds to be used as a test of the suspect's honesty. Unfortunately for you, it's the phony bank examiner who is a crook.

Street Swindles and Other Common Con-Games

Another ingenious swindle involves a caller who says he has inexpensive new appliances for sale. You are requested to meet the salesperson at the loading dock of a retail department store. He or she meets you there, asks you to back your car up to the platform for delivery, takes your money, and is never seen again.

In another very effective swindle, a person approaches you in the street and says you can buy a case of expensive liquor at a low price. You are taken to a store and told you are to wait until he or she returns with the liquor. You are asked to pay for it at that point. Your "friend" enters the store, never to return with either your money or the goods.

Also, avoid street hawkers who appear to be selling expensive goods such as watches, necklaces, rings, bracelets, sweaters, shirts, etc., purchased at bulk discount prices. The peddler's aim is to convince you that you are purchasing expensive, perhaps "hot," merchandise at a bargain basement price when in fact you are overpaying for a nearly worthless item. Besides, it is illegal to purchase knowingly even a single item of stolen property. Also, beware of national brand or designer clothes peddled by street vendors. Most likely you will be overpaying for "knockoffs," or counterfeits, of the original.

There are even cons in which honest citizens are unsuspecting accomplices. For example, the swindler buys a few television sets at regular price from a store and then sells them box-unopened to prominent citizens in the community for cut-rate prices, saying he got the sets from an electronics store that was going out of business. He then uses telephone solicitation to sell hundreds more to the people in the community, who are told when referred to the original buyers that the deal is a legitimate bargain. Of course, he has no more televisions to sell, and the community is collectively out of thousands of dollars.

Another scheme, this one principally to bilk the elderly, is the "pigeon drop." It is usually worked after a person has made a deposit into a savings account and is leaving, passbook in hand. A stranger, approaching the victim, will flash a wad of money, indicate that it has just been found, and ask what should be done. The mark, predictably, will answer, "I don't know." A "passerby" (actually another confidence crook) states that a friend at a nearby bank would know what to do, and agrees to telephone the banker. Upon returning from the phone booth, the group is informed that the money should be split among all of them, providing that it isn't claimed by the real owner by the end of the day. The problem, however, is that a $2,000 fidelity bond is required, "to protect the bank." The pigeon is prevailed upon to provide the bond (with the promise of half the windfall) and awaits the return of the conspirator who claimed to have a banker friend. Of course, no one returns at the end of the day.

Avoid charity fraud. People may masquerade as a representative of a charity, soliciting donations for "needy children" or "cancer research." AIDS and homeless charities may also be targeted, especially in bigger cities where these problems are prevalent. Giving to charity is a selfless thing to do; however, it is best to stick to giving donations to well-established and well-known charities.

Another swindle, one common in large cities, is the multiple rental scam. The con-artist leases an apartment, using an assumed name. Subsequently, the apartment is relet to as many as 50 other people, and the confidence cheat receives a month's rent and a security deposit from each of them.

Another confidence game, "three-card monte," is well known on the streets of New York and other cities. It is ostensibly a game of skill, in which the dealer rapidly moves three cards, and the player attempts to pick a target from among the three that the dealer lays out. Seldom does a player select the proper card. It may be the result of a great deal of skill and dexterity on the part of the dealer, or it may be that the dealer has palmed the target card, and the player is playing a can't-win game. It is an interesting show, with lots of action and occasional excitement. But that isn't all. Frequently, pickpockets mingle among the players and spectators around the dealer and players.

One final note: When attempting to find police assistance, especially if you feel you've just been victimized by a scam, make sure the person you contact is a *real officer.* Con-men often have accomplices who will pretend to be law enforcement agents; their job is to keep the real law out of any dispute, and if possible to swindle even more money from you. Remember, all government agents must have proper ID at all times, and there are absolutely no circumstances when any legitimate authority or police officer will ask for money or valuables or request that you withdraw money from your bank account—*under no circumstances—ever.*

Real Estate Con-Games

Real estate is fast becoming a favorite of the confidence man. The attraction of real estate lies in the fact that the stakes are high. Measured by numbers of six or seven digits, real estate can offer quite a large potential haul for a trickster. One con works this way: The con-artist stands in an upscale residential area, on a busy thoroughfare, and stops people on the street, saying, "Excuse me, but are you the Mr. Green who is to meet Mr. Black here?" Most will say No, but occasionally one will answer "Why?"

The con-artist will zero in on his or her prey, giving the victim a business card, which bears the name of a well-respected real estate firm. (Actually, the con-artist stole the cards from one of those plastic bins that salespeople sometimes have on their desks.) The confidence man explains to the mark that he or she was to meet Mr. Green, who was to sign a contract to purchase "that particular house" on the corner. It must be sold on that day, by order of probate court, so that the estate can be dissolved. If the intended victim expresses any interest, the con-artist will say that the property could be bought at a most attractive price, because with the estate closing that afternoon, there wasn't sufficient time to contact others who had shown interest in the property.

The conversation continues, and the prospective purchaser is inveigled into giving the con-artist a certified check as earnest money. The victim receives the crook's promise that the closing attorney will meet with him or her at the victim's office 2 days later. Only then does the bargain seeker realize that greed has cost him or her a great deal of money.

Another common real estate scam is the time-share or campsite swindle. You are approached by a self-proclaimed agent who informs you that he or she is in contact with a party interested in buying your property. But first you must pay a cash advance or a finder's fee to the agent for the service. Of course, it's a scam; there is no buyer, and your "agent" disappears with the finder's fee.

Repair or Rip-off?

Other common rip-off schemes include "repairmen" or engineers who offer you repair work at unbelievably low prices. A phony engineer might inspect your home and determine that the heating, plumbing, or chimney needs repair. You might be asked to sign a contract and give a down payment, but you'll never see the "repairman" again. An individual might say that he or she has enough material to blacktop your driveway or repair leaks in your roof. The work is done with black oil that never dries, but you have already paid cash, as requested. A "gardener" offers to cover your property with topsoil. Later you learn it is sawdust mixed with motor oil. Use only those businesses that have been around for years or have been referred to you by a trusted source.

Women are perhaps more vulnerable than men to rip-offs by car repairmen and salesmen because of women's presumed lack of knowledge about cars. But, man or woman, you should make sure the repair shops you deal with are registered with your state. They should have a current Department of Motor Vehicles registration certificate. Ask friends and relatives to refer you to a reputable business.

Give the mechanic a written list detailing what's wrong with your car, and keep a written record of all repairs. You will need to supply these materials if you file a complaint and, if you sell your car, these records could increase your asking price. Ask for a written estimate for all repairs. Write down the date, time, price, and with whom you've spoken when authorizing repairs, especially by telephone. The repairman should answer all questions you have. If he fails to, it is probably best to keep looking. If you aren't very knowledgeable about your vehicle and its parts, it's a good idea to bring along someone who is.

After the work is completed, make sure you are given a written, detailed invoice, and inspect your car before paying. If you are not satisfied, speak to the manager or owner. If this proves unfruitful, file a complaint with your state Department of Motor Vehicles. The department will try to settle the dispute by telephone, which is only effective less than half the time. If the department is unable to settle the complaint by phone, it will refer the case to a local office. Other sources of assistance include the state attorney general and the Better Business Bureau. The Department of Consumer Affairs may also provide assistance. In Los Angeles, a major tire dealer was forced to return nearly half a million dollars to customers the dealer had overcharged.

Never accept offers for repairs from people on the street. One very common con involves people in cars who look for autos needing bodywork. They offer these repairs at a low price, and only later do you discover that the materials used disintegrate after a short time.

You should know how to do minor repairs and maintenance on your own. Know how to change a tire and how to check tire pressure with a gauge. Have a can of flat-tire fix that can be used to inflate your tire temporarily if there is a slow leak. Learn how to check the fluids (i.e., oil, antifreeze, transmission, windshield washer, etc.) in your car and how to refill them. Water can be used in a pinch to put into the radiator if your car overheats. You should also keep in your car jumper cables, a flashlight, flares, a tool kit (including a lug wrench to change a tire), and a first-aid kit.

Women need to be especially careful when buying or selling a used car. Do not disclose you are a woman by revealing your first name when placing a classified ad. Car thieves may pretend to be customers interested in buying your car. A common scheme is taking your car for a test-drive and then never returning, or making a copy of your car keys and then coming back to steal the car later.

Never go with a potential buyer on a test-drive, especially if you are alone. Several women have been driven to secluded areas where they've been robbed and raped. Meet in a public place. Never let the prospective buyer know where you live or where you usually park your car. Ask for identification, and make a mental note of his or her description. Keep something of value behind as the buyer's collateral. A thief will try to give you something of little worth. If someone buys your car, insist on payment by cash, and make sure you cancel your insurance immediately. Be sure to remove your license plates and registration decal.

When buying a used car, a reputable dealer is the safest choice. Go during the day, and inspect the vehicle carefully. Pay special attention to the VIN (Vehicle Identification Number); you may be sold a stolen car. Make sure that the VIN matches the title and that it hasn't been tampered with. Be certain the license plate and inspection and emission decals are valid. Be wary if the car has had a recent paint job. Check for proper wheel alignment, rust, leaks, and worn brakes, and look for signs of tampering with the odometer. Start the car, listen carefully, and look for excessive exhaust. Take the vehicle for a test-drive, and have a mechanic or other knowledgeable person examine the vehicle before you make any commitment.

Find out if your state has a "lemon law" that allows you to return the car within a specified period of time if it is not working properly. If you find out you've been ripped off, get your money back. If you paid by check, put a stop-payment on it. If you've taken out a loan, alert your financial institution immediately.

You have to be careful even when going to a certified mechanic. The stories are legend of unnecessary repairs, price gouging, and incompetent work. The standby repairman often preys on the fact that a customer knows very little about how a car runs or how a refrigerator works. Even well-known companies have been found guilty of negligent behavior.

If you are having a repair done, always get a written estimate before-hand, and ask for the old parts back after they are replaced. A scrupulous repairman or mechanic will have no problem with this.

HOW TO PROTECT YOURSELF FROM SWINDLERS

Advice on this subject is easy to give, but implementing it is much more difficult. However, if you can follow a few simple rules, you ought to be safe from the smooth-talking con-artist.

❖ Always look a gift horse very hard in the mouth. Never be rushed into any investment by a smooth talker. Any investment with merit can stand thorough investigation.

❖ Never give money to a stranger offering you a once-in-a-lifetime deal. Remember, the fraud will exploit your weakness—your desire to get a "good deal." A stranger who approaches you with a great deal probably has a great deal to gain from you. (Chapter 28 discusses a variety of financial scams and methods for your protection.)

❖ Walk away from anyone who approaches you with money to share with you. Never withdraw money from a bank, then turn it over to a stranger.

❖ Entrust your repair work to reputable companies or repairers recommended by friends or relatives.

If you've been the victim of fraud, there are places you can turn to for help and information. You can contact such authorities as state and local consumer protection agencies, the local Better Business Bureau, and the state attorney general. If you have a problem involving mail fraud, you should contact the U.S. Postal Inspection Service. If you have a problem with telephone scams, contact the local phone company to see what can be done. A national service you can contact is the National Fraud Information Center, (800) 876-7060. If you're the victim of street fraud, contact the police.

THE PERILS OF DATING SERVICES

The complexity of meeting a mate in this "modern world" may lead you to a dating service. As it gets tougher and tougher to meet someone the "old-fashioned way," a dating service may seem the ideal venue through which to meet people. Be aware, however, of the very serious perils involved in the use of these agencies.

Before disclosing personal information to a dating service, you should investigate the business fully. Some services may be fly-by-night organizations that disappear shortly after collecting your money. Others may collect personal information about you to find out if your home is worth burglarizing.

The best way to find a legitimate service is through recommendations from people you trust. Before committing yourself, check with the local Better Business Bureau, Chamber of Commerce, and Small Claims Court for complaints against the agency. Ask the agency how long it has been in business—obviously, the longer the better. A legitimate business should be able to provide you with references from clients. Be wary about signing any contract, and find out about all fees before making a commitment. Make certain your personal information will be kept confidential and that the service conducts thorough background checks of all its members.

Personal ads are extremely dangerous, as unfortunately the occasional robber, rapist, and, yes, murderer, find these easy ways to meet victims.

CHARLATAN LOVERS

The ultimate con involves a man or a woman who pretends to love you but whose heart is focused on your dollars. It usually begins when your "lover" asks to borrow a little money and ends when your credit cards, jewelry, home, business, and life savings are taken. All of a sudden your lover has disappeared, whereabouts unknown. This type of operation has typically ripped off dozens of partners, usually women. If you happen to locate the impostor, usually you are too heartbroken, poor, and demoralized to pay the legal fees required for legal action.

Common sense, caution, and sound judgment can save you from this painful experience. Experts propose the following signals as a warning that you are dealing with a charlatan Romeo or Juliet:

❖ The man or woman appears slick, too perfect. He or she is extremely attractive and a perfect dresser.

❖ Your partner rarely if ever talks about him- or herself, displaying excessive interest in everything about you. This tactic may be flattering, but it is also unrealistic.

❖ Your partner proceeds rapidly with the relationship emotionally, intellectually, and physically.

❖ You can't pin your partner down on a home or business address.

❖ You learn that your partner has a history of avoiding commitments.

❖ Your partner has no visible means of support and is vague about job and personal resources.

Your best defense against such a partner is a strong offense. Always take care of your personal property yourself; do not be lax or careless with your money or jewelry. Never lend money to a partner whom you have known for only a short period of time and whose history and background have not been definitely revealed. If you decide to invest in your partner's business, work through your lawyer or a business adviser.

Should you be conned, report the crime to the police or the office of the district attorney. Also, immediately report any credit cards that have been stolen. Above all, do not shy away from pursuing the case; your former "lover" will be someone else's Romeo or Juliet tomorrow.

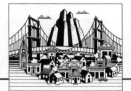

CONSUMER FRAUD, CON-ARTISTS, AND CON-GAMES: A CHECKLIST

1 Get references from friends, relatives, or a consumer service bureau before you contract for service or major purchases. If you decide to use a service, obtain a written estimate first.

2 Retain receipts, warranties, and other related materials in case it becomes necessary to seek replacement, repair, or adjustments of contracted services or merchandise, or to file a complaint.

3 Be especially wary of strangers who approach you on the street with schemes for making quick money.

4 Thoroughly investigate all get-rich-quick schemes before you invest. Don't be tricked by high-pressure salesmanship or a misleading advertisement that threatens you with the notion that the investment will evaporate if you don't act immediately; if a business transaction requires immediate action, pass it up.

5 Never give credit card numbers, or any personal information, over the phone unless you initiated the call and are aware of the business's legitimacy.

6 Advertising can be designed to trick you—watch out!

7 Always read the "fine print." Don't buy on impulse.

8 No purchase is ever necessary in a legitimate sweepstakes.

9 Be wary of mail order or phone sales pitches for schemes that require cash deposits or that require you to call a 1-900 toll charge number to receive the information.

10 Every government worker or repairman should have proper identification and documentation. If they don't, avoid dealing with them.

11 Avoid charity frauds. Donations to well-established and well-known charities are generally the best choice.

12 Make sure the car repair shops you deal with have a current department of motor vehicles registration certificate.

13 Investigate a dating service fully before making a commitment. Rely heavily on recommendations from people you trust.

14 To protect yourself from "charlatan lovers," take care of all your business and property by yourself.

28

INVESTMENT FRAUD AND WHITE-COLLAR CRIME

INVESTORS AT RISK

New-venture underwritings for nonexistent products, diversion of trust funds by attorneys for their personal use, and insider trading in the investment arena are common instances of fraud. Many of them are so infamous that you have undoubtedly already read or heard of them. In one spectacular case, a 23-year-old financial wizard just out of college persuaded experienced investors to give him a total of $10 million for investment in selective stocks. He even sent his clients official-looking statements that resembled those of honest brokerage firms. Instead of investing the money, the young financial "genius" used the funds to purchase two homes, luxury cars, and expensive paintings.

Another case is that of the California man charged with bilking $130 million out of thousands of people investing, they thought, in low-income housing projects through his company, whose slogan was "Good Happens." To add insult to injury, tax shelters were involved, meaning that the investors not only had to face losing their investment, they also had to worry about back taxes they may have owed.

To avoid similar swindles, you must be very careful when you decide to invest your hard-earned cash.

Blue-Sky New Ventures

If it has not happened already, one of these days your phone may ring, followed by a pitch of this kind:

> "Good afternoon, Mr. Wilson. This is Mike Lee of Blue Sky International Securities, Unlimited. Your account representatives at another reputable firm indicated that you are a savvy investor who can spot and act on a great opportunity when you see one. As an established investment firm, we have brought many new ventures public and have made unusually large profits quickly for those privileged to get in on the action before the public offering is completed.
>
> We are currently consummating a deal with what I believe will be our most extraordinary underwriting, a firm called Integrated BioComputerology Services. I don't have to tell you how hot this field is and the overnight fortunes that have been made by outfits like Apple, Compaq, Microsoft, Lotus, and others that started on a shoestring. We are letting a few select clients in on the deal before the public offering is completed the day after tomorrow.
>
> We are inviting special customers like you to participate at our own insider underwriters' and founders' cost of 10 cents per share, and we are even absorbing the customary commission. At the opening, the public's price will be 15 cents, and if this exciting offering goes anything like the many other high-tech firms that we have taken public, the price will quickly rise to 30 cents or more.
>
> I enjoy dealing with astute, seasoned investors like yourself and would like to establish a long-term relationship and prove myself and my firm to you. Let me put you down for just 10,000 shares, a modest commitment of only $1,000. I really want you to have a piece of this action, not simply for the sake of making some important money on this sensational stock but also for what you will come to know as a most rewarding long-term relationship. To beat the opening public-offering prices, you'll have to get a check for $1,000 out to me by tomorrow, preferably by Express Mail. You don't want to take the chance of missing this one!"

Pitches like this come from fast-talking, smooth telephone solicitors in an office crammed with phones and called a boiler room. The first contact that you receive is typically made by a low-paid individual called an "opener." Once you express interest in the pitch by actually committing the $1,000 or requesting more information, you are turned over to a much more accomplished high-pressure sales artist called a "loader." He or she will frequently add to the preliminary pitch some exciting, confidential embellishments that will make the offer seem very plausible and irresistible, and the loader will try to convince you to extend your commitment even further.

You discover too late, after your money is committed, that the entire undertaking was a fraud and that there is little hope of ever recovering your investment. The fact is that under current Securities and Exchange Commission (SEC) regulations, such individuals can solicit by phone without disclosing all the facts in the written offering prospectus. That document need only accompany the first written communication, usually with the order confirmation. Only occasionally does the SEC catch a broker doing a number on a client, whereupon with sufficient evidence, the broker, the firm, or both may be put out of business.

Shell Games

A close relative of the new venture is an existing corporation without any substantial assets—frequently a relatively new business gone sour, as the familiar statistic about 5-year survival rates indicates most new firms do. These nearly bankrupt firms have gone through the significant earlier expenses and delays of SEC registration and underwriting. The essentially dormant company, not yet having taken the formal steps for dissolution, thus becomes a marketable asset in itself, appropriately referred to as a "shell."

Such shells become the basis for many multimillion-dollar swindles in the following way. Stock fraud con-artists acquire the company, apply for a name change through the secretary of state, and then install management figureheads who have no criminal records. The next step after the takeover is to reduce the equity of the shareholders of the original corporation. This is accomplished by declaring a reverse stock split—for example, 1 new share for each 100 original shares.

Using appropriately formulated telephone pitches, like those illustrated earlier, brokers aggressively try to foist the fundamentally worthless stock on unwary investors. With a really good pitch, the investor base may increase geometrically, with the worthless stock continually rising in price. The fraud is completed when the shares held on behalf of the criminal backers are completely liquidated. At this point, the price quickly plummets, leaving the investors holding the worthless stock. Alternatively, the criminal manipulators may manage to pass off the valueless stock in exchange for really valuable assets, or as collateral for a loan.

Numerous scams like this eventually come before the SEC. Although it promptly halts trading in the shell's stock, for most victimized investors the action comes too late to return any of their investments. Most often, the "financial advisers" abscond with the fortune, spend all the money, or end up in prison.

A particularly famous case involved a firm called Texas Uranium Corporation, which, after 3 years of operation, went bellyup. After 10 years of dormancy, the corporation was acquired in 1967 to support a shell con. Texas Uranium was particularly attractive because it still had the legal authority to issue 5 million shares of its stock. After the criminals got control, numerous bogus acquisitions were quickly assigned extremely inflated asset values, amounting to over $5 million, on the shell's balance sheet. As the news spread regarding the quickly rising book value of the company and aggressive acquisitions, the stock price moved sharply higher. By the time the SEC halted trade in 1968, the con-artists had liquidated their shares and amassed a fortune.

The Financial Fortune-Teller

You are at home when you receive a phone call. On the other end is a "Mr. Wingate" who assures you that he doesn't want a cent of your money; only a fool would give money to someone he or she doesn't know, and you're no fool. What he does want to do is give you a taste of his "forecasting abilities" by telling you of a commodity whose value is about to increase dramatically. Sure enough, it increases as promised.

"Mr. Wingate" calls back; still he has no interest in your money. He just wants you to consider his firm the kind of firm you can trust your money with. He gives you a tip that a certain commodity is about to experience a sharp decline. Sure enough, within a short period of time, the commodity's value has decreased.

Who can argue with these results? Certainly not you, so you promise with the third phone call to give "Mr. Wingate" and his "firm" quite a bit of money to invest on your behalf.

What you don't know, as you're helping to make Mr. Wingate a very rich man, is that he originally called 300 people, telling half that the price of that commodity would go up, the other half that the price would go down. When the commodity increased in value, he called the 150 people for whom he'd made the impressive "correct forecast," telling 75 of them that the next commodity's value would decrease, and the other 75 that it would increase.

This means that no matter what, he had 75 people impressed with his unerring accuracy ready to invest. It also means that he had 75 people willing to give a person—whose "forecasting ability" consisted of a phone and a newspaper—enough money so that it was worth his while to work on another 300 people.

Fast-Buck Commodities Futures

Not just the well-heeled but increasing numbers of amateurs are being lured into commodity futures trading. The attraction of these contracts for the future delivery of exciting commodities like gold, silver, platinum, and the like is that they are highly leveraged. Relatively few investment dollars can control sizable sums. By their very nature, futures exercise an almost irresistible appeal to the greedy, get-rich-quick investor. The problem is that unbeknownst to the average investor or novice in this medium, futures trading is a real sucker's bet, with the likelihood of turning a profit well below 10 percent.

As in the earlier examples of securities fraud, commodities fraud is frequently perpetuated by slick, savvy, professional-sounding operators in boiler rooms temporarily located at prestigious Wall Street addresses, or the equivalent at other financial centers. Therein lies part of the danger to the investor: Legitimate commodity futures brokers also operate by phone and have similar addresses. Among other advantages enjoyed by these con-artists is the typically limited grasp of the inexperienced investor in this financial arena. Also balancing the scales in favor of fraud is the complex array of factors that dictate the future price of the commodity underlying the contract. Thus, it is possible to play on the investor's ignorance by identifying a couple of well-known recent events that common sense suggests should make the future price of the commodity worth gambling on.

Of course, the words *gamble* and *risk* never arise in the salesperson's pitch; rather the solicitor will practically guarantee immense profits. As in the earlier scams, things move very quickly. Lest the hot opportunity be lost, the con-artist urges the investor to have bank funds wired to the fly-by-night brokerage firm, with the usual promise that informational literature will be immediately forthcoming. The scam centers on the fact that a genuine futures contract, like those regulated by the Chicago Board of Trade, is not what the investor will be getting. Instead, the investor will receive—if anything at all—an *option* on the touted commodity, that is, a so-called deferred-delivery contract. Unfortunately for the investor, such contracts were banned in 1978 and no longer exist in U.S. futures markets.

PYRAMID SCHEMES, PONZI FRAUDS

Other painful variants on commodities futures fraud also exist. Through a pyramiding scheme or so-called Ponzi fraud, investors may be beguiled by quick profits on some initial trades into committing further hard-earned capital (and spreading the word of their success to friends). The con-artists who set up these Ponzi frauds (named for Charles Ponzi, the organizer, in 1919, of the first such scheme in the U.S.) are, in effect, operating a "bucket shop" in which they invested funds of initial speculators. Some investors are used to pay off others, to set them up for much bigger kills.

Another approach is that employed by some fully licensed but dishonest brokers, in which buy orders are intentionally not executed. If the commodity price then falls, the faked loss is posted to the investor's account, and the broker pockets it. Should the price rise, the broker declares that a clerical error resulted in the order not being processed.

Finally, a consortium of investors can operate over a period of time to manipulate certain future prices, but this takes a level of sophistication and cooperation between brokers and traders that goes well beyond the two simpler schemes just described. As with insider trading, however, the wary investor should never dismiss the possibility.

Almost anyone may be the victim of a Ponzi scheme or hear an irresistibly enticing investment offer pitched by phone from a boiler room operation. Perhaps the phone pitch will even be followed by a written prospectus with pronouncements and disclaimers. By the time you recognize the realities of your investment, the horses will have bolted the barn, leaving you with a significant void in your pocketbook. The account agreement that you long ago signed but barely read—the one with the pro forma, finely printed clause buried on the back, indicating that you would not sue your broker but instead subject all claims to an arbitration board dominated by the investment community—may have left you with little effective recourse.

Land Frauds

Frauds come in many varieties, but perhaps the most enduring of all are land frauds. The United States is a great agrarian nation, and we are conscious of the land. It is no wonder that we have this great attraction to land, nor is it any wonder that the frauds and sharpies gravitate to land-based enterprises.

One typical fraudulent operation offered coal-mining rights on land in a southern state. Promoters had promised as much as 3,000 tons of coal on each of the lots sold. In reality, there was no coal in the field. Part of the success of the operation was due to the efforts of a shill. This person was introduced to potential investors as a satisfied customer who was pleased with his investment and impressed with the reputable management of the operation. Mining rights were sold throughout the United States and overseas. This scam netted the organizers upwards of $3 million.

An almost identical swindle involved supposed coal fields in another southern state. This entrepreneur operated on a grander scale, raking in more than $10 million. The presiding judge termed this the largest fraud he had seen during his tenure on the bench. On a charge of racketeering, the defendant was sentenced to 12 years of a possible 20-year maximum.

THREATS AND COUNTERMEASURES: SOME RULES

As you can see, there are numerous threats and pitfalls to your investment security. The deceptive practices of some investment dealers and brokers, as well as the outright fraud of the criminal, are relatively easy to conceal, because even legitimate investments are complex and relatively uncertain. The already ripe context is enriched by the inherent avarice of the prey. Most investors prefer getting much richer to a little richer, and most prefer it much sooner to a little later. Accordingly, the scams are legion, and not merely a feature of recent history.

And contrary to what most believe, the regulatory agencies—such as the Securities and Exchange Commission, the Federal Deposit Insurance Corporation, and the various states attorneys general and consumer fraud agencies—cannot protect you and your investment. These agencies primarily serve to make sure that full and accurate disclosure of all the relevant investment information is publicly available. They cannot protect you against devious financial schemes; they cannot tell you what is likely to be sound or unsound investment; and even when you've actually been criminally victimized, they can only help after the fact and generally in a way that attempts to enhance as a whole the future fairness of the investment markets to which we are all exposed. For you in particular, this is hardly solace—your money is gone.

Some investors are not deterred from undue risk by even the severe disclaimers of the Securities and Exchange Commission:

> These securities have not been approved or disapproved by the Securities and Exchange Commission nor has the SEC passed upon the accuracy or adequacy of this prospectus—any representation to the contrary is a criminal offense. These securities are highly speculative, involve immediate substantial dilution, a high degree of risk, and should be purchased only by persons who can afford to lose their entire investments.

What is remarkable is that in the face of powerful warnings and such powerful regulatory agencies as the SEC, significant numbers of investors regularly lose large sums through frauds that would make the typical robbery or burglary pale by comparison. And embarrassment, plus the threat of countersuits, will probably dissuade them from becoming a statistic in the complaint records of the criminal courts, regulatory agencies, or consumer protection agencies.

AVOIDING PITFALLS

To reduce appreciably your likelihood of falling prey to investment fraud or deception, you need guidelines on investment security, guidelines that will discipline you to be more prudent and cautious. Do not, on the other hand, be so restrained that you become paranoid and miss important, legitimate opportunities to enhance your future net worth through astute, carefully considered investments.

What you should remember is what you already knew before the "blue sky" and greed took hold: If it looks too good to be true, it most probably is! The markets are ordinarily too large and efficient to allow financial bargains to be anything but highly adventitious and transitory—in short, you usually get what you pay for!

As in life itself, risk inheres in any investment. But a strategy that diversifies by institution, by investment type, by issuer within these financial alternatives, and by commitment over time (rather than as lump sums) should go far in significantly reducing your chances of losing your investment nest egg.

In addition to these general protective rules, you should remember two more: If the investment yield is inconsistent with the general market for that investment risk, then someone probably is misrepresenting the facts. Centuries of lending experience, through wide variations in interest rates and prevailing inflation, have taught us that people can expect about 3- to 4-percent real annualized return on their investment after taxes and inflation; anything more than that should alert you to undisclosed risks.

One final note: Unfortunately, when money is involved, no one seemingly can be trusted. Just because a person is a friend or a relative doesn't mean that he or she can be totally trusted.

A FAIR WARNING

The scams that have been perpetrated on the unwary investor are seemingly without bound. The criminal's inventiveness has produced investment frauds that could fill volumes and keep TV series like *60 Minutes* running forever. Every year, FBI statistics on reported crime reveal that no one is too rich or poor, sophisticated or uneducated, old or young to escape the clever and persistent con. This truth prevails whether the con-artist involves stocks, new business ventures, commodities or land fraud, bogus franchises, invention "marketing," talent "promotion," dead-end "work at home for profit" schemes, religious/medical/charity frauds, and so on.

It is not easy to spot swindlers. They come in all shapes and sizes, from all walks of life. Many swindlers mimic the operations of legitimate firms to the point that, on a cursory glance, it would be practically impossible to spot swindlers. They use any and all means to convince you to buy into their schemes. The reason anybody offering a proposal, legitimate or not, uses a high-pressure tactic is because it often works; you have to condition yourself to step back and say "Wait a minute."

A swindler talks fast and asks questions to keep *you* from asking them. The National Futures Association has prepared a list of questions that will faze a swindler (and that anybody reputable would be willing to answer). The questions include: "Where did you get my name?" "What risks are involved?" "Can you send me a written explanation of your investment proposal?" "Would you mind explaining your proposal to a third party, such as an investment counselor or my attorney?" "Where, exactly, will my money be, and what kind of accounting statements will you provide me?" "Are the investments you offer traded on a regulated exchange?" (Not all legitimate investments are traded there, but no fraudulent proposals *ever are*). If the answers to these and other questions you may have (and ask a lot of them) are vague or unsatisfying, look for other avenues for investment. If you still aren't sure, check with the local police department or Better Business Bureau to see if there are any complaints on file concerning the individual or firm; keep checking, even if it means tracking the individual out-of-state. Your money is too important for you not to be diligent about who is going to invest it. Remember, no investment is risk-free, but you can minimize the risk.

"VICTIMLESS" CRIMES THAT AFFECT EVERYONE

Even if you don't become a direct victim of investment fraud (perhaps you don't even invest), you are still a victim of the widespread problem known as "white-collar crime" that has undermined the very fabric of our society. While rightfully concerned with crime on our streets and in our homes, society often turns a blind eye toward corporate crime, crime that we often think of as "victimless." Because our grandchildren will be in debt as a result of the greed and treachery involved in the savings and loan scandals of the 1980s, we should now maybe take a closer look at the statistics: According to the U.S. Chamber of Commerce, the yearly cost of white-collar crime exceeds the losses sustained by "common" burglary and robbery by several *billion* dollars.

White-collar crime can affect you in more personal ways as well. An example is the accountant who persuaded fellow tenants to go on a rent strike in a luxury apartment building in New York City. He was supposed to open an escrow account with $1.7 million dollars of unpaid rent money. He never did, and instead used the money to open personal accounts and to pay off gambling debts. As voters and taxpayers, we should pay closer attention to the big corporate business dealings and crimes that may not result in sensational headlines. It seems that the larger the amounts of money involved in such crimes, the less likely we are to pay much heed to them. White-collar crime affects everyone, from the businessman to the pool cleaner.

RESOURCES FOR REDRESS

Should fortune not continually shine, and should you believe that fraud has befallen you, you may wish to seek redress through some of the following agencies or their counterparts in your state:

U.S. Securities and Exchange Commission
450 Fifth Street, N.W.
Washington, DC 20549
(800) 942-7040

Federal Trade Commission
6th Street & Pennsylvania Avenue, N.W.
Washington, DC, 20580
(202) 326-2222

Commodity Futures Trading Commission
1155 21st Street, N.W.
Washington, DC 20581
(202) 418-5000

Federal Bureau of Investigation
Justice Department
Pennsylvania Avenue
Washington, DC 20535
(202) 324-3000

Housing and Urban Development Department
Interstate Land Sales Registration
HUD Building
451 7th Street, S.W.
Washington, DC 20410
(202) 708-0502

National Futures Association
200 W. Madison, Suite 1600
Chicago, IL 60606-3447
Toll Free (800) 621-3570
[in IL (800) 572-9400]

Although it is impossible to construct an exhaustive set of guidelines that will anticipate every possible investment risk, the examples and safeguards described in this chapter and the following checklist should serve to reduce your vulnerability to many threats posed by fraud.

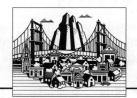

INVESTMENT FRAUD AND
WHITE-COLLAR CRIME: A CHECKLIST

1 If an investment sounds too good, it likely is; do some research before committing your dollars.

2 Never commit funds based on a "cold call" from an unknown broker or brokerage; it may well be a boiler room operation.

3 Beware of the deal that requires a quick response on your part.

4 Be skeptical of securities offered at substantial discounts from the prevailing market investment of comparable type.

5 Be alert to transactions that involve secretive foreign aspects such as off-shore financial institutions.

6 Watch out for unusual delays by brokers in making delivery of your securities or your investment proceeds; you may be caught in a "bucket shop" operation or in the misappropriation of your assets.

7 Be suspicious if transaction confirmations do not arrive promptly.

8 Keep an eye out for evidence of excessive buying and selling by your broker; periodically check through your trades of the past couple of years.

9 Buying and selling should be based on sound reasoning, not the whim of the broker.

10 Seek out good professional investment advice. A good broker is a valuable resource. To find one, ask for a referral from someone you trust who is also experienced in investments.

11 Always check the financial soundness of the issuer of fixed-yield investments in Standard & Poor's, Moody's, or similar agencies, whether the issuer or instrument is a bank or S&L CD, municipal or corporate bond, or other investment.

12 If the net real return (the rate of return minus inflation rate) from a fixed-yield investment is over 3 to 4 percent, examine the investment very carefully before taking the plunge.

13 When buying stocks, determine whether your account representative is a broker or broker-dealer; the latter buy and sell for their own accounts and therefore have a vested interest that may seriously bias the advice you are getting.

14 When first opening an account, obtain the firm's recent financial statements, and be cautious of doing business with those having net capitalization of under $1 million.

---

15 In regard to new accounts at unknown firms, always request evidence that both the firm and the broker are licensed. Inquire about the number of years in business, as well as the experience of the broker and/or lesser-known firms. Get bank references, and check with regulatory agencies.

16 If the brokerage also has an investment banking division, find out the firm's policy about recommending stocks when there is potential for conflicts of interest. Inquire not only about the institution's underwritings but also about senior partners who may serve on the boards of various companies having publicly traded stock.

17 Although deposits in banks and S&Ls are insured by the FDIC and FSLIC, it is wise to obtain a copy of the institution's recent balance sheets, since the government auditor's roster of "problem banks" is not readily available. Certainly, split any joint accounts over $100,000 into separate ones if at the same bank.

18 In regard to "penny stocks" of new ventures, insist on seeing the written prospectus, no matter how sweet the deal seems or the sense of urgency that you are given.

19 Always ask the broker how many shares of penny stocks are outstanding, how many employees the company has, and the company's record of profitability, if any.

20 When you receive the prospectus, look to see if a substantial portion of the underwriting will be siphoned off to pay expenses accrued by the promoters/principals before going public, to pay excessive salaries and the like. Look at the intended use of the funds and the associated planning horizon to see if additional offerings or debt instruments need to be floated soon.

21 Examine not only salaries but also the compensation in the form of stock to be given to officers.

22 Scrutinize the experience of the officers, directors, and promoters; determine their track record in similar deals and in comparable markets. Invest only with well-established investment managers with proven long-term track records.

23 If not in the prospectus, any especially alluring claims about the deal should be backed up in writing by the underwriter/broker. Look not only for what is said but also for what is not said.

24 In new, diversified investment trusts, watch out for the possible unloading into the trust portfolio of one or more "dogs" previously held by the trust organizers; again, obtain and evaluate the prospectus first.

25 Remember that no matter how sophisticated the offering and associated financial jargon may sound, any nitwit or criminal with enough perseverance can float a public corporation.

26 Remember that in most states, anyone, including a charlatan, can call him- or herself a financial adviser (with or without a newsletter), since few states have licensing procedures like those for stockbrokers, real estate brokers, tax attorneys, CPAs, and the like. Whether you deal with a licensed or an unlicensed individual, be hard-nosed, and base your investment decisions on recent historical results, not simply reputation.

27 To reduce risk, use an investment strategy that diversifies by institution, by investment type, by issuer within these financial alternatives, and by commitment over time, rather than just by lump sums.

28 Remember that the key role of agencies like the SEC and Federal Reserve Board is to try to minimize flagrant abuses in their respective jurisdictions. They cannot prevent you from being imprudent or criminally victimized. Their concerns are strongly biased in favor of strengthening the public's confidence in the investment markets and banking system.

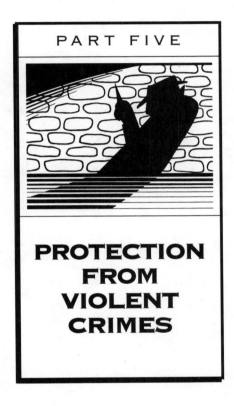

PART FIVE

PROTECTION FROM VIOLENT CRIMES

29

DEFENSES
AGAINST RAPE

Rape is a not a sex crime, but a crime of violence that includes dominating and imposing power or will over the victim. Victims of this crime are primarily women. It is a crime greatly misunderstood by most people, men and women alike. More than any other type of crime, the physical and psychological effects of rape tend to be long lasting. Rape carries with it the immediate physical dangers of being beaten, injured, or killed, as well as the possibility of pregnancy or sexually transmitted diseases, including AIDS. The victim is also subjected to psychological stress and trauma that may last a lifetime. The rape victim often feels humiliated and ostracized. These consequences are compounded by prevailing community attitudes toward rape.

Rape is a crime that affects everyone. No man, woman, or child is exempt from being a victim. In the United States a rape occurs every 7 minutes, and 80 percent of victims know their rapist.

Attitudes toward rape vary greatly. Men have a considerably different view of rape than women. Typical comments—easily identifiable by gender—range from "A woman can run faster with her dress up than a man can with his pants down" to "Castration should be a mandatory penalty for any rape conviction."

Forcible rape is defined as "to carnally know and ravish a person against his or her will." Statutory rape consists of an adult having sexual relations with a person under a legal age of consent (16 in most jurisdictions), even with his or her consent.

MYTHS ABOUT RAPE

Perhaps it is necessary to clear up some misconceptions about rape.

Myth: Rape is an interracial crime.
Reality: In a study conducted in the District of Columbia, the victim and the assailant were of the same race in 7 out of every 8 assaults. A similar study in Philadelphia indicated that 9 of 10 rapes involved two people of the same race. A report in Memphis revealed that 5 of 6 rapes involved people of the same race.

Myth: Men are rarely the victims of rape.
Reality: Researchers estimate that about 10 percent of sexual assaults involve male victims and female assailants. This figure is conservative, because men are especially reluctant, fearful, and embarrassed to report that they have been victimized by rape. A smaller percentage of assaults are committed by women on women, or men on men.

Myth: The major motive for rape is sexual.
Reality: The major motive for rape is power, not sex. Rape is a crime of violence; sex is merely a weapon.

Myth: A healthy woman can avoid being raped.
Reality: Studies show that the rapist uses psychological tactics. Fear is a major weapon. Threat of injury or death easily immobilizes the woman, and she is terrorized into cooperation.

Myth: Rape will never happen to a decent woman.
Reality: A woman does not control whether or not she will be raped. The rapist does. Rape victims are of all ages, social strata, ethnic backgrounds, and appearances.

Myth: The majority of rape attacks are inflicted by strangers in back alleys.
Reality: Researchers estimate that about one-half to nearly 90 percent of the rapists are friends, family members, acquaintances, or social companions of the victim and that about one-third of all rapes occur in the victim's home.

Myth: Virtually all rapes take place after dark. You need not be especially aware or alert during daylight hours.
Reality: Over a third of all rape assaults occur during the day.

Myth: You can almost always tell a sexual offender by his looks.
Reality: Sex offenders display varied personal characteristics, ethnic roots, and appearances. An assailant may be married or single, a friend, relative, or stranger. He may be a school dropout or highly educated. Many

sex offenders are wholesome and good-looking, which allows them to establish rapport with the victim.

Myth: Most rapists attack once but desist from further sexual assault.
Reality: The majority of rapists continue their sexual assaults until they are caught.

PROTECTION OF TEENAGE GIRLS FROM RAPE

The most frequent rape is the assault of a school-aged female by a man of the same race. The assailant is alone, has no weapon, and is probably known to the victim, at least by sight. Perhaps this tells us that the typical rape victim is a little too young, a little too trusting, and a little too inexperienced to take proper safeguards. Obviously, then, we should start our protection with the school-aged females in your home.

Parents should always know where their children are, what they're doing, and with whom. This could be very important in protecting a teenage girl from sexual assault. The following guidelines are also important:

❖ A teenage girl should never entertain her male friends at home without supervision, and early in life she should have learned the importance of not admitting strangers into the home.

❖ She must be taught that there is safety in numbers, but with the caveat that she is safest in the company of other girls. Studies indicate that from 10 to 43 percent of all rapes are gang rapes.

❖ She should be home by the time that most people in the community are asleep.

❖ She should exercise particular caution when she is home alone during the daylight hours, such as after school. She should take special care to see that after-school activities avoid one-to-one relationships or a situation in which she might be the only female in a group.

❖ She should exercise extreme caution in accepting dates. Getting picked up by a stranger is ill advised at the very best. Parents should *always* insist on meeting the dates of schoolgirls living at home.

IF YOU ARE ATTACKED

Since self-protective measures help in the majority of attacks, to whatever extent you are temperamentally and emotionally capable, you should be prepared to defend yourself physically. If you are not serious about, or simply not capable of, inflicting pain or physical harm on your assailant, you shouldn't attempt it. If you are determined to defend yourself, you should remember that your best defense is escape. Remember that legs are to run with and voices are to scream with. High-heeled shoes can be used to kick at an assailant. His natural reaction will be to duck, and his being off balance may give the victim the chance to run.

The best time to make a break for it is as early during the assault as possible. Authorities suggest that the optimum moment to react is during the first 20 seconds. The attacker won't expect an escape then. Also, the less time you are under the control of the rapist, the less likely you are to be hurt or intimidated. Moreover, your chances of escape are better before the rapist gains total control and before he has the chance to throw you to the ground or force you to a secluded spot. The longer you submit passively to his demands, the less likely you are to react later on. Fear of antagonizing your assailant will worsen, and overcoming inertia will become more difficult in time.

Scream as you run, and in case your voice fails you, keep a whistle strapped to your wrist. It will make noise when your voice might not. Some people have suggested that screaming "Fire!" rather than "Help!" might bring assistance more quickly. Yelling will also distract the rapist and alert others to the danger. A powerful, energized, firm, loud scream sends a signal to the assailant that he likely picked the wrong target. Hysterics are not recommended, because this may panic the assailant and will surely communicate to him your fear and vulnerability.

If you are trapped and have little chance of escape, should you fight or not? A woman will tell you to fight; a man will tell you not to. If you do fight, statistics indicate that you *will* be attacked physically—and have your arm twisted or suffer a brutal beating. The best policy is never to fight an assailant armed with a knife or gun, but if his only weapon is superior strength, your chance of avoiding being raped by resisting is probably worth taking. But only you can decide whether and how to resist a rape attack, and since every situation is different, no one can second-guess you. Here are some useful facts that can help you make the decision.

The National Crime Victimization Survey, covering the last 20 years in which statistics were available (1973 to 1992), reported that in 8 of 10 rape attacks, women took measures to protect themselves. Nearly 1 in 4 victims of violent assault physically resisted or captured the offender, 16 percent ran away or hid, 11.5 percent attacked the offender without a weapon, 1.5 percent attacked with a weapon, and the remaining women screamed, threatened, or used another means of self-defense. Victims reported that self-protective measures were helpful in 60 percent of the victimizations, harmful in 7 percent, and didn't make a difference in 11 percent. In 6 percent of the assaults, resistance both helped and hurt, meaning that the offender became more angry and aggressive, but nevertheless an injury or greater injury was avoided. Women fight back in a violent attack in the same proportions as men.

A recent study by Brandeis University of 274 female victims of violent assault found that women who defended themselves were less likely to be injured than those who pleaded with the attacker or who offered no resistance. An earlier study covering a shorter period (1973 to 1987) reported that those who resisted were less likely to be raped than nonresisters. But victims who protected themselves were more likely to be injured (58 percent) than nonresisters (46 percent). If an attacker points a gun at you and orders you into a car and you run, 98 percent of the time he will not shoot. But if you get into the car, your chances of surviving are only 2 in 100.

Should others come to the aid of the victim during a rape attack? In 45 percent of the assaults, measures taken by others were helpful, and in 33 percent they neither helped nor hurt the situation. In only 1 of 10 rapes where others attempted to help did these actions hurt the victim. In most cases, aid made the offender more aggressive and angry, but overall action was more helpful than passivity.

In general, a rape victim *must* resist her attacker. Lacking this, there may be charges of consenting sexual intercourse. However, the resistance need not be physical. To say, "I don't want to do that. Please don't make me do that," clearly establishes resistance. There is, however, the distinct possibility that your attacker will contradict this in court. If, on the other hand, you physically attack your assailant, leaving cuts and contusions on him, you have gone far in establishing your resistance. Of course, this type of action risks retaliation in kind.

You may be able to change the rapist's intentions. He may be reluctant to have sexual contact with you if he believes you have a sexually transmitted disease. You may be able to persuade the rapist that you want to have a sexual relationship with him, but in a more comfortable setting. Pretend to invite him to your place, with the intention of escaping or summoning assistance. Try to make yourself unattractive by telling him you are at the peak of your menstrual period or you have stomach cramps. This may distract the assailant or perhaps cause him to loosen his grip. Some women have vomited or relieved themselves to ward off a persistent assailant, and others have been successful by feigning mental retardation.

Defensive Weapons and Tactics

If you have a weapon, you may even swing the odds in your favor. We have already suggested avoiding weapons such as handguns, knives, tear gas, or Mace. Concealing such a weapon could be a violation of the law, and it might also be taken from you and used against you.

Nevertheless, other items that pose little chance of being classified as concealed weapons might be even more effective, because they can be hand carried or hidden in a coat pocket rather than in a handbag. These include hatpins, a pen or pencil, a corkscrew, pepper, lemon juice in a squeeze bottle, or even a ring clenched in the fist with keys protruding between the fingers, all of which can be used against the attacker's eyes. An umbrella can be a good weapon if used like a spear or sword rather than a club.

However, you should be warned: Many men have had some boxing or other self-defense training, and your assailant may be able to parry your thrust and block your swings. Even so, his reversal from offensive to defensive tactics may give you a chance to flee, and, if you're lucky, you'll at least discourage him from his initial objective. But remember, if you do attack, be prepared to keep it up.

Some authorities will tell you to attack the assailant in the groin area. While this is his most vulnerable spot, he is also likely to protect this area, both through instinct and from a lifetime of training. Instead, go for the pit of the stomach, the throat, the eyes, the temples, or even the kneecap. Other vulnerable and easily accessible parts of the body include the kidneys, solar plexus, pinkie finger, nose, and ears. However, if the rapist should make an embracing type of attack from the front, then a knee to the groin might be effective. Or grab his scrotum in the groin area with both hands, squeeze, twist, and drop to the ground so the full weight of your body is on the scrotum. This technique should disable the attacker.

Some experts recommend a well-placed, closed-fisted thrust aimed at the trachea or Adam's apple, while at the same time using your other hand to yank the rapist's head forward. Correct implementation of this technique is highly likely to disable the assailant. Or cup your hands and with all your force, in one continuous sweeping motion, strike your assailant's ears, and then forcefully press both thumbs into his eyes. This tactic is particularly useful when the rapist is facing you and pressing you toward him.

If you are grabbed from the rear, an elbow to the stomach can be effective in getting you free. Stomping on the attacker's foot, especially with high-heeled shoes, can easily break his foot. Try to hit about halfway between the ankle and the shoes. The pain of this might well discourage any further attack. Even if it doesn't, it might make it easier for you to break free and run. Other aggressive actions include eye gouging, biting, scratching, and kicking. Additional natural weapons include your head, heel, or palm of your hand, thumbs, hips, and forearms. The rapist will usually try to throw you to the ground. Once you are on the ground, your chances of defense are lessened *but not hopeless*. For the best chance of defending yourself, take a self-defense course that is geared to help women defend themselves from such threatening situations.

If, however, you are trapped and so threatened that you cannot escape, you may still be able to avoid attack by doing nothing more than crying, which shouldn't be too difficult under the circumstances. Psychological studies show no particular variations in personality among rapists compared with nonrapists, so there is a chance you can sob your way out of an attack. You might also try to establish some sort of conversation.

Even if you can't talk your way out of rape, you may be able to lessen the physical, verbal, or emotional abuse that might be loosed upon you. One theory concerning a rapist's motivation is that he has not achieved as much in life as he thinks he should. By building up his ego—his feelings of self-importance—you may give him the gratification he seeks and might, prevent him from taking further gratification at your expense.

Your assailant may force you to submit to perverse or humiliating acts, such as oral or anal intercourse. Even after achieving sexual climax, he may continue to force his will upon you. His intention is not sensual pleasure of the sex act but the emotional high of a seriously psychotic individual experiencing total dominance and control over another person. Many rapists would not hesitate to beat, maim, or even murder. A rapist might welcome resistance as a challenge to his right of mastery and increase the fury of his attack. Whatever happens, one thing you can expect is to feel humiliated.

There could be circumstances, moreover, which may make it impossible for you to resist. If, for example, he threatens not you but your child, you may feel that there is no alternative but to accede to his demands. No matter what we, or anyone, may advise you, the decisions you make when face to face with an attacker must be yours, and must be based on circumstances as you see them at the time. Your body will release chemicals in the bloodstream that will help you fight, run, or outsmart. Once the incident is over, and you meditate on what you did and how you might have done otherwise, remember that your actions were dictated by your body as well as your mind, and if you had to do it all over again, it would probably have turned out the same way.

Aftermath: Feelings of Rape Victims

Unlike the victims of most other crimes, the rape victim will experience lingering emotional effects. Here is how a study sponsored by the U.S. Department of Justice described these feelings:

❖ *Fear.* During a rape, victims believe that, in addition to the sexual assault, they are going to be brutally beaten or even murdered. Often the rapist threatens to assault again if the victim goes to the police or threatens to expose the assailant's identity.

❖ *Guilt.* Many women feel guilt after being raped, because they somehow believe they are to blame for having been raped. This feeling of guilt often prevents a rape victim from reporting the crime to the police.

❖ *Loss of control.* Rape victims often feel loss of control over their own lives because they were forced to submit to an act they consider abhorrent. They may reason that "just as the rapist overcame my resistance by force, anyone can persuade me to do anything." It becomes difficult for the victim to make decisions about simple matters.

❖ *Embarrassment.* Rape victims are often embarrassed to discuss the physical and psychological details of the assault. If children are taught that their bodies and sexuality are private matters, they may be reluctant to discuss the assault with medical or law enforcement personnel. Embarrassment is especially prevalent among males who are victims of rape.

❖ *Anger.* A healthier and more appropriate response is anger. The victim has been attacked, demeaned, and humiliated. She may express anger by telling other women about the attack or pressing charges. She may also generalize and extend her anger and mistrust to all men.

❖ *Sense of inferiority.* Victims may wonder why the rapist chose them. These feelings are related to the widespread, but false, belief that those who are raped "asked for it."

These feelings greatly intensify, according to some experts, when the victim is very young or elderly. The naive youngster may not know that rape exists, while the mature woman may have felt that, because of her age, she would not be a likely victim. In either event, the experience could easily prove emotionally disabling, even fatal.

The Rape Trauma Syndrome

The overall effects of rape are now known to be ongoing and long lasting. Every rape victim suffers a clearly defined set of anomalies known as the rape trauma syndrome. The initial stage of the syndrome is characterized by disorganization, often accompanied by anxiety, depression, physical pain, nausea, insomnia, self-doubts, and feelings of guilt.

As this period of self-recrimination abates (usually in no more than a few months' time), it is replaced by what is termed a reorganization period. This is a longer-term disorder, frequently a year or more in duration. In this stage, a victim will undergo changes in habits. Usually these are the result of fear, stemming from the previous attack. Victims may change jobs, retire, or otherwise alter behavior patterns.

It is important that these changes of behavior be recognized for what they are—normal. A victim may, in time, completely overcome the disorder. Proper counseling, of course, is a valuable means for speeding this recovery. Many courts, however, do not currently recognize rape trauma syndrome.

The Decision to Report a Rape

Once a rape is over, only you can decide whether to report it. But failure to prosecute encourages the rapist to try again. There are many reasons a victim may not wish to report a rape, most of which deal with a perception of the attack as a private or personal matter and the reactions of loved ones and friends. One victim failed to report because she believed there was not sufficient proof to convince the police or convict the rapist. Many other victims decline to prosecute, preferring not to be forced to relive the incident throughout what could be a long and perhaps extremely visible trial. Nevertheless, cooperation with the police would probably unearth information that would help solve other rapes.

If you are attacked and you notify the police, your attacker may be punished. You may also protect yourself and other women from future attacks by the same assailant. The police will take you to qualified medical assistance at a facility with experience in treating the types of physical and emotional trauma that you are suffering.

Should you choose to delay immediate treatment, perhaps to locate a friend, physician, or relative whose presence would be comforting, get assistance nevertheless. Call a hospital emergency facility or, ideally, a rape crisis counseling service.

Regardless of how soiled you might feel, don't bathe, douche, or change clothes right after the incident. You may be destroying the evidence necessary for conviction. Your garments, whether torn or not, will probably be required for evidence, so take a change of clothes when you go to seek treatment.

At the hospital, a twofold procedure will be initiated. First, you will receive emergency medical treatment, and second, evidence that could assist in identifying your attacker will be gathered. Afterward, you can have the bath and the rest you need. Then try to resume your normal routine as quickly as possible.

You will probably be spending some time with physicians after the ordeal. There is "morning-after" medication that is somewhat effective in preventing pregnancy. However, its side effects may put you to bed for several days, and the drug itself may be carcinogenic. Also, the availability of other new drugs such as RU 486 could offer further alternatives for rape victims.

You should have an examination for sexually transmitted diseases. Gonorrhea will usually require two examinations, for it is not easily identified in a female, and additional examinations may be ordered by the physician. The test for acquired immune deficiency syndrome (AIDS) likewise will be given many months down the road; at least one follow-up may be ordered. Also, have a comprehensive urogenital examination and, if necessary, psychiatric counseling.

Rape victims often cannot clearly see the attacker, as dark, isolated locations tend to ensure his freedom from interruption. Anything you can remember about his appearance and mannerisms may help to identify him, even if he was masked at the time of the attack. The rape victim should also try to remember everything that occurred and was said. Write down or tape-record these details while the incident is fresh in your mind. In time, your memory will, mercifully, blank out some of the more traumatic incidents, but don't wish for this memory lapse until after you've given your testimony.

Throughout the ordeal following your attack, and perhaps beginning in the emergency room, you may expect contact with the police. Sometimes some police officers (particularly males) may express skepticism. Perhaps this attitude is chauvinistic, perhaps it is an investigatory technique. Regardless of what triggers it, disbelief is something you may encounter. Don't be surprised if your friends (especially the fair-weather variety) derive smug satisfaction from your misfortune. It feeds their unwarranted feelings of superiority.

You may have submitted to the demands of the rapist. This does not mean that you secretly wanted sex; it only means that you didn't or couldn't actively resist the attack. Fear of injury to oneself or to another does not signify consent, nor is it any reason for qualms of guilt. You have committed no crime; your attacker did. Take comfort in the fact that one of four rape victims suffers no disorder from her ordeal.

On the other hand, the majority suffer depression and, to some extent, psychological problems (fear, anxiety, social censure, and sexual dysfunction). It is not unusual for these disorders to exist for a year or even longer. So severe is the emotional trauma of rape victims that they exhibit substantially greater–than–average rates of suicide.

Rape Crisis Centers

Many rape victims are eased through the labyrinth of their ordeals through the excellent assistance of a rape crisis center. If there is a rape crisis center hotline in your community, by all means utilize it. If you don't know about such a service, ask the police or the telephone operator. Typically, these centers perform a variety of essential services. A 24–hour hotline, with a trained counselor, is often available for advice.

You can expect to be referred to community agencies that provide rape victims with assistance. A trained escort-counselor will accompany you through the medical investigation and the various complicated stages of the criminal justice process, including the police investigation, the prosecutor's office, preparation for trial, and all the court proceedings. A taped interview with law enforcement officials will probably be prepared, and this can be replayed to spare you from having to repeat and relive your experience. The rape crisis center also provides in-service training for medical and criminal justice personnel who interact with rape victims. It also provides classes, conferences, literature, audiovisual aids, and speakers to increase community awareness of sex crimes.

Each counselor is trained to understand your physical and mental state, and he or she can assist you in breaking the news to members of your family. Your counselor will offer you calm, reassuring, and unwavering support to help you maintain, or regain, your dignity, self-respect, and self-confidence. After all, the rape incident must not be allowed to dominate your life.

A Day in Court

With any luck, a suspect will be apprehended. Identifying him will be the start of your postrape ordeal. You will be called on to provide information to the prosecuting attorney's office and to testify against your assailant, perhaps before a jury. Whether the arrest of a rapist results in his being brought to trial depends on the quality of the evidence against him. With good evidence, a prosecutor can expect a guilty plea. Otherwise, he will probably take the case to trial. Lesser-quality evidence will increase the probability of a plea-bargained sentence; even-poorer evidence will probably force the prosecutor to drop the case.

It is important to realize that the decision to drop a case against a suspect in no way reflects on the rape victim or her veracity. It is merely the prosecutor's assessment of the available evidence. A reasonable evaluation of the facts surrounding some rapes may lead to the conclusion that the rapes lack the quality of evidence needed to ensure indictment. After all, a rape is most often a craven and furtive act, not a public spectacle with on-lookers who could corroborate testimony.

If you go to trial, you may find that the judge, prosecutor, and opposing attorney (and perhaps the jury as well) are predominantly male. This imbalance may work to your disadvantage, particularly if your appearance and demeanor are not those of "the girl next door." If there were no witnesses to a rape, and there are no visible injuries—and this is usually the case—there may be no way to prove your allegations. In this event, your day in court could turn into a personality contest. Justice might depend on one's appearance or demeanor, or on the preconceived notions of judge and jurors.

The defendant is protected by the law to the extent that past crimes for which he has been charged will not be admissible as evidence against him, except under unusual circumstances. You may not be as well protected, for you have committed no crime. The defendant does not have to reveal matters that might incriminate him. On the other hand, you may be questioned, at least in a few jurisdictions, about your sexual activities. Fortunately, there is a trend toward enactment of laws that exclude the victim's private life from the trial record.

The defense attorney has three primary weapons to gain freedom for his or her client: (1) There was no sexual assault; (2) you have mistakenly identified the defendant; (3) there was no rape but rather sexual relations occasioned by your free will and willing consent.

In some states, corroborative evidence is needed for conviction. This includes witnesses, bloodstains, dirty or torn clothing, and evidence of abrasions and scratches. New rape laws are making corroboration less necessary, but juries may not always convict without some corroboration. Federal courts, and some other jurisdictions as well, require corroboration only in the case of statutory rape or for crimes reported long after being committed. Many times, however, the rape victim herself may provide corroborative testimony. The presence of semen might be corroboration, as might scratches, contusions, and other physical trauma. Laws on corroboration are changing rapidly.

The law stipulates that the accused is innocent until proved guilty of the particular crime for which he is standing trial. If the defense counsel can raise reasonable doubt in the mind of one juror about the defendant's guilt on all of the particulars of the charges, the defendant will have an excellent chance of gaining acquittal.

Even after you have suffered through the assault and the ordeal of the judicial process, the criminal may be set free. The odds are about even that there will never be a trial, and if there is a trial, statistics show that half the defendants are either acquitted or their cases are dismissed.

Of those who are convicted, two out of five will be convicted of a lesser offense. This low conviction rate among those brought to trial is often attributed to the fact that the penalties are so severe that judges or juries are reluctant to convict.

FALSE RAPE CHARGES

Women rarely file false rape charges following consensual sex. Many people believe that over half the allegations of rape are false, but in reality only 2 to 8 percent of these charges are fabricated. One celebrated case involved Cathleen Crowell Webb, who admitted bringing false rape charges against Gary Dotson after he had served 8 years in prison for the alleged sexual assault. Women may invent rape to take revenge on a man who hurt them, or unfounded charges may be brought to appease another male in her life, or a parent, or to account for the presence of a sexually transmitted disease. Petting or foreplay that violates boundaries also accounts for false rape charges. Police are rarely fooled by such ploys, which are sometimes termed partial consent.

SELF-PROTECTION

Unfortunately, your chances of being a rape victim are increasing. Following the suggestions in the relevant chapters of Parts 1, 2, 3, and 4 will decrease the likelihood of your being victimized. Train yourself to be observant so that you can provide a useful description to the police, if necessary. Never walk alone after dark. Be certain to avoid public parks; areas with a lot of trees, bushes, and shrubbery; parking lots; alleys; and deserted areas. Cross the street if you see a group of males approaching you. When waiting for a bus, a traffic light, or a friend, be alert. Your stationary position makes you more vulnerable to attack. If you are on foot and a car pulls up next to you or drives by several times, change direction or run away.

Always be aware of your exact location in case you must contact the police. Follow all instructions and answer all questions posed by the 911 operator. Tell the 911 operator if you require an ambulance. Do not hang up until the 911 operator tells you to.

SEXUALLY TRANSMITTED DISEASES

Any of the diseases that are transmitted through sexual intercourse may be spread by the act of rape. Herpes simplex, gonorrhea, syphilis, and AIDS are all potentially fatal consequences of a rape. All of these diseases can threaten the victim's health and even her life.

Nor does the list of consequences stop there. Sexual partners of the assailed victim are at risk, as are gynecologists, emergency room personnel, and others who may have offered assistance. If the beleaguered woman is pregnant (or becomes so as the result of being attacked), the fetus she carries is at risk from a variety of venereal disorders.

Clearly, the direst of these threats is AIDS. Yet it is a threat that can be used against an attacker. In times past, rapists have tended to disbelieve potential victims who claimed that they were infected with social diseases. Today's attackers may be similarly dubious. However, there is nothing to lose by telling your assailant that you suffer from AIDS. Don't expect him to believe it. Nevertheless, you will have put him on the defensive. Carry a *latex* condom if you feel particularly in danger of rape. This might make your tale of affliction more believable. It would certainly raise doubts in the mind of your adversary.

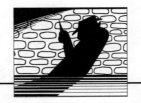

DEFENSES AGAINST RAPE:
A CHECKLIST

1 Practice all personal and home security procedures mentioned throughout this book.

2 Teach school-aged females—who are most often victimized—proper safeguards, particularly in regard to relationships with strangers and the value of locks and other physical security measures.

3 Ensure that a school-aged female entertaining male friends is well supervised.

4 Urge your daughter to travel in a group and to exercise care in after-school activities.

5 Learn some rudiments of self-defense.

6 Run and scream if you think you will be attacked.

7 Don't physically resist or attack an armed assailant. But an unarmed assailant might be vulnerable to physical attack and allow a break for freedom.

8 Carry everyday items for use as defensive weapons: pen or pencil, red pepper, lemon juice in a squeeze bottle, a key ring, or an umbrella.

9 Attack an assailant at his throat, stomach, temples, eyes, kneecaps, or other vulnerable points.

10 Use a knee to the groin if an assailant makes an embracing attack from the front.

11 Deliver a sharp blow to the stomach with an elbow if you are attacked from the rear.

12 Stomp on the assailant's foot, at the instep, as a defensive measure.

13 Try an emotional appeal if escape or resistance is impossible or impractical. By crying or attempting conversation, you may thwart an attack or lessen its severity.

14 Building up a rapist's ego may give him the emotional gratification he seeks, deterring him from seeking physical gratification.

15 Be aware that a date could degenerate into a rape; maintain defenses at all times.

16 Once the incident is over, only you can decide whether to report it. (In general, male victims are more reluctant to report a rape than female victims.) Prosecute only if you are committed to persevere through what could be a lengthy trial that may have a disappointing outcome.

17 Know the number of your community's rape crisis center.

18 Do not bathe, change clothes, douche, or otherwise clean up after an attack. You may be destroying evidence. Take a change of clothing with you when you go to file the report, because the clothing you were wearing might be required for evidence.

19 Write down or tape-record all incidents while they are fresh in your mind.

20 Undergo the required physician's examination, and consider having another from your own gynecologist.

21 The decision to resist or not is solely up to the victim. The decision must be based on circumstances existing at the time of attack.

22 A female must resist a rapist, but not necessarily physically. "Don't make me do it" is a plea that indicates duress.

23 Corroboration of evidence is less important now than it was previously. It is required routinely, however, in cases involving statutory rape and cases that are reported after an unreasonable amount of time has passed.

24 New rape shield laws protect the identity of the victims by providing anonymity. Many of these laws provide for pretrial hearings to determine whether proposed defense evidence is relevant.

25 Seek counseling or other professional help as soon as you are able.

26 Above all, remember that your physical and emotional well-being is the most important concern.

30

ACQUAINTANCE RAPE AND CAMPUS SEXUAL ASSAULT

Acquaintance rape, also known as date rape, is an extremely serious and widespread problem. It occurs when what appears to be a friendly, innocent sexual overture suddenly becomes a sexual attack. Research indicates that between 15 and 30 percent of all women have been raped by an acquaintance. Moreover, up to 88 percent of all rapes involve acquaintances, and between 58 and 80 percent of all rapes were perpetrated by an acquaintance *while on a date.* Far more common than rape by an unknown assailant this type of "friendly" rape is just as horrible and demeaning as back-alley rape.

INCIDENCE

Acquaintance rape can involve relatives, social companions, casual friends, co-workers, and other people familiar to each other. Men of all descriptions and backgrounds have been accused of acquaintance rape, including attorneys, businessmen, physicians, and dentists.

The average age of those involved in incidents of date rape, either as perpetrator or victim, is 18½ years. Research also shows that three-quarters of the men and half the women) involved in acquaintance rape had been drinking at the time of the assault. According to a study of adult acquaintance rape, friends accounted for 20 percent of assailants, husbands 16 percent, boyfriends 14 percent, and other acquaintances such as co-workers, neighbors, and delivery men, the remainder. Because familiarity does not necessarily equal safety, women must therefore always be cautious and alert.

Still there are many misunderstandings and myths about just what acquaintance rape is and when it occurs.

Myth: Forced sex is justified because you dressed seductively, hugged, kissed, touched, and shared close body contact with your date.

Reality: You have the right to dress any way you like and yet not engage in sexual relations. Likewise, having engaged in close physical contact does not mean you have given up the right to decide at what point you want it to stop. Nevertheless, the behavior and dress of all individuals, female and male, should be suitable for the occasion.

Myth: You owe your date sex because he spent a lot of money on dinner, the movies, and an after-hours club.

Reality: Money spent by a man, even in large amounts, on an evening of social companionship does not entitle him to use your body for his sexual pleasure. An expensive date does not constitute a contractual obligation to have sex.

Myth: A woman who rarely goes out alone, especially during evening hours, dresses conservatively, and secures her home from intrusion does not have to be concerned with sexual assault. Only women "out looking for trouble" are raped.

Reality: You certainly decrease the risk of an assault by taking proper security measures and by living a cautious lifestyle. However, most rape involves social companions, friends, or co-workers. Deadbolts and conservative clothing offer little protection from these men.

Myth: Sex relations without your consent is not rape if you willingly had prior sexual relations with your partner.

Reality: Sexual relations against your will, regardless of how close and intimate you have been with your partner, is rape.

Myth: A woman can bring charges of rape only when the assaulter had a weapon and threatened to use it to inflict serious harm on her if she did not comply.

Reality: Any forcible sex, whether or not a weapon was visible, involves intimidation and violence and constitutes rape. You can bring charges against the attacker even though a weapon was not used in the assault.

CHARACTERISTICS OF AN ACQUAINTANCE RAPIST

The best defense against acquaintance rape is the ability to identify and avoid men who are likely to engage in sexual assault. Potential rapists tend to think violence is an acceptable means of attaining goals and resolving disputes. They have an unhealthy obsession with violence on TV and in movies, and may have an obsession with guns. They often have problems with alcohol and/or drugs. They tend to display minimal respect for other human beings generally, and they may be cruel to children and animals. They intrude on the personal space of others, psychologically and physically. These men act "macho"; they exhibit sexist conduct and attitudes. They will be satisfied with nothing less than complete control of their dates' mind and body.

AVOIDING DATE RAPE

Experts say early warning signals for social rape include intimidating stares, standing too close, enjoying your discomfort, acting as if he knows you better than he does, calling you names that make you uncomfortable, constantly blocking your way and following you, touching you in sensitive places "by accident," ignoring what you say, and becoming angry when you disagree with him.

Here are some concrete suggestions for protecting yourself:

❖ Be certain you know the name of every man you date, where he lives, and something about his occupation. Take his phone number, but do not give out your own.

❖ Consult your friends or any other people who know the person before you accept a date with him.

❖ Never invite a man you have met in the street, a bar, or any other public place to be alone with you in your residence or any other private place until you know him.

❖ For your first date, arrange to meet him at the date location, which should be a public place like a movie theater, museum, library, mall, cafe, coffee shop, or restaurant. Insist on a cab or public transportation; avoid driving with him, especially in his car.

❖ Make certain you take along enough money for a taxi and telephone calls.

❖ Offer to pay for part of the date, or arrange to go "dutch," so that you set a tone of equality.

❖ Always maintain a measure of reserve and distance on the first date. This does not mean you should be cold, uncooperative, or impersonal. You can be dignified and at the same time warm, compassionate, and understanding.

❖ Ensure that you are sober on all dates. Alcohol and drugs lower inhibitions and set the stage for unwanted sexual behavior, which can easily turn into sexual assault.

❖ Be wary about strong drugs such as "roofies" or Rohypnol, known as the "date-rape" drug, which can be added to your drink without your knowledge.

❖ Should the two of you decide to go someplace isolated or private on your first date, be sure to tell someone before you go, and be certain your date knows you have done so.

Preemptive Action

Be able to identify danger signals; and be alert for any strange behavior on the part of your date. Is he trying too hard to convince you to accompany him to an isolated location? Has he suddenly steered the conversation towards sex? Is he making lewd statements or describing sexual acts in detail? Is he using foul language? Does he suddenly try to hug, kiss, hold, or touch you without permission or warning? Does he start to push and hit you lightly?

Once you are aware of any of these signals, the next steps are crucial in keeping the situation from getting out of control:

❖ Be assertive and firm in your tone of voice and body language. Trust your instincts. Lethargy and passivity send the wrong signals, especially to a "macho" type. Ambiguous signals tend to confuse your date, making it more difficult to stop sexual improprieties later on.

❖ Do not allow the would-be rapist a small liberty in the hope it will appease him or prevent further aggression. Remember, acquaintance rape, like rape by a stranger, is mainly an expression of violence in with which the assailant seeks to dominate the victim. A token concession is unlikely to stop him.

❖ If you have made a strenuous objection and your date does not stop the unwanted behavior, threaten to call the police.

Confrontation

If these measures have been unsuccessful in dissuading your date from forcing himself on you sexually, there are some additional strategies (already discussed in Chapter 29) that may work as well with an acquaintance rapist as with a stranger.

Use a verbal defense. Try to talk the rapist out of the attack. Use conversation as a stalling tactic. Convince the rapist that you do not want sex under any circumstances with him or anyone else. Explain to him that what he intends is rape. This approach is more likely to be effective with an acquaintance or date than with a stranger.

Invent a surprise. Another strategy is to tell the attacker that you're having your period or that you feel sick. Tell him you are nauseated and are going to throw up. If you can make yourself vomit, do so. Try to make the attacker disgusted. Tell him you have AIDS. Strange or bizarre behavior may also throw a date-rapist off guard. Rant and rave; flail your hands; make sudden body movements; act out hallucinations.

Escape. You should think of these strategies as ways to buy time until you can figure out an escape. As soon as he lets his guard down, run out of the house or apartment or get out of the car. Attract the attention of other people if possible; scream if you have to. Or tell him you have to go to the bathroom and will be right back, then leave through the bathroom window. Telephone for assistance if you can.

The best time for you to attempt an escape is at the very beginning of the confrontation. During the first few seconds or moments, the date-rapist will try to get you under his control. The further the situation escalates, the more important the maintaining of that control will become for the rapist, and the more difficult it will be to pry yourself loose.

YOUNG PEOPLE AT RISK

Acquaintance rape flourishes within the social and dating structures of teenagers. Junior and senior high schools are spawning grounds for sexual assault, because that is where teenagers congregate, socialize, and make choices for dates.

Teenagers are particularly likely not to report sexual assaults because many are convinced no one will believe them, not even their parents, best friends, acquaintances, employers, and co-workers. According to experts, only 1 in 100 rapes by acquaintances results in a police report.

On college campuses, young people of both sexes—most fresh from high school, many away from home for the first time—often live together in co-ed dorms and regularly attend unsupervised parties. They are thrown into situations in which it may seem that acquaintance can escalate into intimacy within minutes. Add alcohol and drugs, and you have an explosive mixture. The student least likely to be a victim of sexual assault is the student who is best informed about it.

How Safe Is Your Campus?

Studies reveal that one in four women is sexually assaulted or raped during her college experience. Seventy-five percent of those assaulted are victims of acquaintance, or date, rape. A survey by *Ms.* magazine found that 15 percent of college students had been victims of rape; another 12 percent experienced attempted rape; 11 percent were sexually coerced; and 14 percent were victims of unwanted sexual touching. These figures may be conservative; they do not include the many students who leave college or transfer to another educational institution after a sexual assault.

According to FBI statistics, 408 rapes were reported in 1992 by the 455 colleges and universities that disclose such statistics. An estimated 306, or 75 percent, of these sexual assaults might have involved acquaintance rape. Because only 5 percent of date rapes are reported, it is estimated that 6,120 incidents of social rape occurred on these 455 campuses in 1992. According to the FBI estimates, nearly 30 times more women are raped than murdered on the nation's campuses.

Reality 101

The campus is a microcosm of society at large, and like that society the campus is not immune from misconceptions concerning rape. In fact, myths concerning rape proliferate because they are passed along within a college community comprising mainly young people who associate with one another on a daily basis. Here are some common myths swirling around the campus:

Myth: Rape occurs almost exclusively at large universities in major metropolitan areas. Your teenager is secure in smaller suburban and rural colleges.
Reality: According to the FBI and other experts on this subject, acquaintance and date rape occur on campuses of all types and sizes in urban, suburban, and rural areas.

Myth: A co-ed who is raped in a parked car or isolated place deserves it, especially if she met her attacker at a singles bar or while hitchhiking.
Reality: No student deserves to be sexually assaulted, regardless of the location she was at or events that preceded the attack. That the assault occurred in an isolated place does not mean consent was given. Only the man who commits the violence is to blame.

Myth: Sexual assault is the woman's fault if she does not resist by screaming or fighting.
Reality: That the victim does not physically or verbally resist does not excuse the rapist or justify the assault. Any sexual relations without consent is rape. In some cases, especially if the woman is not skilled in self-defense techniques, fighting back can result in more serious injury than the rape itself.

Myth: Having unwanted or coerced sex with a classmate, friend, study partner, or date is not really rape.
Reality: Any forced sexual relations is rape, and it doesn't matter whether the man is an acquaintance or a stranger. Acquaintance rape at times may be more traumatic than sexual assault by a stranger because it shatters the bond of trust.

SELF-PROTECTION ON CAMPUS

The two most significant factors associated with campus rape are how often a woman dates and the sobriety (or lack thereof) of her date or acquaintance, as well as herself. The more men she dates, the more likely she will at some time find herself with a man with the characteristics of an assailant. Also, one significant survey reported that 75 percent of men involved in acquaintance rape had consumed alcohol or drugs immediately prior to the assault. Moreover, 55 percent of the victims had consumed alcohol or drugs before the incident. If a woman does drink, she should do so in moderation and stop before she feels dizzy or high. She should find out what her tolerance is before exposing herself to potentially dangerous social situations.

Adherence to the following rules will provide some protection from campus date rape:

❖ Be extremely selective in the men you date. Be aware of any signs that may signal a tendency towards assaultive behavior.

❖ Be on guard when dating athletes or fraternity brothers, particularly first-year students, and especially during your first semester in college.

❖ Avoid parties where alcohol and drugs are consumed. If you must drink, know *and observe* your limit.

❖ Refrain from dating "macho" men who demean women.

❖ Define to your partner as soon as possible—only you can sense the propitious moment—your sexual limits, informing him as to the behavior you consider acceptable and unacceptable. Tell him that kissing, hugging, and touching are not a license for total intimacy.

❖ Terminate your date if the man attempts any form of force or intimidation. Even if the man is a classmate or friend, unwelcome behavior is unwelcome behavior.

❖ Memorize the campus security or emergency telephone number. Write it down and keep it in an easily accessible place as well; if a disturbing situation develops, you may have trouble remembering it.

❖ Ask a female friend or campus security officer to accompany you home after a late-night party if alcohol has made you dizzy or tired.

❖ Never leave a party with a man who makes sexual comments that are unwelcome or that make you uncomfortable.

❖ If your date engages in behavior that makes you feel uncomfortable, be assertive. Tell him if he does not stop, you will end the date.

❖ Leave immediately with a girlfriend if you find yourself one of few women remaining at a fraternity party.

Following these simple precautions will provide initial protection for students who enter college. But also be certain that the college has established an escort service that is available at night and on weekends or that there is a special bus or van shuttle to the dormitories that operates after dark.

Also, the college should have security phones at convenient locations throughout the campus that automatically dial the security office in case of an emergency. Security officers should receive special training on how to prevent sexual assault and deal with its aftermath, including how to manage and treat victims. One often-overlooked measure is for the college or university to establish safe houses or change living arrangements for the protection of victims. A simple step is to change and strengthen the lock to your room.

WHAT PARENTS CAN DO

Engaged in the difficult transition to adulthood, teenagers are often ill prepared for the complexities of campus social life. Discuss with your prospective freshman the issues of acquaintance and date rape and the potential dangers of fraternities, athletes, alcohol, drugs, and parties—especially during the first few weeks of class, the most vulnerable "window" for assaults, when your daughter is unfamiliar with campus lifestyle and policies. Your college-bound daughter should be aware of the warning signs of potentially dangerous behavior and should know never to go to an isolated place with someone she does not know well. Above all, teach your daughter that the dating process is a very serious matter and should not be treated casually.

Consult the FBI *Crime in the United States: Uniform Crime Reports*, found in every major library, for statistics on rape and other serious crimes at the nation's colleges and universities. If the campus your daughter has selected is not listed, find out from the college its crime statistics and compare it to the *Uniform Crime Reports*. Use these data only as a guide, because there are many reasons to choose a particular college. But it is wise to select a campus that has a meaningful rape prevention program, that takes a strong stand against sexual assault, and that mandates meaningful and just penalties for men found guilty of rape.

WHAT YOU CAN DO

Chapter 29 discusses at length the aftermath experience of rape victims and outlines the best strategy to pursue. Whether you report the rape or not, contact your local rape crisis center by calling its hotline. Unfortunately, only 5 percent of victims of acquaintance rape take this very important step. Ask the operator for the telephone number or consult your telephone directory. People at the rape crisis center will know what to do and how to help you.

One major reason victims do not press charges and fail to cooperate with the prosecutor is because they fear disclosure of a past sexual experience or history that may embarrass them or result in long-term harm. Many states have enacted a "rape shield law" that prohibits introducing evidence about a victim's irrelevant prior history. All states should be encouraged to pass this crucial legislation. Remember, it's best to report the incident immediately. The sooner you report the incident, the greater your credibility and the better the evidence will be preserved. (For more discussion of legal prosecution in rape cases, see Chapter 29.)

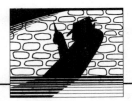

ACQUAINTANCE RAPE AND CAMPUS SEXUAL ASSAULT: A CHECKLIST

1. Be selective in your dating choice. Avoid men who exhibit the personal characteristics of a potential rapist. These include men who espouse violence, who demean and control women, and who are obsessed with guns, drugs, and alcohol.

2. On a date, be alert to behavior that often precedes a date rape, including attempts to take you to an isolated location, physical contact without your permission, and an overemphasis on sex talk and play. If this happens, try to get away from your date any way you can.

3. Have a well-prepared defense plan before you go out, in case your date becomes dangerous. It is important to remain calm and clearheaded when confronted with this situation.

4. Try to talk your date out of the attack, using persuasion or deception—anything that may prove effective.

5. Remember that the most favorable moment for escape is during the first few seconds of the attack.

6. If you decide to resist physically, use any and all tactics, fair and foul, to allow you an opportunity to escape.

7. Never blame yourself for a sexual assault. Rape is the fault of the attacker, no one else.

8 In the aftermath of a sexual attack, get to a safe place or area. Call someone you trust—a friend, relative, or teacher—and tell about the assault.

9 Contact your local rape crisis center.

10 Preserve all evidence, and refrain from eating, drinking, washing, douching, brushing your teeth, and combing your hair.

11 Seek medical help.

12 Seek counseling by highly trained therapists. Join a support group and share experiences.

13 Remember, you alone must make the final decisions involving reporting the rape and pressing charges; however, by doing so you're not only helping yourself, you're also helping other potential victims.

14 If you are attending college, beware of parties where heavy drinking or drug consumption is likely to occur.

15 Be especially alert to "rape hazards" like isolated places, first dates, and weekend parties.

16 Never remain at a party where you are the only female.

17 Be assertive and say No if your date insists on unwanted sexual comments and touching. Terminate the date immediately if the man becomes physically or sexually aggressive.

18 Memorize the telephone number of campus security, write it down, and carry it at all times.

19 Never walk home alone late at night when the campus is deserted.

20 If you are a parent, teach your teenagers traditional values of mutual respect; point out the dangers of peer pressure, drugs, and alcohol. You must serve as a role model.

21 Discuss the dangers of dating and sexual assault with your teenage daughter to ensure that she has a high level of awareness before she goes away to college.

22   Know your daughter's rights should she become the victim of sexual assault, and make sure she knows them as well.

23   Consult FBI statistics on campus crime before choosing a college.

24   Choose a college that is serious about sexual assault prevention and protection.

25   Be certain your college can provide an escort service or special transportation after dark.

26   Check whether your college has automatic-dial emergency phones at convenient locations. If not, insist that they be installed.

27   Insist that college security personnel receive special training in rape prevention and how to deal with a victim.

31

~

SEXUAL HARASSMENT AND STALKING

The manager of a small company repeatedly made suggestive comments to his secretary about her anatomy. On several occasions, he brought pornographic material into the office and displayed it on her desk. When she objected to his behavior, he laughed at her and invited her to sit on his lap. When she refused, he sat on her lap.

Sexual harassment and stalking are each violations of the law. Both involve subtle ways of destroying the confidence, well-being, and security of women who are the primary targets.

SEXUAL HARASSMENT ON THE JOB

The laws regarding sexual harassment are still evolving. Each case is unique, depending on its nature, seriousness, and repetition; a precise definition of sexual harassment must await future court decisions. Harassing actions are prohibited by Section 703, Title VII, of the Civil Rights Act of 1963, and, depending on the nature of your employment, other legislation may apply as well.

Sexual harassment is defined as unwelcome sexual advances, requests for sexual favors, and other verbal or physical conduct of a sexual nature where:

❖ Submission to such conduct is made explicitly or implicitly a term or condition of an individual's employment.

❖ Submission to or rejection of such conduct by an individual is used as the basis for decisions affecting on-the-job status of the individual.

❖ Such conduct has the purpose or effect of unreasonably interfering with an individual's work performance, or creating an intimidating, hostile, or offensive working environment.

Sexual harassment can be inflicted by and against individuals of both sexes, but experts say only a small fraction of sexual harassment incidents involve women harassing men or other women, or men harassing other men.

One major form of sexual harassment involves *quid pro quo*, or "giving something in exchange for something else." This abuse of power occurs when one person holds institutional control over another—for example, a physician over a nurse, a manager over an employee, a professor over a student, or an officer over a lower-ranking officer or enlisted person. Your termination or denial of an employment benefit because you refused to grant sexual favors or because you complained about harassment are illegal.

Similarly, it may be a case of sexual harassment if you've had to resign from your job rather than accept aggressive sexual behavior or an offensive work environment. Unwelcome sexual advances, familiarities, remarks, off-color jokes and comments about people's anatomy, slurs about gender, unwanted touching, spatial encroachments, requests for sexual favors, work discussions that suddenly turn to conversations about sex, and obscene and suggestive letters or notes all constitute sexual harassment. Sexual harassment may also involve visual conduct, such as leering and sexual gestures. This is especially the case when the behavior is unwelcome, coercive, and persistent.

Another aspect of sexual harassment is known as *hostile work environment,* which is created when, for example, superiors or co-workers engage in physical or verbal sexual improprieties that a reasonable person would find unwelcome and abusive. A constant stream of offensive sexual comments, repeated sexual propositions, constant display of pornographic materials, or repeated unwanted touching creates a hostile work environment.

Myth and Reality

Misconceptions concerning sexual harassment are rampant. Only recently has it been recognized as a serious problem, and the law regarding this matter is still evolving.

Myth: Most women seek and desire sexual attention in the workplace.

Reality: Women demand respect and equality in the workplace, not sexual attention.

Myth: Sexual harassment receives too much attention in the media, since it is an extremely rare occurrence.

Reality: Sexual harassment is endemic in the workplace, in academic settings, and in the military.

Myth: Most men who engage in sexual harassment do not really intend to offend women.

Reality: Sexual harassment involves abuse of power and a desire to control the victim. The majority of men who engage in this behavior have a need to subordinate, degrade, and control women.

Myth: Allegations of sexual harassment are often false. Women wish to create problems for men or are acting out fantasies.

Reality: Research has shown that few allegations of sexual harassment are contrived.

If You Are Harassed

These are the steps you should take if you are harassed in the workplace:

Inform the harasser. The first step is to inform the harasser immediately and clearly that you consider his attention, remarks, or behavior offensive and unwelcome and that he is engaging in sexual harassment. Be specific, providing concrete examples of exactly what offended you. Use body language to indicate that you do not want the behavior to continue, like taking a rapid step backwards when the harasser comes too close or suddenly stopping and staring angrily into his eyes. Your primary aim is to have him stop the offending behavior before it escalates. Notification also supports your contention that you were harassed. Rationalizing the behavior, making excuses, or feeling guilty will only encourage the harasser.

Write a memo. If a verbal warning fails to stop the harasser, write him a memo about what he did or said, what you don't like about it, how it made you feel, and the action you will take if he does it again. Deliver the copy in the presence of a witness, or send it certified mail, return receipt requested. Keep a copy of the memo in your personal files away from the office. These actions will counter the harasser's argument that he didn't realize the behavior was unwelcome or that he thought it was good, clean, harmless fun.

Document the situation. The next step is to thoroughly document your situation. Write down everything that takes place; leave nothing to memory or chance. Maintain a precise written record or diary of what happened or what was said: when it was said, the location, your response, and all witnesses, including those who can confirm that you spent time with the harasser. Include a description of how the offensive behavior hurt you and the names of those you told about it. Also, make certain you gather all evidence, including discriminatory cards, letters, notes, and memos sent to you by the harasser, and keep a careful record of all his telephone calls to you.

Document your work performance. Document your performance, showing the work you have done and that you have performed it well. Maintain a record of written materials and verbal statements that indicate positive performance, and keep copies of evaluations by your superior. This is to prevent the harasser from being able to justify a claim that you are raising charges of sexual harassment as an excuse or a smokescreen for poor work.

Report the harasser. Should unwanted comments or familiarities continue, and your verbal and written warnings prove futile, report the behavior to your superior, your union, and your personnel office. Follow your complaint up the company hierarchy until strong action is taken to stop the behavior. If your complaint is ignored and no action is taken, file a formal complaint with the Equal Employment Opportunity Commission (EEOC). You can find a local listing for the EEOC in your telephone directory under U.S. Government listings. Or contact the Resource Management Division, Equal Employment Opportunity Commission, Washington, DC 20507. You have 180 days from the time the behavior occurred to file the complaint with EEOC; otherwise the complaint may be considered untimely.

Go public. Write a letter to the newspaper or contact your local radio or TV news station about your situation. Join a women's support group or a lobbying organization. This may be of assistance to other women who are experiencing sexual harassment, as well as to you.

SEXUAL HARASSMENT IN SCHOOLS

A group of guys corner you in a school hallway, press you against the wall, and tell you what they'd like to do with you. A classmate passes around a note with your name and telephone number that says you're the one to call for "hot sex." Your advisor insists it's OK for a young woman to fall in love with an older man like himself. These are typical examples of sexual harassment that take place in high schools every day.

Sexual harassment in schools involves more than obvious and unwelcome flirtatious advances by teachers or students. Sexual harassment includes: touching and grabbing; sexual remarks, conversations that are too personal, and dirty jokes; obscene gestures; and persistent staring so as to make you feel uncomfortable. Graphic descriptions of women's bodies, pornographic pictures, graffiti, and denigrating language also constitute sexual harassment when they promote a hostile and unequal environment in which women are precluded from attaining their full potential. Statistics show that girls in schools are four times as likely as boys to experience sexual harassment.

What a Student Should Do

❖ Learn and understand exactly what conduct is considered sexual harassment.

- Familiarize yourself with your school's policy on sexual harassment.
- Attend a workshop on sexual harassment.
- If you are harassed, tell a friend about the harassment.
- If the harasser is an adult, or attempts to convince you not to tell anyone, or always bothers you when you are alone, or threatens to hurt you, then *immediately* tell a trusted adult.
- Tell the harasser that the behavior makes you uncomfortable, that you want it to stop.
- Speak to a family member, especially your parents, and ask for their help in lodging a complaint.
- Keep a record of the harassment.
- Avoid being alone with the harasser.
- Write a letter to the harasser detailing exactly what behavior occurred, what it is about the behavior that you object to, that you want him to stop, and what will happen if his behavior persists.
- Report incidents of sexual harassment to your principal, counselor, or appropriate administrator charged with responsibility for this issue.
- Be prepared to press your complaint through the school hierarchy. If your school does not have a written policy and mechanism for handling complaints, speak to your student council, teachers, guidance counselors, and principal, and urge them to formulate guidelines.

What a Parent Should Do

- Discuss your child's feelings about various kinds of sexual attention. Explain what sexual harassment is, and provide concrete examples.
- Raise the issue with your child to determine whether she has been sexually harassed. Explain that certain forms of flirting constitute sexual harassment, even though it may appear to your loved one as unfamiliar, exciting, and flattering behavior. Teenage girls may not necessarily be fully aware of, or informed about, what kinds of behavior demean women.
- Be certain that you are both able to communicate with each other about sexual harassment. It's best for your teenager to learn appropriate tolerance levels from you instead of from his or her peers, who don't necessarily have the right instincts or parental guidance.
- Realize the injury and harm your child feels as a result of sexual harassment.
- Ensure that there will be no retaliation if your child comes forward.
- Be loving and supportive.
- Take seriously all charges of sexual harassment.
- Guide your child through all the necessary steps to stop the behavior.

PROTECTING YOURSELF FROM STALKERS

Stalking involves the unwanted harassment of, following of, and obsession with another person. Most stalking involves harassment, such as repeated and annoying telephone calls and letters, and it may include threats or actual violence against the victim. The worst possible outcome is murder.

Stalking may seem to be an infrequent, far-fetched crime that you only see on the news or in the movies, but it's more common than you might think. According to one study, about 1 in 20 women will be stalked sometime in their lives, either by a former intimate, an acquaintance, or a complete stranger.

Stalkers are psychologically disturbed and in dire need of therapy. Research suggests that over 90 percent of stalkers suffer from mental illness or psychological dysfunction. Stalkers may be male or female, heterosexual or homosexual, but most are men who have been rejected by women. Most murders by stalkers occur because the stalker is unable to accept the end of a relationship with the victim.

Stalkers' Victims

Thirty-eight percent of the victims of stalkers are typical, everyday people; their stalkers are ex-spouses or lovers, acquaintances, or even strangers. About another third of the victims are entertainers, men or women, who aren't very well known. Nearly one-fifth of stalkers' victims are well-known entertainers or sports figures. Similar proportions of stalking victims are executives or supervisors with unhappy employees and psychotherapists stalked by patients.

If you or someone close to you is being stalked, notify the police immediately. You may also get an order of protection from the courts, and keep the police abreast of any and all actions taken. Depending on the law in your state, if you have an order of protection, it may increase an offender's punishment. Report to the police every incident as it takes place. Obtain the name and telephone number of an officer, and request that a file be started. Give the police a photo and all the information you have about your assailant. Ask the police to drive by your home, and have them grade your home's security. Keep a record of events as they occur. Note what happened, the date and time, and your personal feelings. This account may be admissible as evidence in court.

Save and date all evidence—including letters, notes, cards, and answering machine tapes—and take pictures of any damaged property. Wear cotton gloves when opening letters. Hold them at the corners and store them in plastic covers so they may be read without directly touching them. When you have contact with the stalker, note the date, time, what was said, and any witnesses.

An expert on stalking, Park Dietz, warns that arrest without conviction may further incite the stalker. If the stalker suffers from a mild mental illness, the arrest may make him feel threatened. If he is very ill, the arrest may just reassure him of his perceived relationship with his victim. Unfortunately, antistalking laws are not much of a deterrent to psychologically disturbed assailants.

Some Guidelines

Most people can't afford personal protection, such as a bodyguard or a security officer for the home. Nevertheless, here are a few more practical guidelines that will help you protect yourself:

❖ Put a deadbolt on your door, and secure your windows. If the stalker has a copy of your keys, change the locks.

❖ Vary your routes when walking or driving.

❖ Get an unlisted telephone number or caller ID, or screen your calls with an answering machine.

❖ Get a restraining order that places a penalty of fine or imprisonment on your stalker if he keeps contacting you.

❖ Do not try to meet, talk, or reason with the stalker.

❖ Do not return the stalker's letters or gifts. Doing so may incite him further, for one thing, and for another, you may be able to use them as evidence.

❖ Do not respond to his cries for help, such as threatening suicide. The purpose of these attempts is to make you feel guilty or to trap you.

❖ If your assailant is a former spouse or lover, do not reconcile in the hopes of warding off an attack. This only reaffirms his motivation for making you the object of his obsession.

Antistalking Laws

Previously, the criminal justice system offered women who were victims of stalking little protection. A restraining order could be obtained, but if the stalker chose to ignore it, there wasn't much the victim could do. It also didn't help that stalking incidents were commonly viewed by law enforcement as insignificant domestic squabbles.

Recently, major changes have occurred. The first antistalking law was passed in California in September 1990. Since then, all 50 states have passed antistalking legislation. Old laws offered protection only to a victim who experienced direct threats of harm, such as "I'm going to kill you." More recent laws also take implied threats under consideration, such as "If I can't have you, no one else can." Initial infringements of laws usually are misdemeanors, but repeated acts are felonies, and the perpetrators may serve time in jail or prison. When restraining orders are violated, some states immediately classify the crime as a felony. A federal antistalking law is also under consideration. Antistalking laws make it possible to arrest stalkers before they inflict physical harm on their victims. The laws also make a complaint to law enforcement officials much more viable; they are now in a position to do something about it.

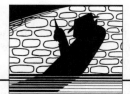

SEXUAL HARASSMENT AND STALKING: A CHECKLIST

1 Be aware that sexual harassment consists of unwelcome sexual suggestions, physical or verbal, that promote a hostile workplace or academic setting and often involve abuse of power.

2 Do not deny that you are the victim of sexual harassment, blame yourself, or feel guilty. Instead, avoid the attack and punish the attacker.

3 Immediately put the harasser on the defensive and on notice that his behavior is unwelcome and that it is sexual harassment. Do not hesitate or delay, or the harassment will only escalate.

4 Provide the harasser concrete examples of his offensive behavior.

5 Write the harasser a memo explaining how his behavior was offensive and how it made you feel.

6 Thoroughly document incidents of sexual harassment. The record should include at the very least what happened and when, where, and how you were injured.

7 Locate witnesses who can corroborate your charges or at least are able to substantiate that you interacted with the harasser at the time and place of the incident.

8 Collect all evidence, including correspondence and telephone contacts from the harasser to you.

9 Maintain a record of your own work performance as proof that it was at least satisfactory.

10 If his behavior persists, report the harasser to a superior, to your personnel office, and to your union.

11 File a complaint with the Equal Employment Opportunity Commission (EEOC) if you feel you are banging your head against a stone wall. Remember, you must do this within 180 days of the harassment.

12 Go public to gain support for your cause.

13 Teach your teenager about sexual harassment.

14 Learn about your school's policy on sexual harassment.

15 If your teenager is harassed, immediately report it to the appropriate authorities.

16 Learn about your local antistalking laws.

17 If you are being stalked, notify the police immediately. Also, get an order of protection against the stalker.

18 Arrest may further incite the stalker. Discuss this option with the responding officer before making a decision to press charges.

19 Keep your own journal of events, and save and date all evidence.

20 Make sure your home is secure, and have your telephone number unlisted.

21 Stalkers need psychiatric help. You cannot help them yourself, especially if you are a victim.

22 Do not try to reason or reconcile with the stalker. These tactics don't work, and you will be putting yourself at further risk.

32

ROBBERY PREVENTION AND DEFENSE

Unlike other crimes, robbery represents a threat to both your person and your property. Robbery is the taking of another's property by force or threat of violence. It is a crime in which there is always a confrontation between the victim and offender. Muggers (street robbers) generally try to frighten or intimidate their victims in order to gain physical and psychological control over them.

Robbery accounts for 35 percent of all crimes of violence. Force without a weapon was employed in 40 percent of robberies. But injuries occur most frequently when no weapon is used, because it is in this instance that a victim is most likely to fight back. Do not be a hero and resist the robbers physically or verbally. While it is true that robbers may use force even if you don't resist, if you attempt to thwart their goals, they will become frustrated and will be more likely to be violent.

Robberies seldom involve people who are known to each other. Studies show that more than three-quarters, and perhaps as many as 90 percent, of all robbers are strangers to their victims.

DETERRING ROBBERY IN SMALL BUSINESSES

If you own a small business or store, keep the premises orderly and clean. A cluttered store gives the impression of carelessness. Make sure that the back room is out of public view, so that the robber is not drawn to property that may be stored in it. Also, the robber will not be certain if someone else is on the premises. Keep a television or radio on in the back room to give the appearance of the presence of others. Be active; move around the store. Maximize the amount of space inside that is visible from the outside by using adequate lighting. Avoid obstructions near the window that might block the ability of passersby and the police to observe what is happening inside the store. Robbers may be reluctant to enter a store with high visibility from outside.

Vigilance Is the Best Strategy

Always greet customers in a friendly manner. This will not only benefit your business but also let potential robbers know that they may be identified later. Robbers seek to remain anonymous and to avoid friendly contact with potential victims. Be alert for anyone appearing to loiter inside or outside the store, seemingly waiting for you to be alone. Call the police to be on the "safe side" if you notice suspicious people.

Careful Planning

Planning how to respond to a robbery attempt is always a wise measure. Every employee—especially those who handle money—should know what to do in the event of a robbery. You should prepare signals so that once a robbery is in progress, you can alert employees who may be in a position to notify the police. Instruct employees not to disclose information about alarm systems, security, the number of employees, or any other information that would assist anyone interested in robbing your store or business. Also, be very selective in the hiring of employees. Many robberies are accomplished with the assistance of an insider, as was the $1 million heist a few years ago of Tiffany's on Fifth Avenue in Manhattan. Once the robbers were apprehended, the police learned that Tiffany's operational security officer was involved in the robbery. He had provided his accomplices confidential information on the security precautions used by Tiffany's to deter robbery.

Handling and Safeguarding Money

Keep a minimum of working cash in your store, especially at night, when most robberies occur. Put larger bills in a drop safe as soon as you receive them. Never allow cash to accumulate in your register. Make bank deposits during the day, varying your route and timing. Take someone else with you, if possible.

Be serious about protecting your money. Display burglar alarm decals in a prominent place. Post signs on the door stating that a second key not kept on the premises is required to open safes. If you belong to a special citizens' robbery prevention program, post signs to this effect inside and outside the store. Since many robberies occur when you open or close the store, try to have someone else present at these times. Robbers case their potential targets and know when only one person will be on hand.

Do not balance registers or count receipts in full view. This actually tempts robbers, customers, and even other store employees. Have cash drawers taken to a secure location to count the money. Record the serial number of a few bills that you permanently keep in the cash register. This can aid the police in tracking down the robbers and help in the identification of your property if it is recovered.

It is best not to rely on firearms. A robber will have the "drop" on you and usually is ruthless and desperate. Alarm systems, electronic surveillance equipment, safes with time locks, and other robbery-resistant items may provide better protection and should be considered for your store.

VIOLENCE PREVENTION PROCEDURES

Though robbery is a crime in which the threat of violence is always present, there are things you can do to lessen that threat.

During a Robbery

Obey the instructions of robbers as quickly as possible. Never argue with them. Robbers are less likely to injure you if you cooperate. The shorter the time it takes the robbers to do their work, the less chance there is for injury or even death. In fact, the average robbery is completed in under 3 minutes. In a small business, remain calm, and reassure your employees and customers. Do not fight with the robbers or attempt to use weapons. By the time you are confronted by a robber, it is too late for such actions. Assume that any firearm is real and loaded. If you need to reach for something, or put your hand in your pocket, or do anything else that the robber may perceive as threatening, tell him before you do it. For your own safety, alert the robbers to any possible surprises, such as an employee working in the back room or a delivery person who may return to the store at any moment.

Take mental notes about the crime and the criminals. Pay attention to the number of robbers, their ages, sex, ethnic backgrounds, appearance, clothing, weapons, voices, nicknames, special characteristics, and unusual behavior or identifying marks. Some stores and businesses have marks on door frames or a wall that aid an employee or witness in estimating the robber's height. This may be easily done by placing two pieces of colored tape at about 5 feet 6 inches, and at 6 feet on the door frame.

One antirobbery technique sometimes recommended is the installation of a doorbell in your place of business. The bell should ring in an adjacent store, enabling your neighboring merchant to notify the police when you are unable to do so. For your neighbor's protection, you can reciprocate.

A word of caution: If the robbers observe you signaling, they will, typically, do you harm. Therefore, signal only if you feel certain it will not be detected by the robber. Surviving the robbery without injury is your number-one goal.

Postrobbery Action

Note the make, color, and year of the vehicle used in the robbery, and the license plate number and state of registration. Check the direction in which the offenders were heading, but do not chase or follow them under any circumstance. The robbers may try to kill you, and the police may even mistake you for the criminals.

Notify the police immediately. Stay on the phone until they get all the necessary information, then remain close to the telephone. Lock the doors until the police arrive. Take inventory of exactly what was stolen, but do not give this information to the responding officers. Reveal this information only to the detectives assigned to your case; the police may talk to reporters, and publicity about a substantial loss may convince other robbers to attack your store, too.

Record the names and addresses of witnesses. Do not disturb any objects the robbers may have touched or held, and avoid discussing the robbery until the police say it is OK for you to do so.

Mugging Defense

Most muggings take place on the street. Thus, the best protection is to be alert and cautious at all times. See Chapter 13 for a fuller discussion of self-defense against street crimes. Be suspicious of strangers, and never trust anyone you do not know. Avoid walking at nighttime, especially in dangerous or unfamiliar neighborhoods. If you must go out at night, walk on well-lighted main thoroughfares. It is useful to carry a small amount of money, say $50, to appease the potential mugger, but large sums should be avoided. Walk next to the curb, and stay away from buildings, alleys, doorways, shrubbery, trees, and benches. Walk at a determined speed, and appear in a hurry to reach a destination. Cross the street if you spot someone suspicious walking toward you or following you.

Be sure that you have adequate change to make a phone call in an emergency; always carry several quarters. If confronted by a robber, use your common sense; maintain your cool and follow the mugger's instructions precisely. After the robbery, call the police. Bear in mind that robbers or muggers initially are after your valuables, but if they should feel threatened by you, it could be very dangerous. Let the robbers or muggers have whatever they ask for, and realize that your primary objective is to survive.

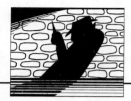

ROBBERY PREVENTION AND DEFENSE:
A CHECKLIST

1 Robbery is a crime in which the offender always confronts the victim, and it is a threat to your person as well as your property.

2 Don't be a hero. Don't resist robbers physically or verbally, or they may be more likely to be violent.

3 To help deter store robberies, keep your business tidy and clean. Walk around and keep busy even when no customers are in the store.

4 Keep your store well lighted and visible from the street.

5 Constantly be on the lookout for suspicious-looking people standing inside or outside the store.

6 Before a crime occurs, set up careful antirobbery plans, including prearranged signals for employees.

7 Do not keep substantial amounts of money in your store, especially at night. Never allow cash to accumulate in your register.

8 Record serial numbers of a few bills, and keep them in the cash register permanently to help police in tracking down the robbers.

9 Try to schedule your bank deposits in the daytime at different hours using different routes.

10 Make it known to the public that you are very concerned about your cash by displaying antirobbery and antiburglary decals.

11 Always open and close the store in the presence of another employee or other trusted person.

12 Your cashiers should not balance or count receipts in public.

13 Use firearms only if you are an expert trained in their use, and only when you have the "drop" on the robber.

14 Always obey the orders of the robbers, and never hesitate to carry them out.

15 Always retain your composure if confronted by robbers, and try to calm your employees and customers.

16 Alert the criminals to possible surprises, such as the appearance of a returning employee.

17 Get a description of the criminals and their vehicle.

18 Call the police without delay after the robbers escape.

19 Determine the amount of your loss, but reveal this only to the detectives who have been assigned to your case.

20 Try to identify witnesses to the robbery, and take their names and addresses.

21 Do not tamper with any evidence.

22 Keep the details of the robbery secret.

23 In your place of business, install a doorbell that rings in an adjacent store. Have your store neighbor act in kind.

24 Select store employees with great care. Many robberies are accomplished with the assistance of an insider.

25 If confronted by robbers on the street, follow their instructions precisely. Remember that your property is worthless compared with the value of your life.

33

ARSON, VANDALISM, AND HATE CRIMES

Fire fighters responded to a suspicious hotel fire. The arsonist deliberately greased stairway and fire escapes, which resulted in injury to 17 fire fighters. This was only one in a series of such fires in the area.

A suburban home was covered in graffiti and pelted with eggs and rocks until several windows were broken. When the group of youths who committed the acts of vandalism were questioned, they responded that they thought nobody lived there.

ARSON

Arson is the willful or malicious burning, or attempt to burn (with or without intent to defraud), a dwelling house, public building, motor vehicle or aircraft, or personal property of another. Only fires determined to be willfully or maliciously started are classified as arson. Fires of suspicious or unknown origin are specifically excluded. But while perpetrators of these crimes may intend merely to destroy property, all too often their crimes result in serious injury and death.

Why Arson Fires Are Set

People deliberately set fires for a number of reasons; personal gain, revenge, mental illness, profit, concealing another crime, vandalism, intimidation, jealousy, and spite are but a few. Revenge is the principal reason that arsonists start fires.

The most frequent arsonists are dissatisfied or former employees who blame their employers for their misfortune. They are particularly dangerous because they have a good knowledge of their workplace, as well as an awareness of the location and schedule of security patrols and fellow employees. In addition, they have easier access than an outsider. Businesses are more prone to arson by an employee during times of labor problems, such as strikes and layoffs.

In addition to the bored juvenile looking for excitement or seeking redress of real or imagined wrongs, the arsonist may be a property owner defrauding an insurance carrier or a homeless drifter looking for an abandoned building to sleep in; when it is cold, homeless people often burn the woodwork for warmth. Property owners, especially absentee ones, inadvertently invite the attentions of this last group. The trash-strewn property with hip-high weeds is an irresistible attraction for an arsonist. If the building is uninhabited, make sure all windows are boarded and entrances securely locked. The less you appear to care about your property, the more likely you are to become a victim of an arsonist.

Extent of Arson

Arson is the leading cause of property loss and damage due to fire, according to the National Fire Protection Association (NFPA), and the number of fires set deliberately continues to rise. The NFPA reports that in 1995, 137,500 suspicious fires were set. Of these, 90,500 were structure fires resulting in 740 fatalities. Direct property losses amounted to approximately $1.6 billion. According to the FBI's *Uniform Crime Reports*, the number of arson reports increased to 102,139 in 1994. The dollar loss of the average structural arson in 1994 was $16,495; for vehicle fires $3,883; and for other fires (e.g., trash and brush fires) $728. Furthermore, because many deliberately set fires go unreported as such, these numbers only begin to reveal the extent of the problem. One reason arson fires may not be reported is that many communities have volunteer fire fighters who are often untrained in determining the cause of a fire.

The dollar cost of arson is just the beginning of the losses: The victims have no place to live, and they probably had not increased their insurance coverage to stay in line with replacement costs. They are usually forced to move to less-satisfactory quarters. In the meantime, the burned-out house that they were forced to abandon will have greatly deteriorated, which will adversely affect the value of all nearby homes. The victims may find the cost of future insurance exorbitant, if not totally unavailable to them.

If arson is widespread, involving blocks of a neighborhood, an entire community can be destroyed. The burned-out homes can diminish the values of sound buildings, perhaps to the point where they cannot be sold at any price. Homeowners can be wiped out and tenants forced to seek a less-troubled neighborhood. The remaining tenantable structures may then be leased to undesirables, putting more downward pressures on the value of neighborhood property.

Who's at Risk?

A business is at an increased risk of arson if one or more of the following factors is present:

❖ Recent unexplained fires in your community
❖ One or more previous suspicious fires at your location
❖ Recent burglaries of your business or businesses nearby
❖ Your business is seasonal
❖ Your business is located in an isolated area or in the inner city
❖ Civic unrest or a riot has occurred in the area
❖ The economy is at a low point and unemployment is increasing

Preventive Measures

Several efforts may be made to reduce the incidence of arson. Some community organizations gather property and insurance information and report suspicious-looking individuals, vehicles, and fires. One such group in Boston, known as STOP, actually uncovered an arson-for-profit ring that had destroyed $6 million worth of property and had set some 35 fires. Thirty-three persons were arrested, including a fire chief, a police officer, insurance adjusters, attorneys, and real estate operators.

Teach your children proper attitudes about fires, and make them aware of the horrible consequences of setting fires. Older kids might be taught to identify fire setters and to organize neighborhood youths to clean up refuse-strewn lots or deteriorated buildings. Encourage civic or business groups to offer rewards for information leading to the arrest of an arsonist. Education and public awareness are key elements in preventing malicious fires. A very successful campaign in Seattle involved athletes, T-shirts, and a contest to name the "Arson Rat."

Arson is often committed in isolated and dark areas, so keep your house and/or business and surrounding property well lighted. Follow the security measures outlined in Part 1 of this book, giving special attention to the information on alarm systems in Chapter 3. Chapter 15 on security in the workplace and Chapter 23 on neighborhood crime prevention are also helpful.

Most incidences of arson occur on weekends or weekdays from 6 p.m. to 6 a.m. As a result, regular working hours are not the only times security is needed.

An automatic sprinkler system is essential, as the lack of one contributes to approximately two-thirds of arson dollar losses and severity of damage. Control access to areas containing flammable materials.

If a suspicious fire has been unsuccessful, be sure to increase future security. About one-fourth of arson attempts may be repeated, with each attempt progressively more dangerous.

Be informed of potential sources of ignition, including storage closets, file cabinets or rooms, mailrooms, and basement. To protect important documents or valuables from fires, install a fire-retardant safe or vault. Train your staff in how to deal with fires.

Perhaps the best advice for dealing better with arson is this: Install smoke detectors. They can be purchased for very little money, and they will provide the early warning that could easily save your life.

VANDALISM

Vandalism is the willful or malicious destruction of private and/or public property. It is a pesky crime, usually committed by bored, playful, or vengeful teenagers. A quarter of vandalism acts are premeditated. Like numerous other offenses, vandalism is a crime of opportunity. The effects of vandalism cost more than $1 billion per year, a large portion of that money coming from taxpayers. Whether you live in an urban, suburban, or rural area, chances are that you have faced some form of vandalism.

Types of Vandalism

Types of vandalism include defacing statues and monuments, breaking windows, destroying public pay phones and parking meters, writing on subway cars and storefronts, tearing pages from school and library books, smashing school furniture, clogging school toilets, turning over tombstones, and ruining business property.

Vandalism also damages your personal property. Many people have awakened to find tire tracks embedded in their front lawns, garden and shrubbery maliciously torn up, or automobile antennas missing. Perhaps you have had the unpleasant experience of cleaning dried eggs off your car and house after Halloween.

A few years ago, a London publication reported an incident of vandalism. A motorist had a flat tire on the expressway. After jacking up the rear end, he was removing the wheel, when he noticed someone opening the hood and attempting to remove the battery. Outraged, the offended driver challenged the opportunistic battery seeker. "Look," replied the latter, "you take the tires if you want—all I need is the battery."

This incident provides considerable insight into the motivation of vandals. In general, the vandal *does* respect the property of others, but only so long as the property is properly maintained. Allowing anything to lapse into misuse or abuse is an open invitation to vandals.

You probably have seen the vacant houses in your neighborhood that remain untouched for months on end. If, however, a single window is broken, almost overnight all of the windows may be shattered, and the structure will be broken open. Soon the building gives every indication of having been thoroughly vandalized.

Besides mere amusement, revenge is the second motive of the vandal. Usually, this type of damage is directed against schools. Often, when a school must enforce discipline, it is to the displeasure of the affected students. A young person may respond to this perceived provocation by plugging a toilet with tissue and disabling the water shutoff mechanism, thus inundating the surrounding area.

A large number of vandals are very young. They may seek amusement, suffer from family or community problems, yearn to be part of a group, or want to look daring in front of friends. Youth unemployment also contributes to the problem. Graffiti artists, often very young, seek recognition and fame among peers. In addition, many consider it an art form. None of this changes the fact that graffiti is a crime.

Some vandalistic actions can become life threatening. Disabled elevators in a college dormitory would be considered by most observers a mild inconvenience. In high-rise apartments for the elderly, the same situation could, under certain circumstances, be tragic. Broken street lighting could lead to rape, robbery, or worse. The offenders rarely consider the possible consequences of what they often consider harmless pranks.

Combating Vandalism

"Since subway cars don't belong to anybody, they may be spray painted." While this kind of thinking is illogical, it is also a widely held belief. Interestingly, when transit officials invited people to decorate the cars, they suddenly became objects that could be appreciated. Subsequent damage was minimized. This change tends to reinforce the hypothesis made earlier, that the vandal *does* respect the property of others so long as it is maintained in a fashion that indicates someone cares about it.

Much of public property is viewed as lacking ownership and is, therefore, especially vulnerable to vandalism. This idea is further reinforced by the often slow repair and maintenance of public property, including schools, housing, and transportation.

In some cases, parents are required to pay for their children's acts. A couple was given a bill for $38,000 after their two teenage sons were arrested for vandalizing over 20 Los Angeles Metropolitan Transit Authority buses.

If the windows of your home or business are repeatedly broken, replace them with unbreakable plastic or glass. Erecting a fence with a locked gate serves as a further deterrent by delineating your property. Make repairs and remove graffiti as soon as possible. Many experts suggest this as the best way to avert continued destruction. Another alternative is a Neighborhood Watch or citizen patrol. For a business, electronic surveillance or a security officer may solve the problem.

Common Targets of Vandalism

Besides schools, vacant structures, and public transportation, the targets of the vandal include abandoned vehicles. These should be hauled away to storage lots or sold through legal channels. Public transportation, like abandoned vehicles, is most vulnerable when not in operation, but proper fencing or security officers can be effective protection against damage.

Following is an examination of a structure, noting possible vandalism targets and suggesting possible protections against them:

❖ Graffiti is an omnipresent problem. Damage by pencil or permanent ink can be discouraged by using rough-surfaced materials that defy this type of marking, but this surface will make it harder to remove spray paints. Perhaps the best way to cope is to use smooth, hard surfaces that can easily be cleaned with mineral spirits or other solvents. Glazed ceramic tiles are especially difficult to scratch and write on. Another option is to paint over the damage as necessary. Certain paints, coatings, and plastic wall coverings help to prevent marking with graffiti.

❖ If glass breakage is a serious and continuing problem, shatterproof or virtually unbreakable substitutes may be called for. However, these products are easily scratched, tend to discolor, and, in the event of a fire, would not stand up as well as glass and might even melt. Persistent breakage might indicate the need for solid doors.

❖ Internal walls may often be broken or dented, even kicked in. Double thickness of wallboard may solve the problem.

❖ Toilet cubicles are vulnerable to a variety of abuse, graffiti being the most common. The usual gaps between partitions and the main walls provide leverage for prying aside the partition entirely. Finally, young people find the rail above the door of the cubicle stall an irresistible trapeze for swinging. Here, high-quality fixtures, stalls, and other items (such as tissue holders and coat hooks) should be utilized throughout. They will be subjected to considerable abuse.

❖ A glass panel, even of frosted glass, in a restroom door provides a considerable deterrent to vandalism by suggesting that someone might witness illegal acts.

❖ To avoid tampering with plumbing fixtures, keep pipes hidden or out of reach.

❖ The floors in bathrooms should be designed to withstand flooding. Installing drains in the floor is a good idea. Spray taps and the removal of sink drain plugs also help to avert this nuisance.

❖ Thermostats, fan switches, and appliance controls are often improperly used, particularly in schools. They should be protected by locks.

❖ Outdoor lighting fixtures should not be located in places where a vandal may have access to them. Keep them high and away from structures that may be climbed to reach them, such as columns or trees.

❖ Finally, if outdoor lighting fixtures are broken frequently, glass fixtures should be replaced with plastic, such as polycarbonate or other sturdy diffusers.

HATE CRIMES

A hate crime is any threat or act of violence that targets an individual, a group, or property, and is motivated by the race, color, religion, national origin, age, disability, or sexual orientation of the victim. Hate crimes often involve vandalism and arson. And, as is the case with those crimes, the motives of the perpetrators are varied and complex, and their conviction and incarceration are difficult to obtain.

These are heinous acts; they undermine the very foundations of our society and of our nation's Constitution, with its built-in safeguards to protect the rights of the individual, preserve respect for human dignity, and help promote tolerance. The impact of hate crimes goes way beyond any specific act, because they foment fear, distrust, enmity, anxiety, insecurity, and confusion. Even if only one individual or group is targeted, this particularly violent form of crime affects us all, personally and collectively.

A Growing Problem

Racial and religious hate crimes have been increasing over the last few years. The FBI reported 7,947 bias-motivated incidents in 1995, compared to some 5,000 similar offenses in 1991. Although part of this increase is the result of a growing number of agencies reporting such incidents, hate crimes are on the rise in many localities.

In Los Angeles, for example, racially-motivated crimes increased by 24 percent between 1991 and 1992. Nationwide, 1,867 anti-Semitic incidents were reported to the Anti-Defamation League in 1993, compared to 1,730 in 1992, an increase of 8 percent. Moreover, Klanwatch, an arm of the Southern Poverty Law Center in Montgomery, Alabama, disclosed that reports of vandalism due to "hate" increased by 26 percent in 1993 over 1992. In 1993, there were 788 incidents of anti-Semitic vandalism, including the painting on property of swastikas and anti-Jewish slogans, and fire bombings of Jewish institutions and public property.

According to the FBI, 57 percent of all hate crimes committed in 1995 were racially motivated. Of these crimes, 62 percent were directed at African Americans. Religious bias was the second most frequent motivation, with Jewish people the most frequent target.

The acting out of racial and religious hatred, and homophobia as well, was also evident in widespread reports of disrupted religious services, cemetery desecrations, cross burnings, fire bombings, and hate-motivated assaults, beatings, and gunshots. At the same time, distribution of hate literature was on the rise, and radio talk shows, which often provided an open mike for hate talk, were winning big audiences and high ratings.

One recent study revealed that 10 percent of bias-motivated hate crimes occur on school property. The number of such incidents has risen also on college campuses (see Chapter 24). Perhaps the most disheartening type of hate crime, however, is that which is done directly and deliberately to our houses of worship. Over the past few years, churches have been spray painted with obscenities, and sacred scrolls were stolen from synagogues, but most shocking of all was the upsurge of church burnings that alarmed the nation in 1996. In the first 6 months of that year, at least 37 churches, mostly black, but some white or multiracial, were damaged or destroyed by suspicious fires. An additional 41 others, according to the Atlanta-based Center for Democratic Renewal, were burned or vandalized in 1994 and 1995.

Months later, many of these cases remained unsolved, but the possibility of a national or even regional racist conspiracy had been ruled out. Still, racial hostility was clearly involved in a number of incidents. And as *Newsweek* reported, "The sheer number of black church arsons now equals the worst years of white racist terror in the 1950s and 1960s."

Where to Seek Redress

You can demonstrate that you will not tolerate hate crimes in your own community or anywhere else by reporting all such incidents, especially those that you or someone you know have experienced, to a government or private agency combating this kind of bigotry.

Nearly every large city has human rights organizations or community relations groups where you can report bias-motivated crimes. In Los Angeles, for example, you can contact the Arab-American Anti-Discrimination Committee, the Anti-Defamation League of B'nai B'rith, the Asian-Pacific American Legal Center, the Community Relations Conference of Southern California, El Centro Human Services, the Gay and Lesbian Community Services Center, the Los Angeles City Human Relations Commission, the Los Angeles Urban League, and the Southern Christian Leadership Conference.

If you are a college student, you should always report a hate crime or any information you may have about its perpetrators, no matter who the target is, to the campus police, the dean, or other designated representatives of your college. If the college attempts to sweep the crime under the rug because of fear of bad publicity, put pressure on the authorities to conduct a serious investigation. Contact student campus organizations, and request that they publicize their opposition to such bias-motivated incidents in the school newspaper or hold joint rallies to combat bigotry.

If you are a victim of an ongoing series of hate-motivated threats, harassments, or acts of violence, you or a government attorney can apply for a restraining order. Once the perpetrator is convicted, you may be entitled to compensation for medical bills, property damage, lost wages, and psychological counseling. Also, you can bring a civil action to recover legal fees and punitive damages. Above all, have the courage to persevere until justice is done and the problem has subsided.

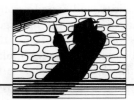

ARSON, VANDALISM AND HATE CRIMES: A CHECKLIST

1 Form community organizations to combat arson and vandalism.

2 Teach your children fire and safety practices and the consequences of malicious destruction of property.

3 Set up groups to distribute educational materials on fire safety and the value of property.

4 Try to prevent arson and vandalism by minimizing the vulnerabilities of your property. This includes installing alarms and smoke detectors, erecting fences, and, if your business is large, hiring private security officers.

5 Well-maintained and cared-for property is one of the best ways to minimize vandalism.

6 Report all hate-motivated threats or acts of violence experienced by you or someone you know to a government or private agency that combats this kind of bigotry.

34

MURDER

Over the last few years, a surge in the number of multiple homicides has captured the nation's interest and concern. Moviemakers, news broadcasters, and talk show hosts have turned their attention to this type of crime. A common misconception is that the multiple murderer is a raving, ranting, vicious-looking, glassy-eyed maniac who randomly selects victims and strikes without warning or mercy. Against this type of random psychotic killer, protection may seem nearly impossible.

It is important to realize that, in reality, most victims are murdered by someone they know, such as a friend, a coworker, or other acquaintance.

Researchers have gathered enough data and knowledge to sort out realities from myths and misconceptions. From all this study has come hard evidence for developing a defense against what earlier appeared to be a totally unpredictable phenomenon.

SERIAL MURDER

Serial murder involves the killing of many individuals over a period of at least several weeks or a few months. Some notorious serial murderers include Jeffrey Dahmer, John Wayne Gacy, the Hillside Strangler, Son of Sam, the Stocking Strangler, the Night Stalker, and the Boston Strangler.

Many serial killers have a childhood history of abuse and rejection by their parents. While still young, they often set fires for fun and torture animals. When they mature, they want to control, dominate, and humiliate their victims, particularly children and women, whom they easily overpower. They become avid consumers of the most graphically violent pornographic pictures, material, and literature. Many of their killings are accompanied by sexual assaults.

The United States Department of Justice's National Center for Analysis of Violent Crime and the Behavioral Science Unit in Quantico, Virginia, both concentrate on analyzing repeat offenders, including serial killers. They serve as a national clearinghouse for multiple killings and provide law enforcement agencies information on violent crimes conforming to a pattern, so that coordinated multiagency investigations can be initiated. The National Center for Analysis of Violent Crime has a database that enables it to compare and contrast by computer individual cases of murder that may be a part of a pattern of serial killings. Once it matches certain cases and a pattern is discerned, the center launches a multiagency investigation.

How Many?

Police estimate that several thousand homicides a year involve serial killers. It is estimated that a new one surfaces each month. According to a Justice Department official, there are probably 100 serial killers operating at any one time in the United States.

A recent study of 203 convicted serial murders reported that 67 percent killed over a period of at least a year. The median number of years for each killing cycle was 4.3 years. The median period for women, who comprise under 20 percent of all killers, was 8.4 years. Three-quarters of the repeat murderers worldwide, captured or known over the last 20 years, operated in the United States. California led in serial killings, with over 50 cases. Texas, Florida, New York, and Illinois were next with between 16 and 25 cases. Iowa, Hawaii, and Maine reported no serial killings through 1988, the time this study was conducted.

The majority of serial murders, 45 percent, involved those killed in their local community or state where they reside or work. Contrary to public opinion, only 28 percent go on a killing spree while traveling long distances. Another 22 percent kill within their own homes, places of employment, or other specific sites. Also contrary to public opinion, not all serial killers work alone; 37 percent of serial killers have at least one partner who abetted in the killings.

The horror of this crime is so great that even the smallest probability of such an encounter sends chills up our spines. Nevertheless, the chance that you or your loved ones will actually meet a serial killer is very small.

Types of Serial Killers

Criminologists have discerned four types of serial murderers. Their motives often involve the pursuit of a personal goal that they have otherwise failed to achieve. The visionary killer acts in response to "voices" or a vision. The hedonistic murderer, seeking a thrill, derives pleasure from torture and death. The attacker, oriented toward power/control, gets satisfaction from the life-and-death control over the victim. Finally, the mission-oriented homicidal maniac focuses on eliminating a group or category of people.

Spree Killers

Another variation of the serial murderer is the spree killer who goes on a rampage of murder, violence, mayhem, and robbery within a very short period of days, or even hours. Spree killers comprise only a small proportion of the nation's serial murderers, although they inflict great harm. Moreover, they tend to be career criminals who are more alienated, marginal, and younger than other serial or mass murderers. Unlike most serial murderers, spree killers usually are unemployed and unmarried. Also, unlike serial murderers, a spree killer's weapon of choice is primarily a gun.

Recognizing the Killer

One problem in protecting yourself and your loved ones is that it is unlikely that you will be able to recognize the serial murderer. The vast majority of such criminals function in the community as law-abiding citizens and kill only when impulse tells them to. Above average in appearance, they usually dress well, speak smoothly, and exhibit charm and intelligence. One psychiatrist characterized them as wearing a "mask of sanity," which is removed only when they strike.

Protection

Obviously, protection against these individuals is very difficult because you are unlikely to recognize their evil designs until it is too late. You can nevertheless increase your security by following the standard practice of being cautious with strangers. If someone you don't know approaches you for no apparent reason or initiates conversation, do not act friendly or personable. Walk away as rapidly as you can. If you cannot avoid a conversation, your response should be terse and to the point. Under no circumstances allow the stranger to continue the conversation and to manipulate you. Never give out your address or telephone number to people whom you cannot be sure to trust. Do not allow anyone into your home whom you fail to recognize or who does not have a specific, legitimate reason for being there.

Avoid situations that put you at the mercy of strangers, like hitchhiking or walking alone in isolated areas at night. Above all, don't be complacent. Convincing yourself that victimization by a serial killer happens to "other" people but not to you tends to make you vulnerable.

Be sure the company you work for has your security as a priority, with good systems and controls that protect you from intruders. Suggest that your company establish an employee assistance program if it does not already have one.

MASS MURDER

It is even more difficult to protect yourself from mass murderers. Like serial killers, these individuals are also filled with rage and frustration. A single event creating stress in the family or the workplace—like losing a job, lover, wife, mother, or other close family member—triggers a sudden explosion of multiple homicide. Most of these acts are carried out with a handgun or rifle.

Mass murderers, like serial killers, are "life-losers" whose converging problems at home and at work drive them to vent their rage and frustration on innocent victims. Many mass murderers have been fired from their jobs or separated from their partners. The murderers blame those closest to them for all these problems. The majority of victims are family members, co-workers, clients, or people who just happen to be in the wrong place at the wrong time.

Be Alert

In situations of this type, there is little more to do than try to run away. Do not try to fight or reason with the killer. These tactics will only enrage the killer and ensure your demise. If you are unable to escape a building, lock yourself in a closet as soon as you hear gunshots or comprehend what is going on.

Early Warning Signs

Be on guard for the warning signs that surface just before these explosive, violent events. For example, a highly verbal worker may suddenly withdraw or become depressed; a cheerful, reliable employee may suddenly turn irritable or begin arriving late for work. Also, be particularly alert for co-workers or employees who suffer from chemical dependency, marital stress, or other exceptional pressures. They should be urged to visit your company's employee assistance program. (Over 10,000 businesses have established these.) If your company lacks a program, suggest this important contribution to employee morale and effectiveness, which could avert a major tragedy. Most important is that your co-worker or subordinate seek professional counseling. Above all, remember to be courteous, fair, and nice to such people. Do not antagonize, insult, or in any way put them down. This strategy will turn the odds away from you as the object of the murderer.

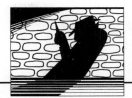

MURDER: A CHECKLIST

1 Be wary of strangers.

2 Be aware that serial killers are hard to recognize. They appear normal and function in the community as law-abiding citizens. They wear what one psychiatrist calls a "mask of sanity" that is removed only when they strike.

3 Never engage in conversation with a person who approaches you for no apparent reason. Walk away as quickly as you are able.

4 Recognize when someone is trying to manipulate you, and resist.

5 Do not give your telephone number or address to strangers.

6 Follow all the suggestions about dealing with strangers contained in this book.

7 Never challenge the killer's instructions or authority.

8 Be on the lookout for such potential signs of possible mass murderers as sudden changes in personality, demeanor, attitude, mental health, marital situation, work behavior, or chemical dependency.

9 Encourage troubled individuals to seek counseling from your company's employee assistance program or from counselors or private therapists.

10 Be sure the company you work for has your security as a priority, with good systems and controls that protect you from intruders. Suggest that your company establish an employee assistance program if it does not already have one.

11 Change your attitude; realize that you could be a victim of multiple murder.

PART SIX

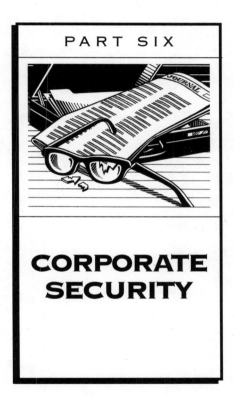

CORPORATE SECURITY

35

KIDNAPPING AND EXTORTION PROBLEMS

In Antioch, California, two gunmen forced their way into a local jeweler's home. They tied the jeweler up, ransacked the house, stole two cars and a 200-pound safe containing jewelry, and took the jeweler's 61-year-old wife with them, leaving a ransom note behind.

Corporate executives, bankers, the well-to-do, and members of their families have been prime targets of extremists, kidnappers, and extortionists in Europe and Latin America for many years. Hostage taking has been recently referred to as "the pest of modern times." These crimes are also occurring with more frequency in the United States.

THE FOUR STAGES OF A KIDNAPPING

Research has indicated that there are four definite stages to a kidnapping. The first stage is the *surveillance stage*. A kidnapper watches his prey to learn the target's daily routine. The second stage is the *invitation stage*. This is when the abductor uses a ruse to stop a potential target's car or to gain admission into his or her home. The third stage is the *confrontation stage*. This is when the "trap is sprung," followed by the *assault stage*. During the assault stage, particularly if the assailant has a weapon or there is more than one assailant, resistance is not recommended. It could be dangerous and possibly fatal.

THE EXTORTION CALL OR LETTER

If you receive an extortion letter, handle it as little as possible, and alert law officers at once. If you receive a phone message telling you that one or more members of your family have been taken hostage, stay as calm as possible. The caller will be extremely nervous and should not be pushed into rash action.

Take detailed notes of the entire conversation—or better yet, make a tape recording. Recordings are extremely valuable to investigators. Even if only an office dictating unit is available, keep it close to your phone at all times. If you can't make a recording, note the exact time of the call, the exact words of the caller, any characteristics such as a regional or foreign accent, and any background noises or music. Have a form handy to help you gain as much information as possible.

If you are at the office, signal your secretary while the call is in progress, and attempt to have the call traced. Ask your local telephone company, in advance, for recommendations regarding the immediate tracing of calls.

Indicate complete willingness to cooperate with the caller. Note each instruction in detail, and even if you are recording the conversation, repeat the instructions back to the caller to ensure they are clearly understood.

If the call is being traced, keep the caller on the line as long as possible. This will help the phone company in its efforts to trace the call. Ask any plausible questions to prolong the conversation: Who is calling? Is this a serious call or just a joke? How do I know it's not a joke? Why have you picked on me in particular? When will I get more instructions?

Ask further questions: What is the hostage wearing? Is he or she all right? What exactly is wanted? Can I speak to the hostage?

If money is demanded, ask in what denominations the bills should be. Where should the money be delivered? When? If the money is to be dropped off, ask how to get to the drop-off point even if you know the route. If money is to be given to someone, ask how to recognize that person.

On the first phone call, try to arrange the simultaneous exchange of money and hostage. If the caller insists on a drop-off point, tactfully try to arrange a person-to-person payoff. Point out the risk of a third person's intercepting a drop-off.

Any ransom money paid should include a minimum of 5- to 10-percent "bait money." The safest type of bait money is probably bills, the serial numbers of which have been recorded.

Offer the caller a code word for identification purposes so that cranks and other potential extortionists are unable to exploit the situation if it is publicized. After the call is completed, notify the Federal Bureau of Investigation and the local police department, regardless of instructions to the contrary. Maintain absolute secrecy, and do not permit any of the facts regarding the kidnapping or demands for ransom to be known to anyone outside the immediate family, except the investigating officers.

Don't handle letters or communications demanding the payment of ransom. Turn these over to law officers as soon as possible. Don't touch or disturb anything at the scene of the abduction. Minute particles of evidence that are invisible to the naked eye may be destroyed.

Be calm, and strive to maintain as normal a routine around the home and office as possible. Place full confidence in the law enforcement officers who are investigating the kidnapping. When kidnappings occur, the first concern of the FBI and other law enforcement agencies is always the safe return of the victim. In addition to obtaining photographs and a complete description of the victim, these officers must have all facts relating to the personal habits, characteristics, and peculiarities of the victim.

ANTIKIDNAPPING STRATEGIES IN THE OFFICE

As a basic company policy, instruct secretaries and business associates not to provide information concerning you or your family to strangers. Have an unlisted home phone number, and list only your address on your mailbox. Avoid displays of wealth or status; advertising your position only invites trouble. Avoid giving unnecessary personal details in response to inquiries from information collectors for use in such publications as business directories, social registers, or community directories. Review your organization's security plans to determine their effectiveness, and make certain that all employees are aware of these plans. Establish a simple and effective signal system in the event of a kidnap attempt. Make sure access to the office is monitored at all times. Have hidden duress alarm buttons installed in the offices to alert others in the building that something is wrong and that proper authorities should be called immediately. Consider hiring bodyguards for you *and* your family, if the situation warrants. Make certain all employees' backgrounds are checked thoroughly.

Vary your daily routines to avoid the habitual patterns for which kidnappers look. Change the times and routes you travel to and from the office. Keep your car locked at all times and the windows raised. Avoid parking where there's poor visibility or in a deserted location. Carry a cellular phone so you can summon help quickly. Keep detailed road maps, and make sure your gas tank is at least half full at all times. Be wary of "stranded" motorists; alert a mechanic or the proper authorities, but don't stop. Consider taking an evasive driving course, and if you're at high risk, consider a bullet-resistant glass or armor. Refuse to meet with strangers at secluded or unknown locations. When leaving your office or home, always advise a business associate or family member of your destination and what time you intend to return, but insist that this information never be revealed except to someone with a legitimate need to know it.

PROTECTION OF CHILDREN

The realization that family members, especially children, are at risk is even more troubling for most executives than awareness of their own vulnerability to kidnapping and extortion. But some protective measures can be taken.

At Home

Make sure that outside doors, windows, and screens are securely locked before you retire at night. Be particularly certain that the child's room is not readily accessible from outdoors. If your home has an intercom system, leave the transmitter in a child's room open at night, or keep the door to the room open so that any unusual noises may be heard. Since leaving the door open removes some fire protection, an intercom is preferable. See Chapter 19 for more discussion of child protection.

If you leave the children at home for a short time, keep the house well lighted and the garage doors closed. Instruct household employees not to let in strangers or accept packages unless they are positive of their source. If you are expecting a package, alert household help to that fact. Try to discourage your children from publicly discussing family finances or routines, and remind yourself not to permit advance publicity for business trips or other occasions when you will be away from your home and family.

At School

Arrange for your children to be escorted to school, and if you feel especially susceptible to kidnapping, do not let them take taxis or public transportation. In one New Jersey town, after a tragic kidnapping incident involving a 10-year-old girl, the parents created a "relay" system in which a parent walks with a group of children for a block or so, followed by another parent, then another, and so on. You don't have to wait until after tragedy has struck to consider implementing a similar plan in your community.

Your prime consideration in selecting a school for your children will be scholastic, but the FBI does suggest a few security policies to check out prior to enrollment. If your child's school doesn't have such policies, bring pressure to bear for their adoption through parent groups, the school administration, or trustees.

Among the policies that the FBI suggests is a rule that before releasing a child to anyone except his or her parents during the regular school day, a teacher or administrative official should telephone one of the child's parents or guardians for approval. When a parent requests by phone that a child be released early from school, the caller's identity should be confirmed before the child is permitted to leave. If the parent is calling from home, the school should check the request by a return telephone call, with the child identifying the parent's voice. If the call is not being made from the child's residence, the caller should be asked questions about such things as the child's date of birth, the courses he or she is studying, or names of teachers and classmates. If there is any doubt, the child should not be released. (See Chapter 24 for more discussion of school security.)

DEALING WITH THE PRESS

After a kidnapping occurs, the press will no doubt be seeking information as soon as the police are notified. While being as cooperative as possible, be sure not to release information that could jeopardize hostages or witnesses, or hamper the police investigation. Only a specifically designated spokesperson should speak to reporters, who should be asked firmly but politely to protect the identities of all witnesses. The press should not be permitted to enter the home or office or to examine the scene of the abduction.

IF YOU ARE A KIDNAP VICTIM

If you yourself are kidnapped, there are a number of things you can do that may save your life. Remember the previous instructions for crisis situations; take a moment to compose yourself; consider your plan; then act on your plan.

Strategies for Survival

Above all, stay calm. Don't threaten anybody. Kidnappers may well be mentally unbalanced, perhaps dangerous psychotics, so don't push them into anything rash. Never fight physically with your abductors: They have probably planned your abduction carefully and will have sufficient manpower to handle you. If your abductors direct you to talk to someone—your spouse or employer, for example—don't attempt heroics.

Cooperate with your abductors as well as you can, but do not tell them what actions might be taken by your family or employer. Assume that you will get out of this situation alive and that everyone connected with your abduction—family, police, FBI—is, first and foremost, working with that objective in mind. Recovery of ransoms or apprehension of offenders is a secondary consideration until the victim is returned safe and sound.

Upon your release, you can best see that justice is served by providing detailed information to the police. So try to determine where you are and to remember everything you can about your abductors and their methods.

Having thoroughly researched facts about you, and having spent a great deal of time in planning the abduction, they will not give you much opportunity to escape. They will transport you to a previously prepared location, designed for the purpose of holding you as long as they see fit. You will almost certainly be prevented from knowing where you are being taken, and it is quite possible that you will be forced to make part of the journey in an automobile trunk.

Particularly if you are held in a dark car trunk, you will require all your concentration and attention to avoid panic. One helpful tactic would be to gather as much information as your confinement will allow. Utilize any of your five senses you can. Hypothesize where you might be going. You will be able to hear and detect odors, and once you are released, these might be important in finding those responsible.

The odds are great that you will be released. Nine out of ten kidnap victims are. If you have the opportunity to leave evidence at the kidnap site (a monogrammed pencil or a business card, for example), you may be providing the police the information that will ultimately result in your freedom. If you are caught in your duplicity, however, it may prove unfortunate. But you are valuable currency to the kidnappers, so there is the distinct possibility that your life will be spared, as long as you represent value to them.

Keep your mind active. Attempt to keep track of time. Even if you are unable to see outside, you may be able to differentiate night from day by temperature patterns or the apparent mealtimes of your captors.

Personalize your area of captivity. Keep your space clean, and insofar as you are permitted, yourself as well. Designate part of your space as a bedroom and sleep there; eat only in your "dining room." If your captors permit you to have the personal items from your billfold, display snapshots of your family.

The Transference Syndrome

Finally, the time will come when you will no longer be a captive. You may escape, you may be ransomed, your captors may be diverted to more important activities, or you may be freed by the police. Far from being relieved by the end of your captivity, you may experience extraordinary reactions. Quite possibly, you will find yourself viewing your captors as your allies and the police as a threat.

Remember the interesting circumstances of a newspaper heiress who was taken hostage. After not being heard from for some time, she was suddenly back in the news, allegedly participating in a bank robbery and admitting being involved in a personal relationship with one of her erstwhile captors. This is a frequent reaction following a prolonged period of captivity. This set of phenomena is termed the Stockholm Syndrome, evolved from the effects observed in 1973 among a group of hostages released from a 5½ day siege following a failed bank robbery in Stockholm, Sweden.

Often hostages will be released to reporters or other representatives of the media. Sometimes the newly released captive will make unfortunate statements, praising the assailants and criticizing the law enforcement personnel who were responsible for the release. Again, this is a manifestation of the peculiar psychological reactions of kidnap victims.

SPECIAL ANTIKIDNAPPING STRATEGIES FOR BANKERS

A kidnapping or extortion plot involving a bank or a banker requires special handling. If hostages are taken, or if a banker is kidnapped offsite and brought to the bank by a criminal, do not trip the alarm. Instead, a prearranged signal—indicating that an extortion is in progress—should be given to another employee. This signal should be well rehearsed and so disguised that the criminal will not be able to intercept it.

The employee recognizing the extortion signal should immediately contact the police or the FBI and give them the address of the hostage's family. If this cannot be reported safely while the criminal is in the bank, it should be done immediately after the criminal and hostage leave. All employees aware of the extortion signal should follow bank robbery procedures regarding observation, preservation of fingerprints, and so on (see Chapter 32).

Ransom money should be paid as directed by the criminal, making certain that decoy money is included. After ransom money is paid, a much higher amount should be publicized because this will often provoke dissension among gang members.

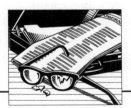

KIDNAPPING AND EXTORTION PROBLEMS: A CHECKLIST

 If an extortion call is received:

    a. Stay calm.

    b. Tape or take notes of the conversation.

    c. Attempt to have the call traced.

    d. Cooperate with the caller.

    e. Have all instructions repeated, even if you under-
stand them.

    f. Repeat the instructions.

    g. Keep the caller on the line as long as possible.

    h. Ask pertinent questions to ensure that the hostage
is, in fact, being held.

    i. Speak to the hostage, if possible.

    j. Determine what, how much, and to whom payoff
is to be made.

    k. If possible, arrange simultaneous exchange of ran-
som and hostage.

2 After the call is received:

    a. Notify the police and the FBI, regardless of the
caller's instructions to the contrary.

    b. Keep all the details of the call secret, except from
family and police authorities.

    c. If a letter, rather than a phone call, was the means
of demand, do not handle it unnecessarily.

    d. Do not disturb the scene of abduction.

    e. Maintain normal routines insofar as possible.

    f. Trust the law enforcement officers involved, and
cooperate completely. Their primary concern is
the safety of the victim.

3 Arrange signals to advise that an extortion call is
in progress.

4 Guard against the release of personal information.

5 Always advise someone when you are to be
expected, but not in such a manner that this information might be compromised.

6 Vary your daily routines, so that you do not establish
regular behavioral patterns.

7 Carry a cellular phone in your car, and be sure that
your gas tank is at least half full.

8 Refuse to meet strangers at remote or unfamiliar locations.

9 Do not leave children alone at home. Leave them in the care of trustworthy people.

10 Teach children good security habits.

11 Avoid obvious indications that children may be home alone.

12 Be careful about safeguarding children en route to and from school.

13 Work for secure practices at your children's schools. Urge the school to maintain personal information files on your child.

14 Don't release information to the press until the kidnapping victim is returned. If this is impractical, release only information approved by the police.

15 If you are a kidnap victim, cooperate and remain calm. Do not offer your abductors information, but gather all details that might assist in their apprehension and recovery of any ransom after your release.

16 Remember to keep your mind active; keep track of time and concentrate on details.

17 On release, refrain from praising the assailants and criticizing the law enforcement officers responsible for your release.

18 In kidnap/extortion threats involving bankers:

    a. Don't trip the alarm if there are hostages.

    b. Signal so that police and FBI can be notified.

    c. Don't disturb evidence.

    d. Include bait money with the ransom.

36

TERRORISM, BOMBS, AND BOMB THREATS

On Friday, February 26, 1993, a bomb blast shook New York City's World Trade Center, killing 6 people and injuring over 1,000 others, while disrupting and displacing hundreds of businesses. It was one of the costliest and most destructive acts of terrorism in U.S. history.

The World Trade Center incident and the bombing of the federal building in Oklahoma City on April 19, 1995, brought home the uncomfortable fact that even U.S. soil is ripe for terrorist activity.

FACTS ABOUT TERRORISM

There are two kinds of terrorism: "discriminate terrorism," in which all victims are potential enemies or combatants, and "indiscriminate terrorism," in which the casual shopper, a planeload of travelers, or the visitor to a nightclub can be a victim. Six basic tactics comprise 95 percent of all terrorist attacks: bombings (which account for roughly half), assassinations, armed assaults, kidnappings, hostage situations, and hijackings. Approximately one-third of all terrorist incidents involve hostages.

Terrorism is not an act of mindless random violence. Terrorist acts are committed with the intention of achieving a goal. Possible goals include the need to attain widespread notoriety while educating society about personal beliefs; to obtain official recognition from a government; to broaden one's power base; to undermine a government's power and morale; to cause a leader to overreact so that he'll look bad to the people of the nation; and to attain widespread notoriety while educating society about personal beliefs—the Unabomber's 18-year series of bombings being a good case in point.

Terrorists are generally young of age: 61 percent are between the ages of 21 and 30; 85 percent of terrorists are male, 15 percent female. Terrorists are not to be mistaken for "guerrillas"; terrorists often come from upper-class families and generally have a better-quality education than the average nonterrorist. Sixty-seven percent of terrorists are single.

When You Travel

Many countries are safe for Americans to visit with little fear of terrorism. Others, notably those on the U.S. State Deparment's list of troubled countries are less friendly and merit extra precautions. When traveling in these countries, one should take steps to avoid being a target, in addition to other precautions for safe travel (see Chapter 16). First of all, don't have an "It can't happen to me" attitude; nobody thinks they'll be involved or targeted. Consider these steps, too:

Don't be an obvious tourist. Watch your clothing; too expensive or "tacky American" can make you a potential target. Remove stickers and personal ID tags from luggage whenever possible. If you have a title or military rank, you might want to consider not using it, and if possible don't dress in a uniform. In short, avoid anything in your appearance that would attract attention. Just blend into the background.

Write down your passport number, the issuing office, and its expiration date. Place a copy in your billfold and your baggage. Use your office address and telephone number on baggage and for hotel registration.

When flying to a troubled land, choose your airline based on its safety and security record and policy, not on economics or comfort. Avoid flying first class; first-class passengers are the most likely to be targeted. Terrorists do not like to seize night flights. Wide-bodied jets are the least likely to be hijacked, and direct flights are less risky than flights with stopovers. If possible, avoid airlines flying the flags of nations involved in hostilities or noncombatant nations supporting those that are at war.

Carry only your passport, credit cards, and a driver's license in your purse or billfold. A little money, of course, is also necessary, but remember to change your U.S. currency to local money as quickly as is practical.

Proceed through the passenger-screening checkpoint as soon as possible after arriving at the airport. Spend as little time as possible in airline ticket areas, cocktail lounges, preboarding screening areas, departure gates, and anywhere in the terminal that is adjacent to large plateglass windows. These areas are either favorites for terrorist attack or are likely to be high-injury locations in the event of explosion or gunfire. The various airline club lounges offer excellent services. In addition to the convenience of a peaceful place to wait, these clubs usually provide another level of passenger screening, an important consideration.

Once in the aircraft, you will have sufficient time to examine carefully the immediate area of your seat. Check the seat pockets, and look under your seat cushion and in the overhead storage bin. These are potential hiding places for explosives and firearms.

In the air, avoid intense, serious discussions, particularly of religion or politics. Avoid mentioning your firm's name or your position to others traveling with you. Napping or reading is a much less provocative way to spend time.

At Your Destination

When you arrive in a troubled country, get your baggage handler to find a taxi for you. Do not agree to carry or watch any briefcase or package for a stranger. Allow baggage handlers at both the airport and the hotel to handle your luggage.

Request a hotel room at the back of the building away from the main entrances. Ideally your room should be no higher than the seventh floor, this being about the highest an aerial rescue ladder can reach.

Be sure that your room is neat and orderly when you leave it. If your possessions are disturbed, you should be able to notice the difference, and this will put you on guard. Leave a TV or radio on when you leave; unwelcome visitors will likely assume you're in for the evening. If you avoid Americanized bars, restaurants, and nightclubs, you will certainly be safer, probably will spend less, and will be able to enjoy the authentic local atmosphere.

Read local newspapers, and learn and use at least some of the local language and customs. Know how to contact the police, your embassy, and consulates. Know where the hospitals are. If you feel the need to smoke, make certain you smoke a local brand of cigarette. In this particular instance, cigarette smoking could be decidedly hazardous to your health, as your smoking preference could easily identify you as a tourist and American citizen.

Overseas Automobile Security

More than 80 percent of all kidnappings and assassination attempts occur while the victim is in an automobile. Always have car keys in hand, avoid spending precious time dawdling outside the car. The car should be as unobtrusive as possible. Always lock the car when leaving it, and inspect it when you return, particularly the undercarriage, wheel wells, and exhaust pipe. You should drive defensively and keep a safe distance between your car and other vehicles. Vary your route to and from work and social points, and at all times keep your gas tank at least half full.

BOMBINGS

Bombings are by far the most common incidents perpetrated by terrorists. Over one-half of all terrorist attacks employed explosive or incendiary bombing devices. Airports and airplanes are often targets of bombs and bomb threats.

Technically known as improvised explosive devices (or IEDs), bombs can be easily concealed because they can be made to look like anything. In a place of business, bombs are typically concealed in garbage cans, file cabinets, under or in desks, and in mailed packages or letters. Plastic explosives are even easier to conceal, because there is no detectable odor and they can be hidden in everyday items, such as clothing, luggage, toys, and cameras. The most common trigger is electrical detonation, but ignition fuses are also used.

Bomb Precautions

Increase physical security at your business or residence, using such tactics as closed-circuit television cameras, alarms, a security patrol, and, if possible, not allowing cars to park within 100 yards of the premises. World Trade Center security officers now closely inspect each employee identification card before permitting entry. Another step you can take to protect yourself is to examine photographs of common bombs.

Be on your guard for suspicious-looking packages, objects, or people who do not belong in an area. If you spot an unusual parcel or similar item, do not touch it, and never yell "Bomb!" This would almost certainly worsen the situation by causing extreme panic. Call the police, the fire department, or the company security force, and then, from a safe distance, warn others about the possible danger.

If you suspect a bomb on a moving train or subway car, alert the conductor. Never pull the emergency brake or activate an alarm; doing so will bring the train to a sudden stop, possibly detonating the bomb. If someone leaves a package or object behind, tell her or him. Treat the object as suspicious if the person fails to respond, denies it is his, or runs away. Note the description of the person, and give this information to the police.

Bomb Threats

Businesses should have a carefully thought-out plan of action in case of a bomb threat. If a bomb is suspected, the last thing to waste vital time on is debating what to do.

The majority of bomb threats are telephoned, so telephone operators should receive special training on how to handle bomb threats. Take all threats seriously until proved otherwise. It is important for the person receiving the call to remain calm and try to gather as much information as possible about the caller and the suspected bomb, such as the type of bomb, time it will detonate, and location. Pay attention to background noises, music, or anything else that might give an indication of where the call is coming from. Ask the caller if the bomb is in a location that you know does not exist, to determine if the threat is valid. Write all information down. Taping calls and caller ID may be devices of assistance if bomb threats recur. As soon as the caller hangs up, notify your employer, then make sure the police, fire department, and any other relevant authority is notified.

It seems illogical for an assailant to forewarn his or her victims, but this may happen for various reasons. The call may be designed to distract attention from an actual bomb location, to keep property damage and/or injuries to a minimum, or, conversely, to cause extreme panic and alarm. In 98 percent of cases, the bomb may be nonexistent; the caller wishes to instill fear. Bomb threats are complicated problems that often require the advice and expertise of trained experts.

Vehicle Bombs

Try not to park your car in an unattended area if you are at a high risk of becoming a bombing victim. Look for unusual objects or wires before unlocking or opening the door of your car. Be alert for anything unusual or out of the ordinary, such as the hood slightly ajar or a window left open when you know you closed it.

Keep your vehicle orderly, so that you may tell if it has been tampered with. Hubcaps are a common hiding place for bombs and should be checked. Marking your hubcaps with paint or a small scratch will help you determine if they have been switched. Check the underside of your car for unusual attachments. Experts also suggest filling up keyholes with soft wax and placing clear tape across doors to determine if someone has gained entry. If you are at high risk, do a complete visual check of your vehicle every time it is left unattended.

Mail Bombs

A mail bomb (also called a letter bomb) is a favorite implement of fear utilized by certain terrorist groups. (It was, for example, the favorite tool of the so-called Unabomber during his long reign of terror.) While other bombs are undiscriminating, the mail bomb is quite discriminating. It is usually addressed to one individual, who is quite likely to suffer injury, sometimes even death.

Several years ago, two such bombs were delivered in London, apparently the work of the same person or organization. One was addressed to the Prime Minister, the other to the U.S. Navy's European headquarters, also located in London. The Navy headquarters bomb detonated, slightly injuring a Navy petty officer. The bomb addressed to Prime Minister Thatcher was defused without incident. However, a similarly addressed bomb did explode several months earlier, slightly injuring an aide.

In another case, an elderly woman opened a package addressed to her brother who had moved out of her residence about 20 years before. A bomb exploded, and the fragments punctured the woman's stomach. No motive was discovered.

Mail–Screening Procedures

Any unusual mail merits careful inspection. Look for the following characteristics if you suspect that something is amiss:

- ❖ Excessive postage
- ❖ Poor handwriting, sloppy typing, or unusual handwriting style
- ❖ Incorrect titles or titles used alone without names
- ❖ Misspelled names or words
- ❖ Oily stains on the envelope or package (which may be caused by explosives)
- ❖ No return address
- ❖ Envelopes that are uneven or lopsided
- ❖ Unevenly distributed weight
- ❖ Extremely large amounts of masking tape or string on the envelope
- ❖ Wire, metal, or aluminum foil protruding out of the envelope or package
- ❖ Mail with an unusual odor, especially if similar to almonds or marzipan
- ❖ Damaged pieces of mail

These precautions are equally applicable to home or office. Companies should check all mail carefully with electronic scanning devices.

If you spot a suspicious-looking piece of mail, don't touch or move it; leave it alone. Open all windows and doors in order to reduce the effects of any blast. Leave the premises, notify the police, and don't return to your home or office until it is absolutely safe to do so.

SPECIAL PRECAUTIONS FOR THE BUSINESS EXECUTIVE

A businessperson needs more protection. Business targets comprise 70 percent of all international terrorist attacks. It is imperative that you keep a low profile. Do not display your name in building directories, on mailboxes, or in any other place accessible to the public. Have an unlisted telephone number. Never display your name or title on a reserved parking space.

Your car should not stand out. Simple, typical, nondescript, standard-model cars are preferable to conspicuous limousines with protective gear. Your vehicle should not display corporate logos, distinctive license plates, or other types of identification.

A firm that specializes in arming vehicles for high-profile, high-risk individuals increased its business by more than 375 percent in 2 years. Arming an automobile can save money for the executive who is paying costly ransom insurance premiums. One major international insurance broker provides such discounts. But even an armored car will prove ineffective unless you practice other standard precautions to reduce your vulnerability. Look for occupied vehicles parked nearby; check to see if you are being followed, and lock your car after each use.

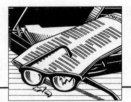

TERRORISM, BOMBS, AND BOMB THREATS: A CHECKLIST

1 To avoid being a target of terrorism when traveling to troubled lands, appear and deport yourself in such a manner that you become "invisible." Act and dress like other travelers, avoid looking American, and blend in with the local population.

2 Before making the trip, leave a detailed itinerary with someone you trust.

3 Use cash or personal—rather than company—credit cards for travel tickets. Consider tourist-class travel.

4 Carry only your passport, credit cards, and a driver's license.

5 Spend as little time as possible in airport areas accessible to the public. Airline club lounges offer good security and excellent services.

6 Avoid intense discussions with other passengers. Topics to avoid include religion and politics.

7 Avoid bars, restaurants, and nightclubs that Americans or other visitors frequent in troubled lands. Avoid using American brand-name items.

8 Thoroughly investigate the accommodations you will use while traveling.

9 Take care in disclosing personal data to other travelers.

10 Use an unobtrusive vehicle for local travel, and check to see that it hasn't been tampered with each time you get in it. Keep the gas tank at least half full.

11 Vary travel routes and flights to make your plans less predictable.

12 Be on guard for any suspicious-looking packages; they may contain bombs.

13 Call the police or fire department if you suspect a bomb.

14 Warn all people nearby of the danger.

15 If someone leaves a package or object behind when leaving a train or subway car, tell him he has done so. If he fails to respond, denies it is his, or runs away, alert the conductor.

16 Take all telephoned bomb threats seriously until proved otherwise. Try to get as much information as possible about the caller and the suspected bomb. Then notify police and fire department at once.

17 Examine your car for unusual objects, wires, or any peculiarities before opening the door.

18 Examine photographs of bombs to familiarize yourself with this danger.

19 Keep a low profile if you are an executive or another likely target for a bomb. Keep telephone numbers unlisted, and don't call attention to your car or parking space.

20 Learn how to screen suspicious-looking mail.

21 Do not touch or move suspicious-looking mail.

22 In buildings threatened by a suspected bomb, open windows and doors to minimize the impact of the explosion.

23 Evacuate the building as quickly as possible, and notify the police without delay.

37

~

COMPUTER AND
HIGH-TECH CRIME

*A board of education computer programmer was recently arrested and charged
with using the school computers to create a racetrack betting system.*

*One company sent a fax that was received promptly and was clear and read-
able. It contained highly sensitive information that had to be withheld from
the competition. Unfortunately, due to a clerical error in transmission, the fax
was sent directly to the competition. Similar horror stories can be recounted by
almost every company.*

*Tom Peter Marlowe was arrested and charged with transmitting sexually ex-
plicit materials via a computer to a 15-year-old girl in Rhode Island. Marlowe had communicated with the girl for about 1 year through electronic
mail. Marlowe was apprehended when he attempted to meet other underage
girls he had contacted the same way.*

If noted bank robber Willie Sutton were still plying his trade, he would be
a computer criminal. Why? For the same reason that he robbed banks in
days past: because "that's where the money is." Today more money resides
in computers than in billfolds. Computers also contain valuable information and intellectual capital that needs to be preserved from disclosure,
misuse or destruction.

Anyone with access to a computer can commit a computer crime. In
one incident, a prisoner serving a 30-year sentence for embezzlement

tampered with computer records at the state penitentiary in order to get an early release. The prisoner also used the institution's computer system to sell 100,000 pounds of cotton grown at the prison for $20,000.

Recently, computers have been used by pedophiles to prey on children, and by pornographers to distribute photographs of a graphic and sexual nature.

THE COST OF COMPUTER CRIME

According to experts, direct costs of computer crime to organizations are nearly $560 million, and indirect costs of computer crime are estimated to be $200 billion. Moreover, the average computer crime nets the perpetrator(s) nearly $500,000. The traditional embezzler, stealing from a manually maintained set of books, nets only about $20,000. Bank robbers do nearly as well: $19,000 for their in-person efforts. Just because no one is pointing a gun at you doesn't mean that the act isn't a crime.

Computer-related activities involve perhaps 10 million people, a number that is certain to increase as time passes. To remain competitive today, companies must rely on computers. About 50 million corporate computers were in use in 1989. By the 21st century, the total should rise to over 200 million computers, mostly connected on networks.

Through such networks, these millions of computer-savvy people could conceivably gain access to the contents of a firm's central computer and the valuable files it holds. For a few thousand dollars, these individuals can purchase a home computer identical to the one they use at work. The central computer may not be able to tell where a message is coming from, only that the access codes are proper. By equipping their home computer with a telephone link, these people could gain access to the computer's information and assets for questionable or illegal purposes.

Certainly the firm will have initiated security measures to protect against the loss of its intellectual property and tangible assets. But what if the computer whiz is more sophisticated than the measures used to protect the integrity of the system?

Far-fetched? Not at all. Several years ago, separate groups of teenagers were able to gain access to data in computers throughout the country, introducing the term *computer hacker* into the general vocabulary. In a relatively short time, they entered more than 60 systems, where they read files, scanned individual medical records, destroyed data, used long-distance telephone lines free, and even "paid" one person's hospital bill. In the fall of 1987, a group of European hobbyists spent 3 months sifting through the files of NASA's scientific work. These electronic snooping hackers confessed their activities, but only after they had reason to believe that they were on the verge of being discovered. A communiqué issued by the group indicated that they had become involved in "industrial espionage, economic crime, East-West conflict, Comecon embargoes, and the legitimate security interests of high-tech institutions." In 1994, three California laboratories specializing in nuclear weapons confirmed that hackers had bypassed their security, penetrated their systems and were using their computers—part of the internet network that connected millions of government, university, and business computers in 156 countries—to store and distribute hard-core pornography. The laboratories were shut down immediately, fearing that the hard-core pornography may have been a smoke screen for an ultrasophisticated espionage organization.

COMPUTER CRIMINAL PROFILE

Studies show that the typical computer criminal is a middle-class male, 18 to 30 years of age, bright, nonconformist, and highly motivated. Such persons view crime as a challenge, and the computer and company as impersonal objects. They may try to hack in from outside the organization, but more often are well-dressed, courteous, ambitious, and hardworking insiders who abuse privileges that have been granted them to illicitly access or destroy corporate information assets. About 15 percent of computer crime incidents involve theft perpetrated by employees, while 10 percent are cases of sabotage usually involving disgruntled workers. By comparison, human errors and accidents account for 50 percent of computer crime losses. Nonhuman computer breakdowns, those resulting from fire, water, and the occasional earthquake, comprise 20 percent of all computer losses.

COMPUTER ABUSE TECHNIQUES

The United States Department of Justice has classified the major methods of computer crime. Many of these schemes have exotic names. They include:

❖ *Introduction of malicious code* like Trojan horses, logic bombs, trapdoors, and viruses. A logic bomb, for example, is a program that on a given date or when a specific event occurs, triggers the destruction of data. Over 10,000 viruses are known which, if they find their way onto your computer, could affect your system, from displaying annoying messages to deletion of hundreds of thousands of records or invoices.

❖ *Telecommunications "phreaking,"*—hacker slang for attacks on phone, PBX or voice mail systems—may result in toll fraud, misuse of systems, or the interception or the destruction of valuable data.

❖ *Using computers to manipulate data* for embezzlement or to commit fraud is quite frequent. One example is when false invoices for equipment or checks are written in favor of the computer operator.

❖ *Supporting or abetting crimes* such as money laundering or drug trading.

❖ *Hardware thefts and software piracy*, including theft of computers, print-
ers, programs, microprocessor chips or trade secrets.

Other criminal specialties that have surfaced over the last few years include "crashers," who purposely damage computer systems, and "cyber-
punks," who threaten to use computers to paralyze the economy or
destroy worldwide communications systems.

Sabotage is one of the easiest ways to attack a computer system. Disgruntled programmers, supervisors, clerks, competitors, political extremists,
or terrorists may attempt to destroy the main physical parts of the system,
critical circuitry, or programs. The sabotage may involve use of explosives,
fire, excessive water, or simply sophisticated programming.

Another form of sabotage occurs when a computer virus is introduced
into the system or network. Like their biological counterparts, computer
viruses are highly contagious and replicate, making copies of themselves,
and affecting the system's operating software or applications programs
running on the system. They may arrive from outside via Internet or
phone connections, be brought in on disks, or even be found on newly
purchased software still in the original package. Untreated, they may
spread rapidly across a network, destroying or compromising data. To
lower the risk of getting a virus, never copy software unless you know and
trust its source, and be sure to use an anti-viral program that can detect
and eradicate viruses before they can act destructively. Since new viruses
turn up at the rate of 20 or more each month, be sure to keep current on
the updated virus profiles provided regularly by the manufacturers of your
package.

Theft of computer services is extremely common. People may use a
computer at someone else's expense. For example, a programmer may use
the computer at his or her primary place of business to mail out bills for a
private business on the side.

To steal property from the company, computer programmers may direct the computer to place orders for merchandise and direct that it be
sent to an unauthorized location. Similarly, they might order the computer
to transfer negligible amounts from each transaction to his or her own account, a technique called "salami slicing." Computer personnel may simply steal data in the form of computer programs or output. This may
involve copying printouts, programs, mailing lists, or other data that would
be of interest to a competitor. Industrial secrets may be pilfered. Stealing
and reselling long distance calling cards has become commonplace.

Of course, computers can be used for much more sophisticated theft,
such as complex financial swindles. False companies can be established, or
misleading information can be provided to investors.

The problem is that there are many ways to penetrate a system without
detection. The computer is particularly vulnerable to electronic penetration, but hackers also use "social engineering" to get access to information

about systems and passwords by seeking help from the computer center, calling and discussing system characteristics with employees, or even applying for a job at the company. Wiretaps using network analysis tools called "sniffers" that were invented to help make networks run better can gather information from lines serving the computer or at nodes of the network. The list is endless.

PROTECTION AGAINST COMPUTER CRIME

It is important to protect the privacy of some information. Even if privacy is not an issue, it is often vital that the information not be changed or destroyed, and it must be available when and where needed. Fortunately, we are not helpless when it comes to preventing or detecting computer crime. We can use powerful cryptology to protect our information assets when they are in storage or in transit over networks, and we have ways to build computer systems and software that protect data while it is being processed. A balanced, cost-effective approach is needed that is based on careful consideration of the risk faced and the impact of a successful criminal attack resulting in disclosure, misuse or destruction of valuable information assets and systems. The following are some basic safeguards to ensure at least a minimum of protection for a computer system.

Employee Screening

Careful procedures should be used for screening employees to determine an applicant's character and integrity, as well as her or his technical qualifications. In-depth interviews, background checks, and fingerprinting are valuable tools for selecting employees who will have access to secured or sensitive information or software.

Division of Responsibility

Set up procedures for a division of responsibilities. No one person should have access to all areas, nor should one programmer have authority to run and modify programs that access sensitive files. A computer operator should not serve as a programmer, nor should a systems manager work as an operator. Rotation of personnel is also helpful.

Computer Center Access

Access to the mainframe computer system or sensitive data by employees should be limited to authorized personnel, and only on a need-to-know basis. All personnel should wear identification badges.

Public tours should be kept a reasonable distance from the equipment to minimize the chance of accidental or malicious damage. Logs recording the time of each visitor's entry and departure should be maintained. Overcoats, luggage, and briefcases should not be allowed in the computer area.

A course in computer security should be a requirement for all employees who have to implement these procedures.

Unambiguous Policies

All instructions to personnel should be in writing to reduce errors in communications. An annual security briefing should be required for all employees. A briefing not only serves as a refresher course but also demonstrates in a highly tangible way that your company is concerned about computer security and that it will not tolerate abusive practices.

Formulate a code of ethics for people working with computer systems and software, and establish penalties for violators. A written code of ethics is a good preventive measure against dishonest employees who may say, "I did not know that 'playing' on the computer was against company policy."

Physical Security

Your main computer facilities should have good physical security. This includes locks, guard systems, alarms, adequate lighting, and few windows. The facilities should be in a relatively isolated area. The computer facility should be constructed of waterproof and fire-resistant materials and have flood control devices. Materials made out of wood, for example, should be avoided whenever possible. A complete security audit and review should be conducted at least once a year. This should include identification of assets and an analysis of vulnerability.

Disaster Plans

Disaster recovery plans should be established and periodically tested. Experience shows that even a minimum of training and drilling may prevent a disaster. You should develop a backup system in case the primary computer system fails. This system should include alternative power sources and alternative computer equipment.

Use special computer safes to store computer tapes, disks, and printouts. Arrange off-site storage facilities for backup tapes and disks. These facilities should be fire resistant and waterproof. Emergency shutdown and recovery procedures for quick start-up should be developed well in advance. These procedures should include practice alerts and dry runs.

Management Responsibility

Information security should be the responsibility of all employees of the organization. Security training and awareness programs should be mandatory at all levels of the organization from executives to clerical staff. Such programs are your best protection against social engineering attacks.

Electronic Protection

Electronic security devices should be utilized—including closed-circuit television systems to prevent the placing of electronic bugs. Also carry out physical inspections to detect listening and other interception devices.

Codes and Passwords

Security codes, passwords, scramblers, and cryptographic devices should be used to screen out unauthorized users and increase computer security. All codes and passwords must be changed periodically without the user's taking any initiative to do so.

Remote Terminals and Networks

Use of remote terminals and networks may be limited by special computer programs. Develop special programs to block unauthorized personnel from using remote and inactive terminals. Limit the number of employees who can access your firm's central files and outside telephone lines from the same terminal or personal computer.

Disposal and Storage

Prepare plans for disposal of stored proprietary information, such as printouts, records, tapes, and disks. Shred or burn papers, and erase unneeded files. Arrange for special computer insurance, because regular insurance policies usually are inadequate for computer protection. Study all legal aspects that may arise as a result of the computer system. This includes computer contracts, leasing, privacy matters, and trade secrets.

HOME COMPUTERS

The use of modems now makes it possible for employees at home or executives on travel to access the office computers. This increases productivity, but also increases vulnerability to attacks from outside. The use of passwords for access control is essential, and call-back schemes included with most modems should be used when possible. Don't forget that laptop computers are an attractive target for thieves and that the data on them may be far more valuable than the computer itself.

E-MAIL

Electronic mail (e-mail) is an increasingly popular alternative to the regular postal service, and even to telephone calls. Over 14.5 million people use e-mail in the workplace, and this number is increasing rapidly.

E-mail is susceptible to many pitfalls, dangers, and breaches of security. Electronic messages can be accessed, intercepted, read, and altered unless proper precautions are taken. For example, e-mail you stored on back-up media for safety can be easily loaded onto another computer for illicit access. Unauthorized individuals may deliberately seek out your private messages. Recently, a *Los Angeles Times* foreign correspondent assigned to its Moscow bureau was disciplined for intercepting and reading his colleagues' electronic mail.

Or consider this scenario. The e-mail message from the company's CEO was direct and unequivocal; the company was undergoing a major reorganization, and substantial layoffs and firings across-the-board should be expected. This message turned out to be a fraud. A prankster engaging in the practice known as "spoofing" decided to cause havoc among company employees. This form of mail forgery is expected to increase over the next decade with the growth in the use of e-mail. A new cryptographic technique known as a "digital signature" can protect the unwary from these forms of electronic assaults. Passwords and encryption systems (which allow coding and decoding) also will help deny the curious from reading what isn't their business.

You should log on to your e-mail only when you are at your desk, so that no other person can receive your messages or send one in your name. Log off your computer when you leave to deny access to anyone interested in snooping. Be sure to change your e-mail password often.

You might also be the victim of electronic stalking. In one bizarre incident, a 32-year-old man was charged with stalking a 29-year-old teacher through electronic mail; he had met her through a video dating service. The electronic stalker never physically assaulted or threatened the woman, but he persistently communicated with her through electronic messages characterized by lovesick pleas and romantic innuendo.

All 50 states have enacted stalking laws, but only one state, Michigan, expanded its laws to include electronic stalking. Recently, a federal bill was introduced in Congress to broaden current stalking laws to ban stalking by e-mail, as well as by telephone.

FAX MACHINES

Rapidity and ease lure people to depend on the fax machine. Employees who traditionally guarded sensitive information by sending it in sealed envelopes marked "eyes only" now transmit proprietary information openly through the fax. The convenience of the fax has transformed business, but unfortunately it increases the vulnerability of information transmitted.

Experts recommend that you secure your fax number as you would your home phone number. Never divulge your fax number unnecessarily, frivolously, or to anyone who doesn't need to know it. Don't let them tie up your machine with junk advertisements, promotions, and personal correspondence. Be extremely security conscience and careful when you send a fax. Think of the potential harm and consequences if the fax were to be read by the "wrong" people. Call ahead to alert the recipient that you are sending the fax. Ask the recipient to confirm that it was received, and verify its contents. Also, verify the origin, date, and number of pages of received faxes.

Some new fax machines use a secret password to scramble a message so that it appears as an unreadable configuration. Only a recipient with the proper equipment and password will be able to reorganize the fax to make it intelligible. This will ensure that the contents are read by the one for whom the fax was intended. The security procedures must be reliable and easy to use, otherwise personnel will avoid implementing the system.

Fax machines often work 24 hours a day, and information on hard copy may be received at any time, including weekends. The fax may remain in the machine receptacle for hours or days until authorized personnel receive and distribute it. This obvious breach of security can be avoided by placing the fax and crypto-equipment in a room that can only be accessed by authorized personnel. It is also now possible for faxes, especially those containing proprietary information, to be securely sealed in tamper-resistant envelopes with only the recipient's name and address appearing on the envelopes. If material is extremely sensitive, it might be best to transmit it via overnight mail.

REPORTING COMPUTER AND HIGH-TECH CRIME

You should establish procedures for reporting criminal acts to the police, district attorney, and other proper authorities. Both the FBI and the Justice Department have dedicated computer crime units. Failure to develop such procedures might delay the reporting process and, in turn, may provide time for the criminal to destroy essential evidence. Investigate all security breaches and suspected criminal acts immediately.

Always prosecute offenders. Failure to press charges and prosecute will only encourage others to commit similar acts. In the past, computer thieves have not been required to "pay the price" as other criminals are. In part, this freedom from punishment has been "computer mystique," a tendency of those who don't fully understand the computer to ascribe near-magical qualities to a machine that is, in reality, no harder to understand than an automobile.

One of the nation's leading experts in computer security estimates that the probability of prosecution in a computer crime is only 1 in 27,000. Even if indicted and found guilty, the computer criminal will, in all likelihood, get off with a ridiculously light sentence. One computer thief, for example, who stole more than $21 million, was sentenced to probation for less than 12 months. Some who hear such reports might be tempted to couple their knowledge of the computer with an intimate knowledge of the firm for which they work, and thus be in a position to divert funds or other assets for personal advantage.

However, the nation's jails are filled with those who have said, "They're not going to get me, because I won't make mistakes." Computer security is getting tighter, and those who fight computer and other high-tech crimes are getting as smart as those who commit them. The would-be computer criminal may join the long list of kings and queens, presidents and dictators, tycoons and executives, and even average citizens who have pitted their abilities against the established order and have paid the price of their vanity.

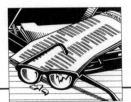

COMPUTER AND HIGH-TECH CRIME:
A CHECKLIST

1 Establish selection procedures for screening all new employees and for in-depth probes for employees who will have access to confidential information.

2 Develop procedures for separation of work responsibilities.

3 Carefully log all suspicious interruptions of computer operations.

4 Only authorized personnel should have access to the computer.

5 All employees should take a special education course in computer security.

6 Write down all instructions to computer personnel.

7 Formulate a code of ethics on computer operations.

8 Be sure your computer facilities have good physical security.

9 Construct your computer facility out of fire-resistant and waterproof materials.

10 Conduct an annual security audit.

---

11 Establish disaster recovery plans, and test them at least once a year.

12 Develop alternative equipment and power backup systems in the event the computer fails.

13 Store all computer tapes, disks, and records in special computer safes.

14 Develop emergency shutdown and recovery procedures.

15 Introduce periodic rotation of computer personnel.

16 Use electronic security devices to prevent electronic penetration.

17 Utilize security codes, passwords, scramblers, and cryptographic devices to prevent unauthorized use of the computer.

18 Limit the number of employees who can access your firm's central files and outside telephone lines from the same terminal or personal computer.

19 Limit the use of remote and inactive computer terminals. Use call-back modems, or install hard-wired security codes when employees must access computers from off-site locations.

20 Destroy all unneeded computer records and printouts.

21 Invest in special computer insurance.

22 Use passwords, digital signatures, and encryption systems to protect your e-mail.

23 Always remain near your computer when it is logged on to your e-mail.

24 Secure your fax number as you would your home telephone number.

25 Notify the recipient that you are sending a fax, and request confirmation that it was received.

26 Secure your fax and crypto-equipment in a secure room in order to avoid security lapses.

27 Send sensitive material via overnight mail.

28 Investigate all suspicions of computer abuse. Press charges and prosecute offenders in all cases.

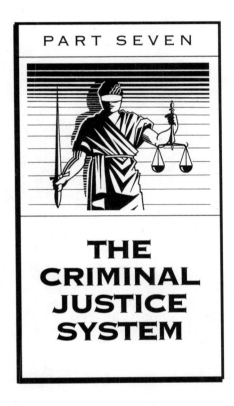

PART SEVEN

THE CRIMINAL JUSTICE SYSTEM

38

~

THE CRIMINAL
JUSTICE SYSTEM:
VICTIMS, WITNESSES,
JURORS

So far this book has concentrated on personal security and crime prevention. This chapter focuses on something nearly as important: what awaits you after a crime has been committed.

THE CHRONOLOGY OF CRIMINAL JUSTICE

Over the centuries, a complex system of legal justice has evolved, requiring constant response to changing conditions. To combat the cost of crime, society has two weapons: laws and those who enforce them.

Crime to Prosecution

Assume that you are walking down the street, and a car stops. The driver demands money from you. You surrender your purse or billfold, and the robber departs. Your neighbor, seeing your difficulty, calls the police at once and gives the information they request. The police see a car matching the description of the one driven by the assailant, and then take the suspect into custody. You make an identification, and a search discovers your property in the robber's possession. The police return most of your belongings to you and give you a receipt for the others, which will be used as evidence against the suspect.

You may be photographed for evidence of the physical assault upon you. When practical, you will be asked to repeat your story for the prosecutor's office, if the police feel that there is probable cause that a crime was committed by the person in custody.

Should the police decline to arrest the individual, the matter would almost certainly be dropped. You couldn't sue the police and force them to arrest the person. You might make a citizen's arrest, but in so doing, you might open yourself to charges of false arrest.

If the Case Isn't Prosecuted

There may be a number of reasons why the prosecutor's office may decline to prosecute. One might be that the arresting officers lacked sufficient cause to arrest, or otherwise violated the suspect's rights. Another reason that prosecution is not pursued is due to insufficient evidence, or a decision that there are other cases more deserving of the attention and the available resources in the prosecutor's office.

Possibly your attacker might not be brought to trial because he or she has an excellent reputation and no previous criminal record. First-offenders frequently are not tried.

A final reason that might prevent your case's coming to court is the possibility that the attacker might be a prominent individual who is owed favors, or is a close relative or associate of such an individual.

Trial and Sentencing

Trials are often disposed of in several ways. Among them are verdicts of guilty or innocent, and plea bargaining. Many trials end in sentencing by the court. Victims may (or may not) be given the right to enter into the court record a statement of the impact that the crimes have had on their lives. Traditionally, victims testify at the trials and bail hearings, but their input before sentencing is a relatively recent concept. These newer concepts are usually permitted at the discretion of the court and may not be allowed in every jurisdiction or courtroom.

Criminal Justice Coordinating Councils

The March 1995 issue of *The Lipman Report* recommends the formation of Criminal Justice Coordinating Councils (CJCCs) as an effective means of fighting local crime. Composed of both public officials and private citizens, CJCC's have greater scope and authority than local commissions composed primarily of private citizens. Member agencies would continue to define and pursue their unique objectives, but because agencies could share information and coordinate strategies, their power, and consequently their effectiveness, would be enhanced.

Local councils could further increase their impact by forming a national alliance. Strengthened by the resources, expertise, and determination of member groups, the alliance would be in a position to influence the nation's policies, programs, and legislation regarding crime.

VICTIMS AND CRIME

If you or a loved one are a victim, review the extremely important suggestions in the chapters on these subjects: child abuse, spouse battering, rape, acquaintance rape, campus sexual assault, sexual harassment, or stalking.

As a crime victim or witness to a crime, or even if you have heard about a crime—especially of a relative, friend, or even an acquaintance—you may experience aftershocks of anger, shock, denial, guilt, sleep disturbances, eating disorders, fright, helplessness, embarrassment, and depression. Psychiatrists refer to these symptoms as "posttraumatic stress disorder" and "rape trauma syndrome."

Be Sure to Report the Crime

If you are a victim of crime, remain calm. Remember that the only way to ensure the arrest of the offender is to call the police. The probability that the offender will be arrested will increase by about 10 percent if you call the police within 2 minutes of the crime. If you have been injured, go to the nearest emergency room for treatment. Then report the crime. If more time has elapsed, notify the police anyway.

Failure to report a crime can mean several things to you. First, there is no way the criminal can be arrested unless the police know that a crime has been committed. Second, the police must allocate their resources wisely. Your failure to report a crime can mean you're not getting your fair share of protection. Third, unless a crime is reported, you usually cannot obtain reimbursement from insurance for losses. Fourth, you may be eligible for an income tax deduction if the crime is reported. Fifth, many jurisdictions have victim compensation programs, but this requires a police report. Last of all, it is your duty. Your assailant may strike again unless you do something. You have an obligation to do what you can to protect not only yourself, but all of us from crime.

You May Be Eligible for Compensation

All states have a crime victim compensation program. In 1984, Congress enacted the Victims of Crime Act, and through 1994 they have allocated $150 million for support of victim compensation and assistance programs. Awards range from $5,000 to $50,000, but most states provide between $10,000 to $25,000 in compensation. About 85 percent of the claims resulted from homicide, rape, robbery, aggravated assault, child abuse, and drunk driving. Domestic violence is also on the list of compensable crimes for most states, but only a fraction of all claims are for this offense, because victims are often reluctant to report domestic violence to police, nor do they always cooperate with the investigations.

If you suffered physical or emotional injury or monetary loss because you were a crime victim, a family member or dependent of a crime victim, or an individual who happened to be present during the crime, you may be eligible for compensation. If you paid for medical or burial expenses for a crime victim you may be entitled to receive reimbursement.

Most programs also pay for loss of earning power, property damage, support, counseling, and rehabilitation services. Some states allow compensation for victims who suffer undue financial hardships; other states pay moving or relocating expenses and the cost of a course on self-defense, if you are in imminent danger. In most states, you are eligible for an award if you are totally innocent and did not contribute to your victimization. But you must report the crime to the police, usually within 3 days, and cooperate fully with the investigation. The deadline for filing a compensations claim in most states is 1 year, but verify this matter, because deadlines vary from 180 days to 3 years. Ask the police or prosecutor's office for an application for your state's compensation program. Generally, the offender does not have to be convicted for you to receive payment.

SEEKING CIVIL REMEDIES

Increasingly, crime victims are using civil litigation against their assailants as a means of restitution. They seek compensation for financial losses, such as lost wages, counseling and hospital expenses, and property loss. A civil settlement may be awarded even if the defendant was found not guilty of the crime. Time limits for filing suits vary from about 3 months to 3 years.

Third parties may also be liable for their failure to provide "reasonable and adequate" protection from crime. Such institutions as businesses, hospitals, hotels, and government agencies may have contributed to the possibility of a crime occurring by their negligence in security. Check with your attorney or a local prosecutor to determine liability.

While it isn't possible for a civil suit to undo the crime or its effect, civil suits do help compensate for expenses and give victims a greater sense of control over their lives. Such suits also help heighten public awareness of the need for increased crime prevention.

The criminal may be sued for income and property. Portions of wages, benefits, tax refunds, and government payments can be awarded to the victim. Real estate, personal property, financial holdings, and bank accounts are also possible resources for satisfying civil judgments.

Civil remedies on behalf of child abuse victims may be sought against negligent third parties who failed to prevent the abuse from occurring. These third parties often include schools, day-care facilities, camps, churches, and youth groups. The statute of limitations may be extended for victims of sexual abuse because of the delayed discovery rule. The effects of the abuse may not be fully determined until much later, as the victim may have repressed memories of abuse.

Women who have been victims of rape and domestic violence may seek civil remedies.

In Court

Now you are ready for your day in court. This will not be an easy task. You may have experienced apathy, aloofness, and bureaucratic behavior on the part of the police, and you very well may be in for more of the same once judicial proceedings begin. You will arrive at a large, strange building, perhaps with many entrances, with many people walking around. You may even encounter the criminal who victimized you, nervously pacing up and down the court corridor.

Whatever you do, avoid contact with the defendant, and do not get involved in conversation. Criminal defendants or their friends and relatives have been known to intimidate, threaten, and harass victims. If this occurs, report the incident to the prosecutor immediately. Threats away from the courthouse should also be reported to the prosecutor, the police, or both.

One of the most depressing and infuriating aspects of your court experience is the ease with which your trial may be postponed. You may take time off from work, arrive at the courthouse, wait around for hours, and then learn that the proceedings have been delayed. These delays may occur over and over again during the trial, and they may last for months.

Lesser problems include difficulty with parking, finding your way around inside the courthouse, and uncomfortable waiting conditions. You might even find it difficult to determine the status or progress of your case. Try to find someone in the prosecutor's office who is willing to update you on your case. This may be the best single way to mitigate frustrating experiences. Otherwise, you can contact your victim/witness assistance program for help and support.

Courthouse Security

An increasing concern, especially for women, is courthouse security. In a courthouse hallway on the morning of March 9, 1994, at 9:15 a.m., Milwaukee bus driver Shirley Lowery was stabbed to death by her estranged live-in companion. Lowery was in the process of requesting a 2-year injunction against her former lover when the fatal attack occurred. The incident took only a few seconds, and the few court officers on the premises were powerless to prevent the violence. The entrances to the courthouse were not protected with metal detectors.

The fear generated by Shirley Lowery's horrifying death caused numerous other Milwaukee women who were seeking restraining orders to withdraw their petitions. Similar reactions on the part of women have occurred throughout the country because of an epidemic of violence in the nation's courthouses.

Whether it be family court, divorce court, or criminal court, incidences of violence on courthouses premises are on the increase. If you must go to court to seek a restraining order because your ex-partner is stalking and/or threatening you, insist that he undergo a thorough search every time he enters the courthouse. Also insist that the court have an adequate staff of court officers trained to deal with emergency situations. Be sure you are guarded every second you are in the courthouse. Whomever you are facing in court (whether a criminal defendant or an ex-spouse) should never be permitted to confront you. If your courthouse does not have metal detectors, insist that they install them. If they don't do so, contact your newspaper and local radio and TV news stations.

Don't get too caught up in the symbolism of "the court" as a place where justice prevails and the bad are punished; the courthouse itself is a building, nothing more and nothing less. Too many criminals and defendants don't leave their violent and destructive tendencies outside; as with any situation, be prepared.

The Witness Stand

Now you are ready to testify. Your evidence can make or break the case. Review your testimony before your court appearance. Picture in your mind what occurred, so that you recall details. You may make notes, but do not memorize your testimony, because it will appear staged.

Remain alert and calm, and never lose your temper. Be attentive and listen carefully to each question. Answer all questions precisely, but never volunteer information. Of course, you have a right to explain your "yes" and "no" responses. The more objective your testimony, the greater its value. Above all, be yourself. Judges, jurors, and attorneys, like most people, appreciate sincerity and integrity.

Taking the witness stand is not an easy matter, especially if you are unaccustomed to public speaking. But if you follow these simple instructions, you may be sure that your testimony will be greatly improved.

Victim Assistance

Victim/witness assistance programs are intended to lessen the impact of crime and judicial procedures on the innocent, while maintaining the constitutional guarantees for those accused. Each community provides different types of crime victim services, but most include sexual assault centers, child abuse treatment centers, domestic-violence shelters, and victim/witness centers. These programs usually provide emergency and long-term support to victims and their families. Services may include counseling, temporary shelter, clothing, food, transportation, and medical care. Assistance may also be provided throughout all criminal justice proceedings and for filing your crime victim compensation program. Additionally, many programs notify your friends and relatives and intervene with your employer to minimize loss of pay and benefits due to your absence from work. If you or someone you love or know has been the victim of crime, call The National Organization of Victim Assistance (NOVA) for immediate support, referrals, and help: (800) TRY-NOVA. NOVA will provide information for serious forms of criminal victimization, including homicide, rape, assault, robbery, burglary, child abuse, spouse battering, stalking, and sexual harassment.

A useful development is block clubs or Neighborhood Watch groups that provide assistance to victims (see Chapter 23). According to the National Institute of Justice, one of the finest programs of this sort is the Philadelphia Block Watch, which provides many support services for crime victims. These include reassuring the victims, staying with victims, listening to their fears and anxieties, extending practical assistance like lending victims money or baby-sitting, accompanying victims to court, aiding victims in obtaining the proper type of help, helping victims make informed decisions, explaining the criminal justice system and what to expect from it, and providing liaison with the police and the prosecutor. A similar program to aid victims can be established by any community.

WITNESSES AND JURORS

Witnesses testifying in a criminal court proceeding, like the victims of the crimes they witnessed, are innocent of any wrongdoing. And, like crime victims, they are often ill prepared to deal with all the confusing and complex intricacies of the judicial system. As has been pointed out, however, it is possible to receive much-needed counseling, practical help, even protection if need be, through one of the innumerable victim/witness assistance programs that have been established in recent years.

There is still another group of individuals called on to play a vital role in the functioning of the courts. Neither victims nor witnesses of crime, they are the people who are summoned for jury service. For many of us, this is a more familiar service.

When you are called for jury duty, be punctual, and follow instructions carefully. If for some reason you are unable to serve on the jury during the scheduled time, notify the jury commission, which may be able to postpone your jury duty or excuse you. Try to get some idea of how long you will have to serve: 2 to 3 weeks is not unusual.

Before serving on the jury, you will be screened by the attorneys for both sides. The defense attorney and prosecutor both attempt to select jurors who are likely to sympathize with their side. Don't be insulted if you are rejected.

After you have been selected for the jury and the trial begins, concentrate on the proceedings and try to follow the case. Listen to and weigh all underlying conflicts; above all, be objective. Never discuss the case with anyone (even other jurors) until the judge instructs you to reach a verdict. Don't read newspaper stories about the case, listen to radio commentators, or watch TV news programs; this could result in a mistrial.

Although you will be paid for serving on a jury, the fees are usually very low. Therefore, try to make arrangements with your employer to share the financial burden. Your participation is important.

Always remember that the jury is the foundation of our criminal justice system, one of the basic safeguards in our fight against crime.

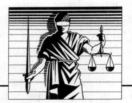

THE CRIMINAL JUSTICE SYSTEM: VICTIMS, WITNESSES, JURORS: A CHECKLIST

1 Always report a crime, even if you are only a witness.

2 Seek medical treatment if you have been injured.

3 Remember as many details as you can about the crime scene and the criminal, including all unusual occurrences and characteristics.

4 Try to record the names and addresses of all witnesses.

5 Record what property was lost, stolen, or damaged.

6 Note the name and shield number of the investigating police officer, and also record the special police report number assigned to your case.

7 When a suspect is apprehended, be sure to press charges.

8 Be aware, if you are a witness, that you may have to deal with some of the complexities of the criminal justice system as victims do. Seek help and guidance from one of the many victim/witness assistance programs established in recent years.

9 Be careful when preparing your written complaint.

10 If you are unable to appear at the trial on the scheduled date, notify the prosecutor's office immediately.

11 Find out whether your state has programs for victim compensation or restitution and whether or not you are eligible for benefits.

12 Investigate the possibility of filing a civil suit as a means of restitution. A civil settlement may be awarded even if the defendant was found not guilty in a criminal trial.

13 Notify the prosecutor's office or the police if the suspect or the suspect's associates attempt to threaten or intimidate you. Insist that the courthouse staff be trained to deal with emergency situations.

14 Be sure to contact the prosecutor's office or special victim/witness hotlines if you find your case has been delayed or postponed.

15 Try to establish a steady contact in the prosecutor's office who can inform you about the proceedings.

16 Prepare your court testimony carefully.

17 Retain your composure, and never lose your temper on the witness stand.

18 Speak slowly and in a loud and clear voice when presenting testimony. Answer questions precisely but do not volunteer information.

19 If you do not understand a question, ask that it be repeated.

20 Your testimony should be precise, objective, and truthful.

21 Always appear in court at the scheduled time if you have been selected for jury duty.

22 Notify court authorities if you cannot serve on the jury on the scheduled date.

23 Be alert and listen to all the trial proceedings.

24 Do not discuss the case with anyone, and avoid all exposure to news coverage about the trial, because this could cause a mistrial.

25 Make arrangements with your employer to assist you financially, because fees paid to jurors are relatively low.

26 Always remember that jurors play a vital role in the criminal justice system. Your participation is one of the important steps you can take to protect yourself from crime.